Rangeland Management

McGraw-Hill Series in Forest Resources

Henry J. Vaux, Consulting Editor

Allen and Sharpe An Introduction to American Forestry
Avery Natural Resources Measurements
Baker Principles of Silviculture
Boyce Forest Pathology
Brockman and Merriam Recreational Use of Wild Lands
Brown and Davis· Forest Fire: Control and Use
Chapman and Meyer Forest Mensuration
Dana Forest and Range Policy
Davis Forest Management: Regulation and Evaluation
Duerr Fundamentals of Forestry Economics
Graham and Knight Principles of Forest Entomology
Guise The Management of Farm Woodlands
Harlow and Harrar Textbook of Dendrology
Heady Rangeland Management
Panshin and de Zeeuw Textbook of Wood Technology Volume I—Structure,
    Identification, Uses, and Properties of the Commercial Woods of the United
    States
Panshin, Harrar, Bethel, and Baker Forest Products
Rich Marketing of Forest Products: Text and Cases
Shirley Forestry and Its Career Opportunities
Stoddart, Smith, and Box Range Management
Trippensee Wildlife Management
    Volume I—Upland Game and General Principles
    Volume II—Fur Bearers, Waterfowl, and Fish
Wackerman, Hagenstein, and Mitchell Harvesting Timber Crops
Worrell Principles of Forest Policy

Walter Mulford was Consulting Editor of this series from its inception in 1931 until January 1, 1952.

Rangeland Management

Harold F. Heady

Professor of Range Management,
Department of Forestry and Conservation
Associate Dean,
College of Natural Resources
University of California, Berkeley

McGraw-Hill Book Company

New York   St. Louis   San Francisco   Auckland
Düsseldorf   Johannesburg   Kuala Lumpur   London
Mexico   Montreal   New Delhi   Panama   Paris
São Paulo   Singapore   Sydney   Tokyo   Toronto

Rangeland Management

1 2 3 4 5 6 7 8 9 0 KPKP 7 9 8 7 6 5

Library of Congress Cataloging in Publication Data

Heady, Harold F.
    Rangeland management.

    (McGraw-Hill series in forest resources)
    Includes bibliographies.
    1. Range management.   I.   Title
SF85.H39   636.08'4   74-18100
ISBN 0-07-027693-5

This book was set in Times Roman by Creative Book Services, divi-
sion of McGregor & Werner, Inc. The editor was Thomas A. P.
Adams, and the production supervisor was Judi Frey.
Kingsport Press, Inc., was printer and binder.

To Eleanor, my wife,
who has become a range manager

Contents

Preface

Rangeland Management focuses on practical management of the world's range-lands. It combines results from research, descriptions, and field examples to stress widely accepted principles, on the one hand, and variations in their application, on the other. It is intended for intermediate-level university students who have had basic courses in botany and zoology. A background, from formal university studies, reading, or experience, in the ecology of renewable natural resources would be especially helpful prerequisite subject matter for studying the management of rangeland.

This book is intended as a text for a course in the management of range vegetation and animals. A university degree in Range Management includes several courses. Rangeland Management is not intended to be the text for courses in range ecology, range resources, range plants, range inventory and planning, range economics, range policy, or other topics. These subject areas warrant development and use of separate texts. *Rangeland Management* will serve those students in allied fields such as agronomy, animal husbandry, forestry, and wildlife who sample a single course in range.

Range workers, who may not be acquainted with the rapidly expanding range literature, will find that many reviews in this book do not give final answers to rangeland problems. These discussions show that all answers are not available, provide opportunity for professionals and students to analyze their specific problems in comparison with those cited in the text, and give teachers a basis for emphasizing their particular fields.

Three groups of chapters draw attention to the influences large herbivores have on their environment, to the management of grazing animals, and to the direct manipulation of range vegetation. Throughout these divisions emphasis is given to much more than domestic livestock, which constitute only one user, one influence, and one product from rangelands. Wild animals also are range animals, and so is recreational man in many ·aspects of his rangeland activities. Numerous references stress the multiple users and products of rangeland.

Part One separates the grazing process into several parts. Each chapter, the one on physical effects, for example, describes a single type of influence by animals. These chapters separate animal impacts to emphasize that grazing is a complicated ecological factor, that an understanding of the parts promotes a better synthesis of the whole, and that separate aspects of grazing are used differently in the management of rangeland systems. The several grazing factors are among the few environmental influences on vegetation which man can manipulate.

Part Two employs the basic concepts of the grazing process in describing four broad ways that animals can be managed. For example, one way to manage animals is to successfully select and change mixtures of animal species. Doing this depends to a large extent upon matching food habits with food availability. One animal mixture might be used to develop a different food supply that is necessary for other animals. These chapters emphasize the dual goal of animal management, animal products and the feedback influences of animals on their habitats.

Part Three groups the chapters on direct vegetational manipulations that do not require the use of animals. These chapters constitute most of the subject matter called *range improvements*. Each chapter stresses how, when, and where the practice is used, illustrates formulas for application, and discusses relationships with other practices.

Overall, the aim of this book is an analysis of rangeland-management systems, I hope with sufficient information on principles for worldwide interest and enough detail to be useful in the pasture.

I-cannot express completely and adequately my appreciation for help received in writing this book. James Bartolome spent hours searching in the library for numerous well-known publications and others extremely difficult to find. He checked and rechecked literature citations, names, spellings, and grammar. We argued many points, and his ideas resulted in helpful revisions. My debt to him is gratefully and gladly expressed. But others have helped, too. During my many years of teaching, graduate students have honed my ideas and criticized my expressions. I have learned much from them that has been included in this book. My visits to experiment stations, pastures, ranches, and ranges where management has been developed or applied have taken the time of many people in over 20 countries. Their displays of results, responses to questions, and, sometimes, disagreements with viewpoints have taught me rangeland management on a worldwide basis. I find it impossible to list all of these people. Nevertheless, they have encouraged me to write *Rangeland Management* and I am thankful to them. However, I am most deeply grateful to my wife, who was most helpful as companion and recorder on many field journeys and as litterateur during the writing.

HAROLD F. HEADY

Rangeland
Management

Part One

Grazing Animals as Ecological Factors

Chapter 1

Rangeland Grazing

Rangeland occupies approximately 47 percent of the earth's land surface, farming takes 10 percent, commercial forests grow on 28 percent, and ice covers 15 percent (Williams et al., 1968). All areas except the ice-covered regions produce forage for domestic and wild animals, water, and recreational facilities. Rangeland supplies additional products and values such as minerals, construction materials, medicines, chemicals, fuel, areas for preservation of endangered species, and anthropological sites.

RANGELAND DEFINED

Rangeland vegetation includes shrublands, grasslands, and open forests where dry, sandy, saline, or wet soils; steep topography; and rocks preclude the growing of commercial farm and timber crops (Fig. 1-1). Range vegetation may be naturally stable or temporarily derived from other types of vegetation, especially following timber harvest and brush clearing. Cultivation gradually infringes upon and takes land formerly used for range purposes, but abandonment of cropland

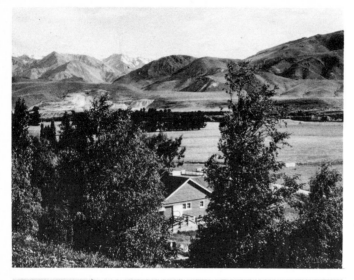

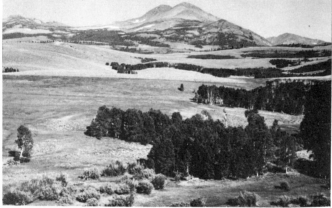

Figure 1-1 Rangeland.

returns other areas of natural vegetation and range grazing. Varying economic and social pressures result in continual land-use changes. Thus, rangeland areas and rangeland products exist as a part of man's total land-based system, but there are indistinct and changing boundaries among various uses of the land.

RANGE MANAGEMENT DEFINED

Range management is a land management discipline that skillfully applies an organized body of knowledge known as *range science* to renewable natural-resource systems for two purposes: (1) protection, improvement, and continued

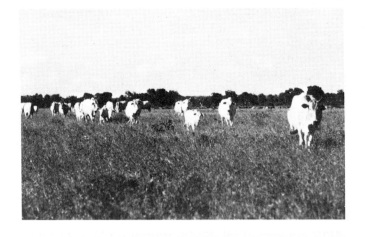

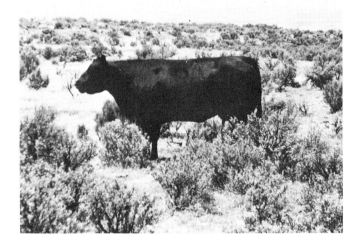

welfare of the basic range resource, which may include soils, vegetation, and animals; and (2) optimum production of goods and services in combinations needed by mankind. The range management profession has certain objectives that distinguish it from other vocations. The central objective of range management is to manage land to produce forage that will be used by domestic and wild animals. Emphasis is placed on a wide variety of natural rangeland ecosystems instead of on farming techniques such as planting of annual crops, irrigation, and cultivation to control weeds. Yet, management of rangeland includes agronomic practices such as noxious-plant control, seeding of grasses and legumes, and fertilization. However, these crop-improvement techniques when applied to rangeland generally are aimed at rehabilitating or approximating natural systems and at achieving permanent results with one application. The manager aims to renew and to sustain his wildland resources rather than to obtain high production through annual cultivation.

Management in the range context implies selecting from among alternative techniques for optimum production. Ecological principles underlie most of the decisions made by the range manager concerned with extensive natural and derived ecosystems. For example, he manipulates forage production by altering numbers and kinds of animals as well as the times and locations of their grazing. The mingling of rangeland ecosystems with traditional agricultural and forestry systems at the business-enterprise level necessitates consideration of and selection from among a wide array of managerial alternatives. Close relationships with other professions keep decisions pertinent to the needs of society as a whole. Thus, the range manager is a highly skilled practical ecologist and the person most knowledgeable about the resource under his supervision (Lewis, 1969).

THE RANGE ECOSYSTEM

Range systems consist of many interacting environmental forces, local combinations of organisms, and the impacts of management. These systems remain mostly under the control of the overall environment, although man alters populations of organisms on the land and varies the rates of physical inputs. Picturing *management* within the encirclement of natural processes in the diagram (Fig. 1-2) indicates environmental control.

Rangeland Development

The three boxes at the bottom of the outer ring in Figure 1-2 depict the interacting state factors of Jenny (1941). He suggested that soil is a function of parent material, relief, climate, and organisms. Over time, mature or well-developed soils result. The process is labeled *soil development* in Figure 1-2. Major (1951) applied Jenny's concept to vegetation and developed the thesis that vegetation depends upon the same state factors as does soil. *Primary succession* describes the development from pioneer to relatively stable communities of plants and animals. Mature soil and climax communities continue to be located at a specific topographic place on a particular physiographic base and to receive an energy combination that the universe provides for that spot. Jenny (1958) called this natural ecosystem a *landscape*. The vertical arrows in Figure 1-2 suggest a time scale for development and deterioration but not necessarily the same scale for vegetation, soil, and range condition. The range landscape system is complicated further because each range site or location, even a square decimeter or smaller, has its separate set of organisms, inputs, and responses. These vary continuously through space as well as time.

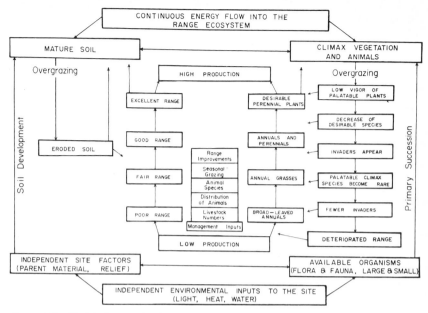

Figure 1-2 Model of a rangeland ecosystem.

The outer ring in Figure 1-2 depicts an evolutionary and geological development from a random to an ordered landscape and suggests that the system constitutes an outer environmental control within which man must live. For the range manager, environmental control determines the natural ecosystem that he depends upon, tolerates, and manipulates as best he can. He faces a challenge to understand the local specifics for each box in the diagram and the rates of change among them.

Rangeland Deterioration

The early range-resource user entered this system after it was well developed. Most areas had mature soils and climax vegetation, only temporarily set back because of an occasional natural catastrophe. Man destroyed the natural vegetation and animals to make room for food crops, he harvested timber for fuel and shelter, and he replaced wild herbivores with his domestic animals. Too many poorly managed animals overgrazed the ranges, causing deterioration of vegetation through several commonly accepted stages (Fig. 1-2). The most palatable plant species were selected first, continually grazed, and closely defoliated; this practice caused reduced vigor, lessened seed production, and, eventually, plant death. Usually the space vacated by desirable species became the expanded home of less desirable species. If overgrazing continued, these species gave way to annual invaders, many of which were weeds introduced from other continents. The palatable climax species became rare, and continued overgrazing reduced the invaders also. Deteriorated ranges resulted in ever-widening patches of totally bare soil, beginning where animals naturally congregated.

Disappearance of soil-holding mulch and plant roots permitted erosion, which further destroyed the land. Erosion is characteristic of overgrazing. Except on steep slopes and fragile soils, erosion came after considerable vegetational deterioration had occurred and did not proceed as far as exposure of parent material. In Figure 1-2, *eroded soil* and *deteriorated range* are located at different horizontal positions, showing the difference in degree of deterioration.

An extensive summary of range problems in the western United States by the U.S. Forest Service in 1936 established the fact that overgrazing had already destroyed more than half of the range forage resources and that deterioration was continuing on three-fourths of all rangeland at that time. Little more than 50 years of high livestock numbers, uncontrolled grazing on public lands, and lack of knowledge or care for the land mainly caused the destruction. In addition, extensive droughts and drastic price fluctuations combined to result in the periodic presence of surplus cattle and sheep on the western ranges. Times of droughts and peak livestock numbers varied from place to place. Conditions in California illustrate the stress on rangelands. From 1880 to 1900, the wildlands of the state were subjected to the severest overgrazing from the highest livestock numbers, the greatest acreage plowed, the least informed forest practices, and the most extensive promiscuous burning of any time in history. The conservation movement that led to the formation of the forest reserves was an outgrowth of that destruction, but the destruction continued on nonforest lands until the next conservation movement, in the 1930s, which developed after widespread land disaster due to severe drought, overextended cultivation, and economic depression.

Rangeland Improvement

The range manager may begin his efforts to halt destructive processes and increase yield at any stage of range condition and with various procedures; hence the management techniques in the center of Figure 1-2 are shown without arrows connecting to the adjoining circle. Whichever technique is used first, to what intensity, and where constitute major land management decisions. However, control of animal numbers and distribution is of major importance and usually first to be applied. Establishment of seasonal grazing plans and alteration of kinds of animals often come later. *Range improvements,* such as brush control, terracing, and seeding, are placed at the top of the management pyramid in Figure 1-2 because their success depends in part upon control of animals.

Secondary plant succession from bare soil, such as near a watering point or in an abandoned field, usually begins with broad-leaved annuals, changes to dominance by annual grasses, becomes a mixture of perennials and annuals, and finally returns to climax vegetation. Sampson, in 1919, was one of the first to describe these stages for meadows in the western forests, and his descriptions of secondary succession following relief from overgrazing continue to be pertinent to management of forest ranges. Many others have described patterns of species dominance and successional stages for numerous vegetation types. Gradually stages in secondary plant succession became the foundation for range-condition evaluations (Dyksterhuis, 1949).

The parallel nature of four secondary-plant-successional stages and four range-condition classes is suggested by their horizontal placement in Figure 1-2. Because of variable site conditions, types of vegetation, evaluations by technicians, and management objectives, condition classes are not always comparable to successional stages. The horizontal positioning of three boxes in Figure 1-2 *(high production, desirable perennial plants,* and *excellent range)* somewhat below the original climax implies that the newly regenerated conditions are different from the original vegetation. For example, new plants may have been added to the vegetation, animal populations changed, and perhaps minerals added to the system. In fact, net productivity may be higher on the regenerated range than on the original range because of continued managerial actions.

The diagram emphasizes that grazing, as an ecological factor, causes the major vegetational changes. Overgrazing destroys vegetation and soil. Those management practices that manipulate animals depend upon benefits from grazing. Therefore, at different levels, grazing both destroys and improves rangeland ecosystems. Analyzing the separate effects of grazing animals (Part One of this book) promotes their use as managerial tools (Part Two).

THE GRAZING FACTORS

Grazing animals exert an influence upon the productive rangeland system by their defoliation of plants through eating and physical damage, by their digestive processes, and by their movements. Separation of this total influence into individual factors fosters an understanding of grazing impacts and promotes informed rangeland management based upon manipulation of range animals. To use his grazing animals as tools to attain production goals, the manager must know the impact of grazing upon the land. Consideration of animals only as products is not enough.

Figure 1-3 shows these reciprocal relationships between land and animals as arrows from vegetation through the grazing factors (large circle) to animals and from animals to vegetation. Grazing also affects the decomposers and the soil. The range manager has two sets of manipulatory tools. One aims at controlling range vegetation by altering the grazing factors, and the other applies such items as seeds and fertilizers directly to the vegetation-soil complex.

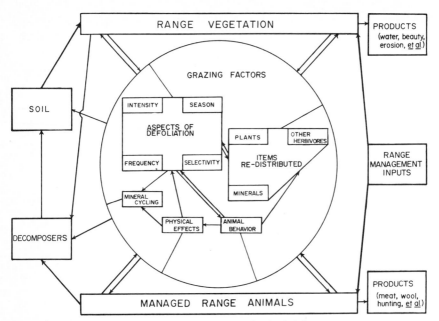

Figure 1-3   Vegetation influences range animals, and animals influence the range through a number of interacting grazing factors.

Individual Effects of Grazing

When a grazing animal eats, it selects certain plants or plant parts and removes them to a definite degree or intensity. This event occurs at a specific season in the phenological development of the plant, and it may be repeated at frequent intervals. The act of grazing is mostly one of defoliation, although not all defoliation is due to grazing.

Grazing includes four aspects of defoliation: intensity, frequency, seasonality, and selectivity. These factors influence growth and reproduction of the vegetation being grazed. Managed animals influence distribution of vegetation by their continual spatial rearrangement of minerals, plants, and other animals. Accumulations of minerals where animals bed stimulate some plant species more than others. Animals move plants whose seeds attach externally to their bodies or survive passage through their digestive tracts. Predators follow their prey, and parasites usually arrive with their hosts.

Each species of range herbivore has its own peculiar behavioral pattern that determines part of its total impact on the habitat. Sheep often graze into the wind, many species prefer specific types of cover, some establish territories, and herding instincts are common. Animals exert a physical impact by trampling, which damages plants, makes trails, loosens sealed soil surfaces, and covers seeds. Other physical actions by animals include the burrowing activities of rodents and the mixing of organic materials with mineral soil by invertebrates.

Slight to nearly complete decomposition of plant material in digestion by herbivores occurs rapidly and speeds mineral cycling. The reduced state of chemical bonds in dung and urine makes the minerals more quickly available for use by plants and hence by another herbivore than are minerals from slowly decomposing, ungrazed plant materials.

The grazing factors are shown in Figure 1-3 as a highly complex set of interacting processes, but they do not influence each other to the same degree. For example, one aspect of defoliation can hardly happen without the others. Cycling of minerals depends upon defoliation, but the recycled minerals influence grazing only after being returned to the soil and reabsorbed by plants.

Effects of Grazing as a Whole

Range managers have little data on many individual relationships in the grazing process. In general, the total grazing influence, or the large circle in Figure 1-3, has been the center of attention and the internal operation of the grazing process has been minimized. Studies of individual factors have concentrated on animal response. For example, data on the influence of forage selectivity on the nutrition of domestic animals can be found for more situations than can data on vegetational responses to selective grazing.

Perhaps, from a practical viewpoint, separation of grazing factors is not necessary because every animal is always a whole animal. A cow, for example, tramples plants while selectively grazing forages to a certain intensity. Thus its grazing effects are confounded. Another viewpoint is that separation of grazing factors is important because different animal species graze and behave differently, so vegetation responds differently to them. Better understanding of these various aspects of grazing should give knowledge useful to the manager who must make decisions about stocking rates, kinds of animals, seasonal grazing, and many other range inputs. The following chapters analyze these separate grazing factors.

LITERATURE CITED

Dyksterhuis, E. J. 1949. Condition and management of range land based quantitative ecology. *J. Range Mgmt.* 2: 104–115.

Jenny, H. 1941. *Factors of soil formation.* New York: McGraw-Hill.

———. 1958. Role of the plant factor in the pedogenic functions. *Ecology* 39:5–16.

Lewis, J. K. 1969. Range management viewed in the ecosystem framework. In *The ecosystem concept in natural resource management,* ed. G. M. Van Dyne, pp. 97–187. New York: Academic Press.

Major, J. 1951. A functional, factorial approach to plant ecology. *Ecology* 32: 392–412.

Sampson, A. W. 1919. Plant succession in relation to range management. *U.S. Dept. Agr. Bull.* 791.

U.S. Forest Service. 1936. *The western range.* Senate Document 199.

Williams, R. E., B. W. Allred, R. M. Denio, and H. A. Paulsen, Jr. 1968. Conservation, development, and use of the world's rangelands. *J. Range Mgmt.* 21: 355–360.

Chapter 2

Intensity, Frequency, and Season of Defoliation

Plants react to defoliation in numerous ways. Moderate degrees of live-herbage removal may stimulate one species to produce more branches or seed but severely reduce another in size and growth rate. However, all range plants can be grazed to some degree. The manager's purpose is to find the heaviest degree of defoliation that maintains production levels.

Fortunately, range plant and animal species have evolved an interdependent relationship in which defoliation is as much a part of the system as is the need for herbage by grazing animals. Natural selection operates both to provide herbivores with food and to permit plants to maintain their continuous needs regardless of defoliation if it is less than some critically destructive amount. The fact that plants palatable to one kind of animal or another dominate the world's grasslands and commonly occur in shrublands and forests suggests that adaptive processes through natural selection operate to foster both the eater and the eaten.

Grazing and defoliation can get out of balance, as illustrated by overpopulation of wild animals and overgrazing by domestic animals. These stresses, either natural or man-caused, speed selective processes. The range manager aims to control stress from overgrazing or overpopulation and its consequent defoliation. Therefore, he must define and understand the effects of herbage removal.

DEFINITIONS

Herbage removal entails an amount, a time in relation to phenological development of the plant, and a frequency if defoliation occurs more than once (Alcock, 1964). Herbage removal also involves selection of the plants being defoliated (Chapter 3). These four aspects of defoliation (Fig. 2-1) are confounded in general usage in experimentation and grazing management. Unfortunately the concept of intensity includes elements of frequency and seasonality of defoliation. This analysis defines and uses these terms as follows.

Intensity of Defoliation

The degree to which herbage has been removed is called *the intensity of defoliation.* Commonly, *intensity of range use* has been defined as *the proportion of the current year's forage production that is consumed or destroyed by grazing animals* (Range Term Glossary Committee, 1964). Intensity may be expressed qualitatively or quantitatively as a proportion of the plant weight or height that has been removed. In clipping experiments, where the investigator harvests and weighs the removed materials, the calculation of proportion of material removed depends upon some measurement of the remaining stubble. The investigator obtains the measurement of the proportion of weight that has been removed only with sacrifice of the whole plant. If animals harvest the forage, direct measurements of amount removed become extremely difficult and the investigator must rely upon measurements of ungrazed plants to reconstruct the portion that has been eaten.

Because of these difficulties and the fact that plant regrowth begins from the material left unharvested, intensity of herbage removal is defined in terms of the amount or length of herbage remaining on the plant. Commonly, for grasses, it is expressed as the average stubble height or weight of plant materials per land unit. For shrubs, the average length of twig or proportion of current growth that remains on the plant after grazing or treatment defines *intensity.* As grazing animals depend upon the amount of material removed and the plants upon the herbage remaining, it would seem that attention to material left is as important as attention to material removed.

Frequency of Defoliation

The definition of frequency of herbage removal is *the interval of time between defoliations and the number of these occurrences.* In a clipping experiment, frequency might be expressed as weekly herbage removal to a constant stubble height occurring between certain dates. In grazing situations, frequency of defoliation becomes the rotation schedule for schemes that use large numbers of animals

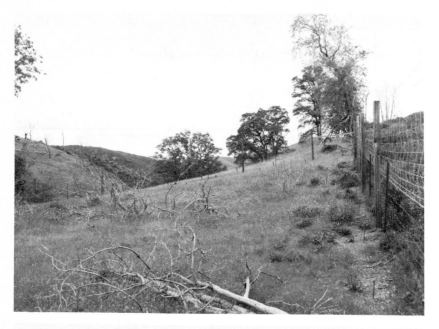

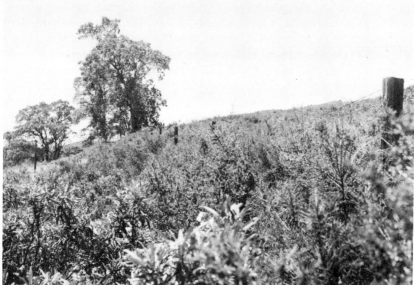

Figure 2-1 Upper photo was taken in June, 1953, following many years of intensive browsing on California chaparral by sheep and deer. Lower photo shows shrub growth after 14 years without browsing.

in small areas for short grazing periods. With light and continuous grazing, frequency of defoliation becomes difficult to determine.

Clipping studies may be the preferred procedure for separating effects of frequency from those of intensity of defoliation. For example, repeated clipping at the same stubble height but at different time intervals would hold intensity of defoliation constant and vary frequency. By definition, intensity of defoliation does not differ as the interval of time between defoliations changes. Some studies describe increasing numbers of clippings as greater intensity of herbage removal. Undoubtedly plants clipped more than once have less photosynthetic tissue than those clipped once and in this sense are subjected to increased intensity. However, in this example, intensity effects are confounded with frequency and seasonal effects. Only by careful attention to these concepts can adequate determinations of effects of degree and of timing of defoliations be distinguished. Recommendations in this book concerning numbers of animals and seasonal grazing schedules use information about these separate effects.

Season of Defoliation

The definition of *season of defoliation* is *herbage removal at different times measured along the growth curve of the plant.* Some grasses and most forbs are highly susceptible to defoliation and lose vigor when growing points are removed at any time. Others show little effect in terms of dry weight and seed produced. Sensitivity of some plants to defoliation increases rapidly when the flower stalks begin to develop and decreases rapidly as the plants approach maturity.

Growth patterns determined under field conditions are subject to much variation resulting from irregularities in weather. Growth in terms of calendar dates has general meaning but minimal predictive value for another year and location. Therefore, the investigator must define the growing cycle of the plants precisely in order to relate effects of herbage removal to plant development. He may accomplish this by measuring normal growth at frequent intervals and constructing a growth curve to serve as an experimental control or standard. The response of the species to various herbage removal treatments can be measured as deviations from the expected growth curve.

DETERMINING EFFECTS OF DEFOLIATION

Investigators in hundreds of experiments have used clipping, grazing, or both treatments to study effects of defoliation. While this chapter is not the place for an extensive review of methods, a brief description of experimental techniques is needed to facilitate understanding of the results.

Clipping Studies

Clipping has been the principal technique used in the study of defoliation. Most investigators have applied clipping to single species grown in pots under fluctuating greenhouse or lathhouse conditions. In recent years, controlled-environment chambers have replaced the greenhouse. Other pot-type studies have depended upon the natural environment, with supplementary water supplied as needed. The substrate upon which the plants were grown has varied from closely controlled nutrient solutions and untreated but uniformly mixed soil in pots to planting in field plots. One investigator rationalizes that growth conditions must be controlled and measured if responses are to have predictive value for other situations, while another investigator grows his plants in as nearly natural an environment as possible with the aim of immediately determining practical responses.

Clipping treatments differ as much as growing conditions do. Treatment variables include clipping height, time of first clipping, frequency of clipping, time of last clipping, and type of material removed. These variables have been defined by calendar dates, growth stages, and occasionally both items. For example, one study might stipulate that plants be clipped to a defined stubble height every two weeks while another might require clipping only when regrowth reaches a certain height.

Measurements of plant response to clipping nearly always include dry weights of material removed and a final weight of crowns and roots at the end of treatments. Pots or boxes facilitate measurement of root responses because whole plants must be harvested. A pot contains all the roots, it contains only the roots of the plants treated, and these roots can be removed easily from the container. Other measurements include length, width, and thickness of various parts; color; degree of branching; reproductive responses; ratios of various plant parts; longevity; changes in plant form; vigor; and chemical composition.

A pot experiment that includes comparisons of three species, three intensities of defoliation, and three clipping frequency regimes, replicated five times, requires 135 pots plus replacements. This experiment entails a sizable effort but includes only a small portion of the possible permutations and needed information.

Although results are available from many clipping experiments, few are comparable and seldom do they repeat testing of the same hypothesis. The general principles that regulate plant responses to defoliation remain unclear in many instances. A suggestion for procedural improvement specifies that the growth curve for an untreated set of plants be determined in each clipping experiment as the normal from which various defoliations cause deviations. Clipping of a new replicate set of previously unharvested plants at each two-week interval throughout the growing season gives a measure of cumulated growth. The plotted data produces the typical normal growth curve (Fig. 2-2). Clipping of the same replicates again (at the same stubble height as earlier clipping) at plant maturity yields measurements of regrowth. A third clipping at ground level gives stubble

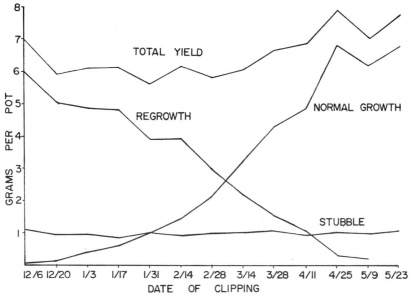

Figure 2-2 Mean oven-dry weights, in grams, of *Avena barbata* resulting from clipping a new set of replicates on each date to determine normal growth. On May 23, all plants were clipped to a 4-centimeter stubble height for measurement of regrowth and to the soil surface for stubble weights *(Savelle, 1966).*

weights. The sum of these three weight measurements—accumulated growth, regrowth, and stubble weight—for each treatment date provides an estimate of total response from the first clipping. The data and curves provide a basis for evaluating various other treatments of intensity, frequency, and season of defoliation.

Grazing Studies

Effects of defoliation by grazing animals have been studied in many experiments with stocking rates. Usually these experiments specify grazing with a constant number of animals for a certain period of time or until a certain degree of forage utilization has been attained. Interpretations of degrees of defoliation usually depend upon the difference between measurements taken before and after grazing or inside and outside of small areas protected from grazing by cages. A glance at Figure 1-3 suggests the complexity of using grazing animals for the study of defoliation effects. Grazing animals confound all of the grazing factors so that the investigator cannot determine the relative importance of, for example, frequency and intensity of defoliation without the influence of trampling. As most grazing periods are relatively long in range studies, no accurate measure of either frequency or season of defoliation can be obtained.

Effects of Clipping Versus Grazing

Several differences exist between the effects of grazing and clipping. Livestock tend to remove plant parts and defoliate species selectively while clipping tends to be uniform. Only with extremely heavy use by livestock does an even stubble height develop. Grazing animals usually take repeated bites to harvest an individual plant, but the time interval between the bites may permit regrowth. Different animals graze by pulling, breaking, or biting at random heights whereas cutting with shears is uniform. Even with heavy continuous grazing of pastures, individual plants may escape defoliation for a time; clipping treatments have tended to be at constant time intervals and at a uniformly severe intensity. If the amounts and kinds of foliage removed by clipping and grazing are the same, the effects of both are likely to be the same (Jameson, 1963a), but that is an unlikely situation.

Therefore, clipping and grazing affect range vegetation differently. Grazing animals do more than defoliate. They trample, move seeds and minerals about the landscape, and select what and where they eat. Clipping does not duplicate these effects on soil and litter. Therefore, clipping should be considered as a means of studying the defoliational effects of grazing, not the whole set of grazing factors. In this context, clipping is a sensitive and valuable tool that can yield more information about defoliation alone than can a grazing trial.

Leaf Area Index (LAI)

The ratio of living leaf area to ground surface is *the leaf area index.* For any given pasture composition, LAI increases with growth and decreases with defoliations and leaf shed. Employment of the LAI emphasizes the proposition that defoliation should be guided by the need to achieve maximum conversion of solar energy to plant products because pasture plants use light for photosynthesis (Humphreys, 1966). Optimum LAI may be regarded as indicating the leaf area resulting in maximum net photosynthesis. Lower than optimum LAI values suggest that there is insufficient foliage to use the available light. Higher than optimum values result in less or no increase in productivity because of increased shading of lower leaves in the canopy (Williams, 1966).

Defoliation, as measured by decreased LAI, can be considered an alteration of photosynthetic systems of individual plants and plant communities. If it is so, changes in LAI measure changes in productive efficiency and indicate deviation from ideal patterns and amounts of foliage. However, systems of defoliation, species, growth stage, and environment change relationships between LAI and growth rate. As Vickery at al. (1971) stated, the varied responses of net production to defoliation, measured by changes in LAI, were to be expected. Most work with LAI has been done with pasture species where LAI alone has not become an adequate guide to management (Brown and Blaser, 1968).

The range manager has less opportunity than has his pasture counterpart to control LAI effectively. His dry ranges always have sufficient light for plant growth. The short, rapid growing season gives little time for manipulation. In comparison, meadowlands where the herbaceous canopy can become thick and tall, and warm-season tropical and subtropical grasslands, present opportunities for the use of LAI as a guide to defoliation practice.

EFFECTS OF DEFOLIATION ON PLANT MORPHOLOGY

Defoliation, including removal of perennial stems, alters normal structural changes that occur during the development of plants. Removal of terminal buds from young Christmas tree branches often causes several lateral buds to germinate, foliage to increase, and the tree to thicken. Hedging of browse plants by animals and development of an even underline of foliage on shrubs and trees attest to morphological responses by plants to herbage removal. Lawn mowing results in an increase in grass tillers, leaves, and percent of ground cover below the clipping height.

Because of their great importance on rangeland, grasses are emphasized in the following discussion of form control by defoliation.

Grass Morphogenesis

The apical promeristem of a grass stem consists of an ever-expanding cone with cells being displaced laterally as the central point enlarges by cell division. Organs such as leaves and spikelets arise as primordial ridges immediately below the apex. Each leaf extends vertically from a ridge to quickly enclose the shoot apex. Soon a meristematic collar separates leaf blade and sheath. Where leaf sheath and stem join, a node, and perhaps an axillary bud or adventitious roots, develops. Cell division at leaf collars and nodes finishes early, and major apparent growth thereafter is by cell elongation. Of necessity, each new leaf forms above and inside the older leaves, and all remain rolled or folded together until elongation of the stem internodes separates them. Therefore, grass leaves originate in a linear sequence and expand in order by elongation (Fig. 2-3).

Grasses have a segmental growth form, and each unit is known as a *phytomer* (Evans and Grover, 1940). A phytomer consists of an internode, a leaf, and a node with or without an axillary bud and adventitious roots. A series of phytomers, one upon another, constitutes a whole plant. Leaves and internodes are limited in growth, but buds produce new phytomers. The separate existence of a phytomer series terminates with seed production. *Tillering,* germination of axillary buds, proliferates new vegetative and reproductive materials. Elongation of internodes elevates only fertile culms in some species, lengthens vegetative stems in others,

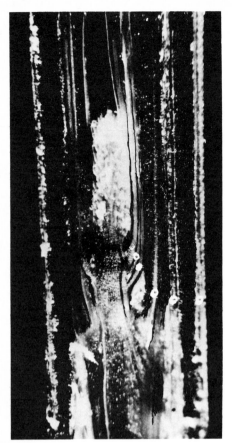

Figure 2-3 Longitudinal section of *Setaria macrostachya* showing the developing inflorescence and six sheaths (marked with white dots). A single axillary raceme is present on the right side between the third and fourth sheaths. The panicle length is 2.0 millimeters and the stem width is 2.6 millimeters. *(Photo by D. R. Cable.)*

and may do both in still different species. Height and display of foliage and inflorescence, arrangements of leaves, number of nodes, timing of the period of elongation, and perhaps size attained appear to be species characteristics (Rechenthin, 1956). However, they can be altered. Defoliation by grazing and cutting changes the architectural display of foliage and reproductive parts from taller, open arrangements to lower, compact, horizontal positions.

Initiation and Development of Culms

Major control of culm initiation and elongation in grasses apparently rests with the species. Branson (1953) suggested that one group of grasses maintains a high proportion of vegetative culms with growing points in or near the soil, another group has a high proportion of vegetative culms with elevated growing points early in the growth cycle, and the third group develops inflorescences on most stems. However, elevation of the fertile apices may be gradual for much of the growing period in one species or rapid in another following an early period with abundant leaf growth but little stem elongation. Examples of plants in the three groups are as follows.

Group I Infertile apices numerous and in or near the soil	Group II Infertile apices numerous and soon above the soil	Group III Fertile culms more numerous than the infertile; apex elevation varied
Andropogon gerardi	*Agropyron smithii*	*Agropyron desertorum*
Bouteloua gracilis	*Bromus inermis*	*Agropyron spicatum*
Buchloe dactyloides	*Panicum virgatum*	*Andropogon scoparius*
Hilaria belangeri	*Sorghastrum nutans*	*Bromus mollis*
Lolium perenne	*Sorghum halepense*	*Elymus canadensis*
Poa ampla	*Themeda triandra*	*Festuca octoflora*
Poa pratensis		*Hyparrhenia hirta*
Sitanion hystrix		*Annual grasses*
Stipa comata		
Tristachya hispida		

Defoliation effects are closely associated with removal of meristematic tissues. Frequently, growth of roots and culms has been inversely proportional to the intensity of clipping in experimental studies (Branson, 1956). As intensity increases or stubble height becomes lower, the chances increase for apical meristems to be removed. However, Group I grasses and certain of the Group III species may be defoliated through much of the early growing periods without danger that the growing point will be removed. An example of the different responses that result from defoliation is given below for *Agropyron desertorum* (Cook and Stoddart, 1953).

Clipping position	Type of subsequent growth
1 Below uppermost culm node while still in sheath	1 Only from axillary buds at culm base
2 Above uppermost culm node	2 Culm continues to develop
3 Between seedhead and uppermost culm node	3 Culm continues to develop but is headless
4 Upper part of head removed	4 Culm continues to develop with part of an inflorescence
5 Leaves below collar; culm apex intact and enclosed in several sheaths	5 Culm and seedhead develop; leaves without blades
6 Leaves above collar; culm apex intact and enclosed in several sheaths	6 Culm and seedhead develop; leaves with stubby blades

Comparisons of three South African grasses illustrate extreme patterns in the elevation of shoot apices (Booysen et al., 1963). *Hyparrhenia hirta* buds initiate in the spring, and remain at low level until midsummer, when the apex becomes reproductive and the internodes elongate. Buds of *Tristachya hispida* begin growth in the spring but remain close to the soil until the following spring, when the apices become reproductive. Growing points of *Themeda triandra* elevate in midsummer but do not become reproductive until the second summer. The growing points of *Themeda* are vulnerable to grazing for at least nine months, but repeated clipping or grazing tends to lower the apex height and to favor plants with self-protecting basal buds (Rethman, 1971).

When a culm enters the reproductive phase and begins to elongate, no new leaves will be produced. Removal of the apical meristem prevents further development of the culm and stimulates axillary buds at the base (Jewiss, 1972). Grasses in general require a new culm if new leaves are to develop. *Andropogon scoparius* and *Bouteloua curtipendula* have 10 to 15 basal nodes with potential buds in the first 2.5 centimeters of culm, and others, for example, *Sorghastrum nutans* and *Agropyron cristatum,* as few as two to four such nodes.

Defoliation that removes the growing point and stimulates new tillers from rhizomes, stolons, and low buds on vertical stems does not necessarily result in greater biomass production. Total yield of *Avena barbata* may be little influenced by a single defoliation (Fig. 2-2). Late removal of the growing point may be too late in the season for regrowth of fertile culms (Sims et al., 1971). Evidently late clipping and frequent clipping tend to reduce flowering and maintain plants in vegetative stages of growth. Maintenance of culmless vegetative growth by heavy grazing during the boot stage may be highly desirable for species such as *Sitanion hystrix* which have undesirable awns at maturity. Many pasture management systems use frequent grazing and mowing to prevent flowering and resultant dormancy of the forage species. Normally, vegetative material has a higher nutritive value than has mature herbage.

Many species resistant to defoliation (1) maintain vegetative buds in or close to the soil surface, (2) do not elevate the apical meristems more than 2 or 3 centimeters until rapid elongation and flowering take place, (3) produce numerous fruiting stems, and (4) have the capacity to initiate abundant new culm development from basal buds.

EFFECTS OF DEFOLIATION ON GROWTH

The good health of plants depends upon their ability to maintain normal physical and chemical processes. Many studies have included treatments and measurements to characterize normal growth and the influence of defoliation on growth. Jameson (1963b) reviewed over 420 papers on the responses of plants to harvesting, and there now are many more.

The Carbohydrate Cycle

The concept that disappearance or persistence of grazed plants correlates with amount and percentage of plant food reserves has been propounded and reviewed many times (Jameson, 1936b; Cook, 1966). Overharvesting, either by cutting or grazing, generally reduces the nonstructural carbohydrates in roots and perenniating stem bases. However, quantities of movable carbohydrates such as sugars, dextrins, fructosans, and starch fluctuate through normal cycles in relation to developmental stages of pasture species. Separation of induced from normal changes in carbohydrate status remains difficult.

Structural carbohydrates are omitted from discussion here because they rarely become energy sources for plant development and are not subject to rapid fluctuation in quantity. Following Weinmann (1947), this discussion uses the term *total available carbohydrates* (TAC) for the group of carbohydrates commonly referred to as *food reserves*.

TAC compounds originate in the leaves or other sites of active photosynthesis and may be stored there, but, more frequently, roots, rhizomes, and lower stems accumulate TAC reserves. The places of TAC accumulation are the points of origin for new growth. In woody plants, accumulations occur in or near aerial buds as well as in stems and roots. As plants begin to grow, the reserves closest to the growing point are used before more distant food materials begin to move. For example, the upper leaves of grasses furnish the foods used for elongation and seed development. Lower leaves may be parasitic in the sense that they use more food than they produce. In general, energy foods formed closest to a meristematic center are used by that center.

The seasonal cycle of TAC concentrations has been described as a succession of three conditions (Humphreys, 1966): (1) a gradual decline during the dormant season due to continued respiration, (2) a rapid decline with the onset of new growth, continuing until photosynthetic products become greater than immediate needs, and (3) a sharp rise during maturation and onset of dormancy. Probably there are minimum amounts of TAC shortly after initiation of growth and maximum amounts at the beginning of dormancy. Normally, this cycle is stated in terms of TAC concentration as percentage of dry weight or as milligrams per gram.

Not all species follow this generalized cycle. TAC declined in roots of *Agropyron spicatum* until 45 percent of foliage height was reached (McIlvanie, 1942), but in *Bromus carinatus* only until 10 percent of the height was attained (McCarty, 1938). In *Elymus cinereus*, TAC declined to less than 5 percent at growth initiation, rose to nearly 8 percent at the early boot stage, and declined again during head development (Krall et al., 1971). *Agropyron spicatum* has a midseason high in TAC and a decline during seed maturation (McIlvanie, 1942). *Agropyron desertorum* reached two lows of TAC contents in roots, one at the beginning of growth and the other during the flowering stage (Hyder and Sneva,

1959). In contrast, *Purshia tridentata* exhibited a single low point in TAC at the end of seed formation (McConnell and Garrison, 1966).

Some herbaceous species appear to be storing TAC during seed development while others are using stores at that time. Storage in lower culms and roots normally occurs during maturity of the foliage and at a time when TAC in the leaves is declining. Fall regrowth reduced reserves in *Oryzopsis hymenoides, Stipa comata,* and *Sitanion hystrix* (Coyne and Cook, 1970). Rapid growth of new tissue at any time normally indicates low or decreasing TAC content.

Many herbaceous plants in mountainous and alpine areas use stored food for growth before snowmelt, show lowest TAC levels in crowns and rhizomes before flower bud formation, and attain a large store of reserve food at fall dormancy. Flowering shoots on alpine herbs commonly reach peak carbohydrate content at the bloom stage (McCarty and Price, 1942; Mooney and Billings, 1960).

Deciduous woody plants appear to reach greatest storage at the time of leaf fall (Kramer and Kozlowski, 1960), long after seed maturity for many species. Thus, variations in the TAC cycle are related to types of measurement, species of plant, growth cycle, part of the plant considered, and site where the plant grows.

Effects of Clipping upon TAC

Defoliation causes a TAC fall in both roots and crowns, and many workers believe that its effects are more drastic when TAC levels are low (Humphreys, 1966). After studying several cool- and warm-season grasses, including bunch and sod types, Crider (1955) claimed that root growth stopped for 6 to 18 days following a single clipping of half or more of the foliage anytime during the growing season. Eight desert shrubs and grasses had reduced TAC in crowns and roots in the winter after single clippings at four different times during growth. Regrowth the next season appeared correlated with autumn TAC levels (Trlica and Cook, 1971).

After reviewing many publications on carbohydrates in plants, (Cook, 1966) concluded that 20 to 25 days on the average, elapsed, between a single clipping and increase of TAC levels in roots. Donart and Cook (1970) claimed that normal TAC levels often were restored by the time regrowth of several species on mountainous summer range had reached 20 percent of the expected total growth. The interval for herbage regrowth and TAC replenishment increases in length as plant maturity approaches. Apparently, recovery of roots lags behind top growth and any reduction in root quantity signifies less root depth.

Reserve foods provide the energy needed for the initial production of new photosynthetic tissue whenever and as often as new growth occurs. Excessive and frequent defoliations in most studies have resulted in nearly complete exhaustion of stored TAC. Defoliation approaching the time of normal late-growing-season accumulation magnified the effects. Generally, early clipping had little effect on food reserves at plant maturity. If only small amounts of both producing green tissue and foods remain, new leaves develop slowly until new TAC from new green tissue again overtakes the needs in the production of new growth. Short, heavy grazing treatments and repeated grazing of the same area by animals may cause as severe defoliation as does clipping. Although some species replenish reserves and grow faster than others and much variation occurs due to site, plants should be given at least three weeks between grazings during the rapid growth period, with six weeks perhaps a safer guide.

Critical TAC Levels

Much of the evidence that lower TAC levels cause certain plant responses remains circumstantial. It associates variation in reserve food status with differing degrees of good health or vigor of plants. Cook (1966) claimed that management should not aim for the highest levels of TAC but should take care not to exceed critically low levels. These levels remain elusive because threshold levels of TAC in plants that die or are at the level of death seldom have been measured. By using unlighted growth as the technique, Ogden and Loomis (1972) showed that *Agropyron intermedium* did not recover when total water-soluble carbohydrates (sucrose and fructosans) were reduced to approximately 1 percent of the plant's dry weight.

Some evidence suggests that excess TAC respires away (May and Davidson, 1958) and that high concentrations of photosynthates inhibit photosynthesis (Moss, 1962). Humphreys and Robinson (1966) described defoliation treatments in which root mass and TAC in roots and crowns varied by factors of about 4 but total shoot growth varied by only 8 percent. Thus, variation in species response to defoliation may be related to the location of cutting, age of axillary buds, age of remaining green tissue, root environment, and physiological restriction on TAC movements as well as to TAC amounts. Much remains to be determined concerning critical levels of TAC as affected by defoliation, especially that done by animals.

Other Nutritive Components

Defoliation influences other nutritive components of plants in addition to carbohydrates. Herbaceous and woody species tend to lose crude protein, phosphorus, and other minerals but to gain in structural carbohydrates as the growing season progresses. Stimulation of new growth by clipping and grazing tends to retard maturity and to decrease the proportion of structural materials. Therefore, percentages of crude protein, phosphorus, and potassium increase as intensity and frequency of defolition increase. Young twigs of *Purshia tridentata* have higher percentages of proteins, fats, and soluble carbohydrates than do older stems (Aldous, 1945). Total amounts of these components may be lower if biomasss decreases more than the compensation resulting from their percentage increases. Changes in vitamins, hormones, and other compounds that result from defoliation, and their effects on the well-being of the plants, are poorly known.

Herbage Yield

When lower stubble heights of grasses and less twig length in shrubs indicate that intensity of defoliation has increased, production of herbage decreases. For example, Canfield (1939) reported the 10-year average yield of *Bouteloua eriopoda* as 9.8 grams per square meter when clipped at the 2.5-centimeter height and 19.5 grams per square meter at the 5-centimeter height (Table 2-1). Although magnitude of yield differences varies between species, many investigators have obtained similar results as to the effects of intensity and frequency of defoliation on production.

Defoliation close to the soil surface with short intervals between clippings relates directly to decreased biomass of tops and roots of most species in tall and middle-height grasslands. Exceptions, such as increased production at certain levels of defoliation, have occurred with short species of grasses and those that maintain growing points near the soil surface. Short grasses in Kansas produced more with light and moderate use than with no defoliation (Albertson et al., 1953). Removal of the terminal bud on shrub twigs often results in two or more branches and increased growth (Shepherd, 1971) but less flower and fruit growth (Garrison, 1953).

Removal of 90 percent of the current growth from desert shrubs killed many of them. Even 50 percent removal in late spring and summer for three years caused significantly lower yield than that from unclipped plants. After seven years of rest, recovery in most species was proportional to degree of vigor deterioration during the clipping (Cook, 1971).

Browse species in moist climates usually seem to be favorably affected by moderate clipping in certain stages of growth. Lay (1965) showed that browse production increased with a number of species when 25 or 50 percent of the current year's growth was removed in either fall or winter. Garrison (1953) obtained similar results from *Purshia tridentata, Ceanothus velutinus, Chrysothamnus nauseosus, Holodiscus discolor,* and *Cercocarpus ledifolius.* Topping of tall *Purshia tridentata* plants to a 0.9-meter height increased yield of new growth for at least four years (Ferguson and Basile, 1966).

Foliage removal has more influence on yield at some seasons than at others. Defoliation effects on *Elymus cinereus* gradually became more severe with advancing growth until the late boot stage, after which time the combined yield of growth and regrowth increased to a high at flowering (Fig. 2-4). Sincle clippings that removed three-quarters of the foliage at boot stage also resulted in reduced yield the following year. The authors suggested that *Elymus cinereus* can be grazed prior to the boot stage if no more than 50 percent of the herbage is removed (Krall et al., 1971). Clipping at the boot stage was too late for new culms to complete the normal growth cycle. This was clearly the most critical time to defoliate the species.

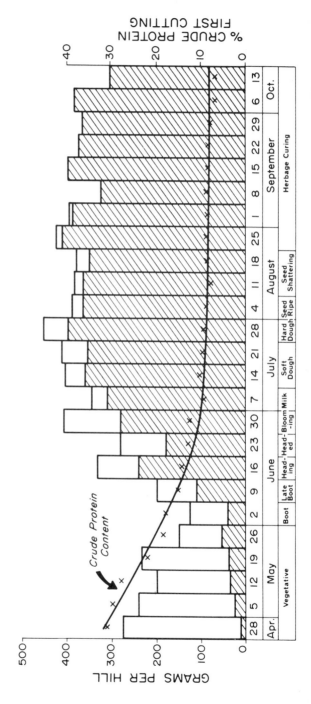

Figure 2-4 Yield at time of a single clipping (hatched bars), regrowth yield at plant maturity (plain bars), and crude protein content of *Elymus cinereus* in 1966 at Bridger, Montana (*Krall et al., 1971*).

Table 2-1 Ten-year average annual yield in grams per square meter of *Bouteloua eriopoda* clipped at two intensities and four frequencies *(Canfield, 1939)*

	Intensity	
Frequency	2.5-cm ht.	5-cm ht.
Two-week	9.83	19.54
Four-week	11.07	21.44
Six-week	9.37	32.09
End-of-season	9.65	34.34

Clipping of *Agropyron spicatum* at early bloom reduced its yield to 15 percent of the controls (Blaisdell and Pechanec, 1949) and greatly reduced flowering the next year (Heady, 1950). Repeated heavy defoliation at the boot stage may eliminate this species from the vegetation within three years (Wilson et al., 1966).

Several species that may be grazed early if care is taken to stop defoliation in time for them to mature a seed crop include *Elymus cinereus, Agropyron spicatum* (Stoddart, 1946), *Agropyron desertorum* (Cook et al., 1958), *Balsamorrhiza sagittata* (Blaisdell and Pechanec, 1949), and *Mertensia arizonica* var. *leonardii* (Laycock and Conrad, 1969). Numerous species with this type of response form bunches in growth habit and belong to the highest successional stages.

Clipping after plants have ceased growth is generally believed to do no harm to the plants. However, Anderson (1960) found that removing herbage of prairie vegetation in September decreased yields the next year from 3,900 to 2,650 kilograms per hectare. Conrad (1954) found that delayed removal of aftermath from mid-September to late October increased the next year's yield by 38 percent. Curtis and Partch (1950) obtained a sixfold flowering stalk increase in *Andropogon gerardi* and 60 percent more height growth by removing old growth in mid-March. These may be indirect effects that operate through changed environment rather than direct stimuli from clipping.

PROBLEMS IN DEFOLIATION PRACTICE

Many studies relating to intensity, frequency, and timing of defoliation confound the treatments and even confuse the terminology. Increased frequency of defoliation may be called *increased intensity* and time of cutting referred to calendar dates or days since planting, all without reference to the phenological sequence of growth stages. The separate effects of intensity, frequency, and season of defoliation seldom have received attention in any study. Regardless of these criticisms, defoliation studies with individual plants and plant communities have contributed to an understanding of grazing effects. Although contradictory results make every generalization risky, a number of solid conclusions can be stated.

Removal of living tissue will cause varied responses according to intensity, frequency of removal, and phenology of the plants at the time. Defoliation according to any one of these three factors or any combination of them can cause plant deterioration, no obvious effects, or even stimulation, depending upon level or timing of application. Plant responses to severe treatments have shown decreased (1) aboveground biomass, (2) culms or woody branches, (3) seed, (4) height of leaves and culms, (5) length of twigs, (6) quantity of nutrients per land unit, (7) root biomass, (8) root length, (9) TAC storage, and (10) vigor. Overdefoliation causes winter killing, drought injury, and changes in botanical composition of range vegetation. All these results vary by species present and by site.

Senescence and decreased nutritive quality of lower leaves in a thick grass stand due to abundant, tall, flowering stems may be remedied by cutting or grazing. New growth is more leafy and higher in proportion of nitrogen than is old growth so defoliation usually improves quality of forage for livestock. This tradeoff with losses from overdefoliation requires careful synchronization of grazing pressure with pasture growth. Manipulating animal grazing with the aim of developing nutritive feeds requires small pastures, long growing seasons, and species that tiller easily or branch profusely. Extensive areas and short growing seasons effectively reduce application of such a management restraint on rangeland.

Perennial grasses vary in sensitivity to herbage removal, but a majority of them sustain little damage if early defoliation ceases in time for them to complete seed maturation. From early boot stage in some species to late flowering in others appears to be the most sensitive time for defoliation. Species of legumes, other forbs, and shrubs differ as widely in response to defoliation as grasses do.

Resilience to defoliation in a species means that other factors exert prime control over growth. They may have high photosynthetic capacity, protected meristems, ability for rapid shoot and leaf differentiation, a low degree of apical dominance, a high ratio of leaf area to leaf weight, and other characteristics contributing to vigor. The importance of most of these adaptations to management and grazing use of range plants remains poorly defined up to the present time.

LITERATURE CITED

Albertson, F. W., A. Riegel, and J. L. Launchbaugh, Jr. 1953. Effects of different intensities of clipping on short grasses in west-central Kansas. *Ecology* 34: 1–20.

Alcock, M. B. 1964. The physiological significance of defoliation on the subsequent regrowth of grass-clover mixtures and cereals. In *Grazing in terrestrial and marine environments,* ed. D. J. Crisp, pp. 25–41. Oxford: Blackwell.

Aldous, C. M. 1945. A winter study of mule deer in Nevada. *J. Wildl. Mgmt.* 9: 145–151.

Anderson, K. L. 1960. An effect of fall harvest on subsequent forage yield of true prairie. *Agron. J.* 52: 670–671.

Blaisdell, J. P., and J. F. Pechanec. 1949. Effects of herbage removal at various dates on vigor of bluebunch wheatgrass and arrowleaf balsamroot, *Ecology* 30: 298–305.

Booysen, P. de V., N. M. Tainton, and J. D. Scott, 1963. Shoot-apex development in grasses and its importance in grassland management. *Herb. Abst.* 33: 209–213.

Branson, F. A. 1953. Two new factors affecting resistance of grasses to grazing. *J. Range Mgmt.* 6: 165–171.

———. 1956. Quantitative effects of clipping treatments on five range grasses. *J. Range Mgmt.* 9: 86–88.

Brown, R. H., and R. E. Blaser. 1968. Leaf area index in pasture growth. *Herb. Abst.* 38: 1–9.

Canfield, R. H. 1939. The effect of intensity and frequency of clipping on density and yield of black grama and tobosa grass. *U.S. Dept. Agr. Tech. Bull.* 681.

Conrad, E. C. 1954. Effect of time of cutting on yield and botanical composition of prairie hay in southeastern Nebraska. *J. Range Mgmt.* 7: 181–182.

Cook, C. W. 1966. Carbohydrate reserves in plants. *Utah Agr. Expt. Sta. Resources Series* 31.

———. 1971. Effects of season and intensity of use on desert vegetation. *Utah Agr. Expt. Sta. Bull.* 483.

———, and L. A. Stoddart. 1953. Some growth responses of crested wheatgrass following herbage removal. *J. Range Mgmt.* 6: 267–270.

———, ———, and F. E. Kinsinger. 1958. Responses of crested wheatgrass to various clipping treatments. *Ecol. Monog.* 28: 237–272.

Coyne, P. I., and C. W. Cook. 1970. Seasonal carbohydrate reserve cycles in eight desert range species. *J. Range Mgmt.* 23: 438–444.

Crider, F. J. 1955. Root-growth stoppage resulting from defoliation of grass. *U.S. Dept. Agr. Tech. Bull.* 1102.

Curtis, J. T., and M. L. Partch. 1950. Some factors affecting flower production in *Andropogon gerardi*. *Ecology* 31: 488–489.

Donart, G. B., and C. W. Cook. 1970. Carbohydrate reserve content of mountain range plants following defoliation and regrowth. *J. Range Mgmt.* 23: 15–19.

Evans, M. W., and F. O. Grover. 1940. Developmental morphology of the growing point of the shoot and inflorescence in grasses. *J. Agr. Res.* 61: 481–520.

Ferguson, R. B., and J. V. Basile. 1966. Topping stimulates bitterbrush twig growth. *J. Wildl. Mgmt.* 30: 839–841.

Garrison, G. A. 1953. Effects of clipping on some range shrubs. *J. Range Mgmt.* 6: 309–317.

Heady, H. F. 1950. Studies on bluebunch wheatgrass in Montana and height-weight relationships of certain range grasses. *Ecol. Monog.* 20: 55–81.

Humphreys, L. R. 1966. Pasture defoliation practice: A review. *J. Aust. Inst. Agr. Sci.* 32: 93–105.

———, and A. R. Robinson. 1966. Subtropical grass growth: 1. Relationship between carbohydrate accumulation and leaf area in growth. *Queensland J. Agr. and Ani. Sci.* 23: 211–259.

Hyder, D. N., and F. A. Sneva, 1959. Growth and carbohydrate trends in crested wheatgrass. *J. Range Mgmt.* 12: 271–276.

Jameson, D. A. 1963a. Evaluation of the responses of individual plants to grazing. *U.S. Dept. Agr. Misc. Pub.* 940: 109–116.

————. 1963b. Responses of individual plants to harvesting. *Bot. Rev.* 29: 532-594.

Jewiss, O. R. 1972. Tillering in grasses—its significance and control. *J. Br. Grassland. Soc.* 27: 65–82.

Krall, J. L., J. R. Stroh, C. S. Cooper, and S. R. Chapman. 1971. Effect of time and extent of harvesting basin wildrye. *J. Range Mgmt.* 24: 414–418.

Kramer, P. J., and T. Kozlowski. 1960. *Physiology of trees.* New York: McGraw-Hill.

Lay, D. W. 1965. Effects of periodic clipping on yield of some common browse species. *J. Range Mgmt.* 18: 181–184.

Laycock, W. A., and P. W. Conrad. 1969. How time and intensity of clipping affect tall bluebell. *J. Range Mgmt.* 22: 299–303.

May, L. H., and J. L. Davidson. 1958. The role of carbohydrate reserves in regeneration of plants. 1. Carbohydrate changes in subterranean clover following defoliation. *Aust. J. Agr. Res.* 9: 767–777.

McCarty, E. C. 1938. The relation of growth to the varying carbohydrate content in mountain brome. *U.S. Dept. Agr. Tech. Bull.* 598.

————, and R. Price. 1942. Growth and carbohydrate content of important mountain forage plants in central Utah as affected by clipping and grazing. *U.S. Dept. Agr. Tech Bull.* 818.

McConnell, B. R., and G. A. Garrison. 1966. Seasonal variations of available carbohydrates in bitterbrush. *J. Wildl. Mgmt.* 30: 168–172.

McIlvanie, S. K. 1942. Carbohydrate and nitrogen trends in bluebunch wheatgrass, *Agropyron spicatum,* with special reference to grazing influences. *Plant Physiol.* 17: 540–557.

Mooney, H. A., and W. D. Billings. 1960. The annual carbohydrate cycle of alpine plants as related to growth. *Am. J. Bot.* 47: 594–598.

Moss, D. N. 1962. Photosynthesis and barrenness. *Crop Sci.* 2: 366–367.

Ogden, P. R., and W. E. Loomis. 1972. Carbohydrate reserves of intermediate wheatgrass after clipping and etiolation treatments. *J. Range Mgmt.* 25: 29–32.

Range Term Glossary Committee. 1964. *A glossary of terms used in range management.* Denver: American Society of Range Management.

Rechenthin, C. A. 1956. Elementary morphology of grass growth and how it affects utilization. *J. Range Mgmt.* 9: 167–170.

Rethman, N. F. G. 1971. Elevation of shoot-apices of two ecotypes of *Themeda triandra* on the Transvaal Highveld. *Proc. Grassland Soc. S. Afr.* 6: 86–92.

Savelle, G. D. 1966. Report of results obtained from clipping four species of annual range plants. Unpublished report.

Shepherd, H. R. 1971. Effects of clipping on key browse species in southwestern Colorado. *Tech. Pub.* 28. Colo. Div. Game, Fish, and Parks.

Sims, P. L., L. J. Ayuko, and D. N. Hyder. 1971. Developmental morphology of switchgrass and sideoats grama. *J. Range Mgmt.* 24: 357–360.

Stoddart, L. A. 1946. Some physical and chemical responses of *Agropyron spicatum* to herbage removal at various seasons. *Utah Agr. Expt. Sta. Bull.* 324.

Trlica, M. J., Jr., and C. W. Cook. 1971. Defoliation effects on carbohydrate reserves of desert species. *J. Range Mgmt.* 24: 418–425.

Vickery, P. J., V. C. Brink, and D. P. Ormrod. 1971. Net photosynthesis and leaf area index relationships in swards of *Dactylis glomerata* under contrasting defoliation regimes. *J. Br. Grassland Soc.* 26: 85–90.

Weinmann, H. 1947. Determination of total available carbohydrates in plants. *Plant Physiol.* 22: 278–290.

Williams, W. A. 1966. Range improvement as related to net productivity, energy flow, and foliage configuration. *J. Range Mgmt.* 19: 29–34.

Wilson, A. M., G. A. Harris, and D. H. Gates. 1966. Cumulative effects of clipping on yield of bluebunch wheatgrass. *J. Range Mgmt.* 19: 90–91.

Chapter 3

Selective Defoliation

Each herbivorous species or individual, wild or domestic, large or small, selects a daily ration from available plants. All grazing includes elements of choice ranging from obligatory grazing on, or choice restricted to, a single plant species or genus to display of little food preference for any species. The plants preferred are said to be *palatable*. As used here, *preference* refers to animal reactions and *palatability* to plant characteristics. Separation of these two concepts aids analysis and understanding of the grazing process, although they are inseparable in food selectivity. Forage selectivity results from a highly complex interaction among three sets of variables operating over time: the plants being eaten, the animals doing the grazing, and the environment of both.

Each animal lives, grows, and reproduces on the food it selects, so animal responses to selective feeding constitute a large and important study discipline. Digestibility trials; chemical analyses of feeds; and determinations of intake, nutritional requirements, nutritional imbalances, growth rates, reproductive rates, and many other animal responses belong to interdisciplinary understanding between the interests of rangeland and animal management. At the same time an animal takes food for nutritional needs, it exerts an influence upon further production of food. Therefore, selectivity is an animal influence upon the habitat, a factor closely related to intensity, frequency, and season of defoliation (Fig. 1-3). This chapter emphasizes analysis of selectivity and its importance as an influence of animals on the range.

EXPRESSIONS OF SELECTIVITY

Selectivity of herbage expresses the degree to which animals harvest plants or plant parts differently from random removal. The Range Glossary defines *selectivity* as *the grazing of certain plant species to the exclusion of others* (Range Term Glossary Committee, 1964). Ratios between the proportion of any species, part of

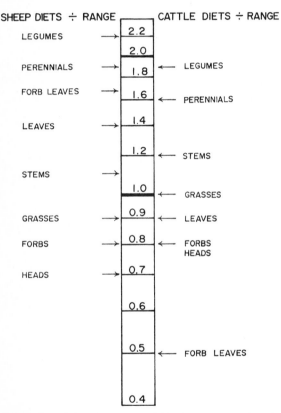

Figure 3-1 Selectivity ratios exhibited by sheep and cattle for plant groups. Ratios shown on the central axis express dietary composition in proportion to range composition. Those parts of the diet near the top of the scale were highly selected while those near the bottom were rejected *(Van Dyne and Heady, 1965).*

plant, or group of plants in the diet and the proportion of that item in the herbage available to the animal were used by Van Dyne and Heady (1965) as expressions of relative preference (Fig. 3-1). The term used here is *selectivity ratio*. The two percentage compositions used to calculate the ratio should be determined by the same procedure, for example, the point system on both fistula material and clipped vegetation from the same pasture. Selectivity ratios effectively show differences in food habits (Table 3-1).

Most statements about selectivity have been based on measurements, ocular estimates, or general observations of the amount or percentage of material removed from a pasture, referred to as *actual use*. Comparisons, if any were made, were with amount of herbage that should have been removed with ideal grazing, referred to as *proper use* and *proper utilization*. When the range is used properly, one species may have 60 percent of current growth removed but a less preferred species only 40 percent. These are expressions of forage preference when the whole range is correctly utilized, rather than of selectivity as defined above.

Another definition of selectivity simply ranks species in the order they were preferred and utilized by animals. Diet alone does not indicate selectivity because it does not compare what is eaten with what is available to be eaten.

METHODS OF STUDYING SELECTIVITY

Degree of use on each species in a stand as a measure of selectivity has been determined by comparison of herbage weights per unit area from paired grazed and ungrazed plots. These techniques may employ small cages, exclosures, and sizable livestock-free areas to eliminate grazing. Commonly, determination of the degree of herbage utilization constitutes the principal aim of studies using ungrazed plots, and measurement of selectivity or some aspect of forage preference is secondary.

Another approach to gathering data on food selectivity centers on observation of feeding animals (Bjugstad et al., 1970). The observer records the time an animal grazes on a species or the number of bites it takes to obtain a frequency of use for each species or for certain vegetational types. Various watching techniques have been used with tame animals, where the observer maintains close proximity to the animal, and with wild animals, where field glasses permit close examination of the eating process. Tamed white-tailed deer, mule deer, red deer, and antelope permit exceptionally close observation of feeding (Wallmo and Neff, 1970). Reichert (1972) described the procedure for taming mule deer to the point of keeping them on a leash during feeding. Most observational studies of this type aim to characterize food habits, digestion, and animal behavior as much as to quantify selectivity.

Feeding two foods at a time to penned animals quickly shows which is preferred and permits ranking the foods. Pairing a third food species first with one

Table 3-1 Selectivity ratios exhibited by several animal species for numerous dietary items. *(Ratios were calculated from data given in the sources cited.)*

Animal	Plant species or group	Selectivity ratio	Season	Location	Source
Cattle	Sporobolus airoides	7.1	Yearlong	New Mexico	Herbel and Nelson (1966)
	Bouteloua barbata	6.4			
	Bouteloua eriopoda	1.7			
	Salsola kali	1.3			
	Gutierrezia sarothrae	0.2			
	Scleropogon brevifolius	0.2			
Cattle	Phalaris tuberosa	2.6	Summer	California	Van Dyne and Heady (1965)
	Stipa pulchra	2.2			
	Trifolium spp.	1.9			
	Bromus spp. (annual)	1.0			
	Avena barbata	0.6			
	Aira caryophyllea	0.5			
Sheep	Phalaris tuberosa	10.0	Summer	California	Van Dyne and Heady (1965)
	Stipa pulchra	3.1			
	Trifolium spp.	1.8			
	Bromus spp. (annual)	0.9			
	Aira caryophyllea	0.4			
	Avena barbata	0.3			
Sheep	Grasses	1.5	Summer	Utah	Smith and Julander (1953)
	Forbs	1.7			
	Browse	0.5			
Angora goats	Grasses	0.7	Winter	Texas	Malechek and Leinweber (1972)
	Forbs	∞			
	Browse	1.6			

Table 3-1 Selectivity ratios exhibited by several animal species for numerous dietary items. *(Ratios were calculated from data given in the sources cited.)*

Animal	Plant species or group	Selectivity ratio	Season	Location	Source
Angora goats	Grasses Forbs Browse	0.7 8.3 1.0	Spring	Texas	Malechek and Leinweber (1972)
Angora goats	Grasses Forbs Browse	1.1 8.0 0.7	Summer	Texas	Malechek and Leinweber (1972)
Angora goats	Grasses Forbs Browse	1.0 4.0 0.8	Fall	Texas	Malechek and Leinweber (1972)
Mule deer	*Quercus* spp. *Cercocarpus breviflorus* *Garrya wrightii*	1.7 1.3 0.3	Yearlong	New Mexico	Boecker et al. (1972)
Mule deer	Grasses Forbs Browse	0.3 3.3 0.4	Summer	Utah	Smith and Julander (1953)
Mule deer	Grasses Forbs Browse	5.9 2.4 0.3	Spring	Utah	Smith and Julander (1953)
Pronghorn antelope	Grasses Forbs Browse	0.2 2.8 10.9	Yearlong	Alberta	Mitchell and Smoliak (1971)
Pronghorn antelope	*Artemisia tridentata* *Artemisia tridentata* *Artemisia tridentata*	4.1 3.6 2.9	January February March	Montana	Bayless (1969)

Table 3-1 Selectivity ratios exhibited by several animal species for numerous dietary items. *(Ratios were calculated from data given in the sources cited.) (Continued)*

Animal	Plant species or group	Selectivity ratio	Season	Location	Source
Bighorn sheep	*Lupinus* spp.	24.8	Winter	Wyoming	Oldemeyer et al. (1971)
	Agropyron spicatum	2.2			
	Chrysothamnus viscidiflorus	2.3			
	Artemisia frigida	1.1			
	Astragalus spp.	0.2			
Rocky Mountain goat	Grasses	1.6	Summer	Montana	Saunders (1955)
	Forbs	0.6			
	Browse	0.1			

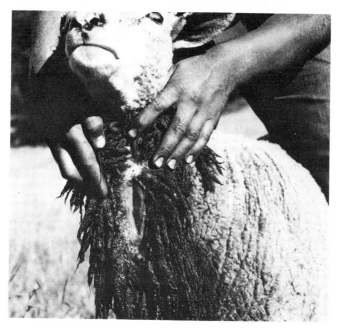

Figure 3-2 This shows one of the first successful esophageal fistulas in sheep. Swallowed food dropped into a collection bag or passed to the rumen when a cannula was secured in the fistula.

and then with the other allows ranking of three species. Examples of this technique include preference ranking for several species of browse by penned deer (Nichol, 1938) and for forage plant selections by livestock. Placing grazing animals on plots of single herbage species or cultivars and giving them free choice in cafeteria fashion gives results similar to those obtained by pen feeding.

Retrieval of eaten material for measurement of any kind was next to impossible before the surgical establishment of fistulas became successful. The initial installment of esophageal fistulas in sheep (Torell, 1954) permitted the collection of relatively unchewed but animal-selected and -eaten material with apparently minor influence on the animals' natural grazing habits (Heady and Torell, 1959). Point sampling, in this instance a crosshair in a binocular microscope of about 15 power, provided frequency data and percentage composition of species and parts of plants in each fistula-collected sample (Fig. 3-2). Within a few years, the fistula technique became a frequently used procedure for collecting dietary material grazed by tame animals (Van Dyne and Torell, 1964). Its use with grazing wild animals still remains difficult because fistulated animals require frequent care and close supervision. Rumen fistulas are used mainly for digestion studies and seldom for determinations of food habits.

Sampling and analysis of stomach contents of killed animals has given abundant information on the food habits of wild animals. These partially digested materials have been separated into their various components by estimations, hand picking and weighing, point sampling, screening, and flotation procedures. Major criticisms of stomach sampling stem from biased high estimates for nondigestible material, small numbers of animals sampled, and sacrifice of animals.

The frequency, size, and pattern of different plant cells such as epidermal, guard, cork, and silica cells varies by plant species. Undigested stomach contents and fecal material often have a high proportion of cuticle with attached cell walls and fibrous tissues. Cutin in the cell walls and cuticle is unaffected by digestive enzymes. These conditions permit determinations of diets on a qualitative basis by determination of the frequency of the different kinds of material in the feces. The method does not indicate the quantity of the separate species eaten by an animal. Regardless, the technique has gained wide use in the determination of food habits of those animals that cannot be fistulated or slaughtered (Martin, 1964; Zyznar and Urness, 1969).

Relatively recent work on gas production with in vitro digestion using chromatographic techniques yielded new data and added the factor of digestibility to selectivity of feeds (Oh et al., 1968; Hanks et al., 1971).

PALATABILITY FACTORS

Palatability factors are those attributes of plants which alter their acceptability by grazing animals. They may stimulate a selective response by animals or they may prevent the plant from being grazed (Heady, 1964). Factors causing palatability are not completely understood; for example, nutritive and chemical contents correlate with palatability in many instances but in others they do not. Palatability of a given plant species changes, sometimes for unknown reasons, but probably because of changing characteristics that an animal can recognize by its senses of touch, taste, and smell (Cowlishaw and Alder, 1960).

Chemical Composition

Many studies correlate palatability with various plant chemical components. It is commonly accepted that forage high in crude protein is highly palatable to cattle and sheep (Hardison et al., 1954; Cook, 1959; Blaser et al., 1960; and many more). Forages high in sugars or with sugars added correlated with high palatability to cattle (Plice, 1952) and deer (Mitchell and Hosley, 1936). High proportions of fats or ether extracts usually correlated with high palatability (Hardison et al., 1954; Blaser et al., 1960). Livestock accepted the grass cultivars highest in phosphorus and potassium before those with low contents of these minerals (Leigh, 1961). Percentages of lignin and crude fiber increase when crude protein, the more simple carbohydrates, and fats decrease; therefore, negative relationships between palatability and content of lignin and crude fiber are as common as positive relationships between palatability and content of other compounds.

Plice (1952) found that manure-affected plants in a pasture were higher in crude protein, calcium, potassium, iron, fat, nitrates, and vitamins than were unaffected plants. The latter contained more silica, aluminum, phosphorus, tannin, chloride, and sugars. Any type of added artificial sweetener, such as sugar, saccharine, or sodium cyclohexyl sulfamate, increased the palatability of the manure-affected plants. These results suggest that the taste of sweetness and not the presence of sugar itself determines palatability. Molasses sprayed on dry grass improves acceptance by animals and furnishes them an energy supplement as well (Wagnon and Goss, 1961).

Of the commonly determined chemical ingredients, high crude protein correlates most frequently with high palatability. However, several investigators suggested that total nutritive value relates to palatability more consistently than does any single part of the feed (Cook et al., 1956; Cook, 1959). Definitive work that separates the influence on palatability of the several feed components remains undone. In effect, most studies have correlated groups of compounds, rather than single items, with palatability.

Confusion arises because numerous unpalatable species contain as much as, or more, nutrients than those readily grazed. Therefore nutrient value alone does not explain palatability of plants to animals. In 1964, Nagy et al. demonstrated that essential oils of *Artemisia tridentata* reduced rumen bacteria, fermentation, and appetite in deer and cattle. Volatile fatty acids supply a major source of energy to ruminants, so not all essential oils can be antagonistic to rumen functions. Only the oxygenated monoterpenes from *Pseudotsuga menziesii* were found to inhibit sheep and deer rumen organisms (Oh et al., 1967). Essential oils from other aromatic plants may be even more inhibitory (Oh et al., 1968). Animals avoided those plants with volatile oils that caused rumen disorders; this event suggests that digestibility is an important prerequisite of palatability. Greenhalgh and Rei (1967) showed that digestibility and palatability had about equal effects on intake of two nontoxic feeds, straw and alfalfa. Undoubtedly proper functioning of the rumen and other parts of the digestive tract influence selectivity of feeds.

Many conflicting results have been reported in studies aimed at explaining palatability according to differences in chemical contents. Usually, palatability for sheep and cattle is indicated by high over low crude protein, phosphorus, and gross energy and low over high crude fiber (Arnold, 1964a), but no completely consistent relationships have been found. Perhaps the best positive indicator is crude protein, unless the feed contains an inhibitor to digestion or a substance toxic to the animal.

Proximate chemical analyses in digestion trials and feed analysis have yielded proportions of crude protein, crude fiber, lignin, etc., which are hardly recognizable by their smell or taste. Conversely, other compounds not found in the usual analysis stimulate these senses. Unclear relationships between palatability and the compounds of proximate analysis should be expected because these relationships are more associative than cause and effect.

Proportions of Plant Parts

Grass and forb leaves contain greater proportions of fats, crude protein, and simple carbohydrates and less lignin and crude fiber than do stems. Fruits and seeds vary among species, but they usually have a relatively high content of crude protein, fats, and carbohydrates. Although chemical contents may not be the reason for differences, leaves, flowers, and seeds are generally more palatable than stems are. In the dry season, when stems may be the principal material available, sheep and cattle continue to show preference for other plant parts (Van Dyne and Heady, 1965):

	Percentage of diet in late dry season		
	Stems	Leaves	Inflorescence
Cattle	77	8	15
Sheep	70	19	11

Most grazing animals select leaf over stem and green material over dry. The proportions of plant parts influence the palatability of forages.

Growth Stage

As herbaceous plant materials mature, they generally decrease in palatability and in nutritive value. The whole plant becomes higher in fiber, and the leaf-stem-fruit ratio changes toward a higher proportion of stems than in young material (McIlvanie, 1942; Cook and Harris, 1950). Succulence decreases and harshness of foliage increases (Springfield and Reynolds, 1951). Pigden (1953) showed that position and extent of lignification in each grass species characterized advancing maturity, curing qualities, and palatability. Deer in the southeastern United States take twigs when they are succulent, in the spring and summer, but avoid them in the winter (Cushwa et al., 1970). Systems of management that prevent accumulations of mature plant materials tend to maintain these species in highly palatable condition.

Palatability of other species gains as the growing season progresses. The selectivity ratio for *Medicago hispida* from new growth to maturity illustrates changing palatability of this species as it becomes older (Heady and Torell, 1959):

February 1	0.15
March 5	0.82
April 1	1.08
May 2	2.25
July 9	2.45

Arnold (1964a) showed this trend for increasing palatability as growth stage advances in several legumes and attributed it to changing odor.

Animals alter their preferences to meet changes in palatability. For example, juvenile sage grouse maintain a diet of succulent forbs by selecting one species after another paralleling the development of the plant species (Klebenow and Gray, 1968).

External Plant Form

Palatability usually is reduced by the presence of awns, spininess, hairiness, stickiness, coarseness of texture, and unfavorable odor from external glands on the plant. Glabrousness and succulence tend to enhance palatability. Growth habit or position of the various plant parts affects accessibility and palatability.

Kind of Plant

All plant species vary in their palatability (Fig. 3-3), presumably due to difference in chemical composition; plant growth stage; and proportions of leaves, stems, and fruits.

Although a few species of plants dominate each range type, many species occur within the daily travel range of large herbivores. At any one feeding, only a few of these plants will constitute the diet. During a longer time period, all available species are likely to be grazed to some extent, as was found in the southern New Mexico desert grassland (Herbel and Nelson, 1966) and in the California annual grassland (Van Dyne and Heady, 1965). The less abundant species can add considerably to animal responses but may go unnoticed in analyses of available forage. For example, *Ramalina reticulata,* a lichen, may be missed as an important component of the forage because it grows on trees and is consumed immediately after falling.

Associated Feed Elements

The availability or proportional botanical composition of a species in the vegetation influences its acceptability. Three investigations of the effects of proportional availability on selection of plants have been conducted. Plants with low palatability were selected to a greater degree when they composed a small rather than a large proportion of the stand (Tomanek et al., 1958). Cook (1962) found that increases in the proportion of a palatable desert plant led to increased use of it and increases in the proportion of unpalatable species resulted in less use of them. Cowlishaw and Alder (1960) found that the presence of highly unpalatable species or materials decreased the selection of palatable species. Associated feeds alter the palatability of any other food item in the diet.

Hurd and Pond (1958) showed that, on mountain ranges in Wyoming, preference for *Stipa columbiana* was greater and preference for *Danthonia intermedia* was less in the *Artemisia* type, a grass-shrub cover, than in a grass-forb

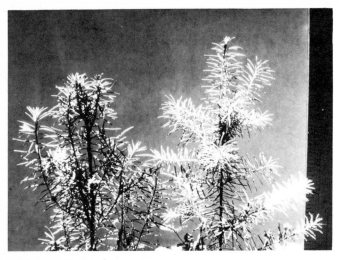

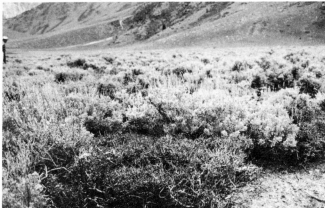

Figure 3-3 Examples of palatability. Upper photo: two seedlings of
Pseudotsuga menziesii growing side by side, one browsed and the other
untouched. *(Photo by G. Connolly.)* Lower photo: *Purshia tridentata*
closely hedged and *Artemisia tridentata* lightly browsed in eastern
California. Opposite page, upper photo: *Themeda triandra* grazed and
Elyonurus argenteus ungrazed in southern Africa. Opposite page, lower
photo: irregular grazing on seeded *Lolium* in Australia.

cover. Annual species on one habitat showed different acceptances by sheep when
the species occurred together in different proportions (Heady and Torell, 1959).
Such relationships are common with many species.

Normally, as availability of forage decreases, so does selectivity. Where
forage is abundant in relation to the grazing pressure, animals express their
preferences freely. As feed becomes less available, the more palatable portions
disappear first, then animals must eat less palatable forages (Arnold, 1964a; Van

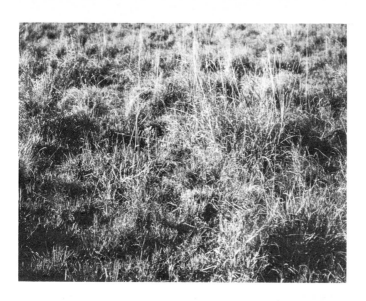

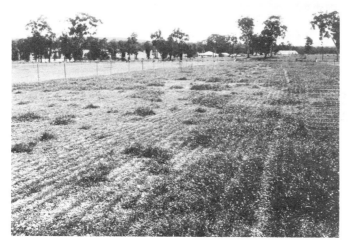

Dyne and Heady, 1965). While one or a few species may be preferred at one time, usually most species will be eaten to some degree, and over a full season all may be selected.

PREFERENCE FACTORS

Animal reactions that regulate food acceptance have been classified into three interrelated systems (Young, 1948). One of these systems includes stimuli within the animal body which bring on desires for beginning and ending of eating. The second system conditions the animals through evolutionary development of feeding habits on a long time scale and through learning on a short time scale. The third system affecting food preference comprises the animal's environment. These three systems operate a chain of events that includes recognition of food, movement toward the food, appraisal, eating, and leaving the food source. Preference for a food may be exhibited at any point in this series. Unfortunately, these stimulus-response mechanisms in food selection are not well understood for ruminant grazing.

Internal Animal Factors

Animal preferences for foods are stimulated by the senses of sight, smell, taste, touch, and perhaps hearing, in special instances. In a series of experiments with sheep on pastures, Arnold (1966) impaired their sight, smell, taste, and touch separately and in combinations. Blinkering sheep changed their behavior but did not alter their preference for certain forage species. Arnold concluded that sight allowed them to recognize food items and to orient themselves with their surroundings while smell, taste, and touch in the lips each were important in determining the acceptability of some forage species but not others. Apparently each plant stimulates these three senses differently.

Longhurst et al. (1968) showed that deer use smell to make their initial selection of forage. If they like the smell, they taste. If they like the taste, they feed upon the plant. Once the plant is learned, feeding proceeds without initial testing. Hearing is used when fruits are falling but, like sight, has little importance in determining preference.

A very small amount of data exists on the influence of physiological state of an animal on preference for foods. Changing conditions of breeding, pregnancy, lactation, fatness, fear, excitement, fullness of the intestinal tract, and hunger influence animal behavior, grazing time, and amount of forage intake by animals (Arnold, 1964b). Consequent changes in food preferences would be expected, but whether they exist and how they operate have not been explained.

Learned and Evolved Behavior

Previous grazing experience influences the selectivity of foods. Sheep reared on range and pasture were compared as to their preferences for forages after a three-week equalizing period for stabilization of rumen organisms by pen feeding. Those sheep reared on irrigated pasture ranked *Medicago sativa* first in preference, but others raised without *Medicago* selected their previous diets. However, these differences soon disappeared. Differences between preferences for generally unpalatable species lasted longer (Arnold, 1964a).

If the motivation in selective grazing is adequate nutrition, animals should consume highly nutritious but unpalatable feeds before less nutritious but palatable materials. Little evidence exists that grazing animals have nutritional wisdom enabling them to select the best available diet (Arnold, 1964a). Precise rectification of salt deficiency seems to be an exception. Several workers have demonstrated, however, that forages actually eaten contain a higher nutritive content than the average of the pasture from which they were selected (Weir and Torell, 1959).

Restricted food habits, such as that of the walkingstick *(Diapheromera velii)*, which feeds only on *Psoralea tenuiflora* (Ueckert and Hansen, 1972), may have evolved through double natural selection: the grazer becoming more and more specific for food and the producer withstanding the pressure or even evolving a symbiotic need for the consumer. The grazing animal must have an instinct or a hereditary nutritional wisdom to select the foods it can use. This selection process would seem to be a self-regulating mechanism, whereby materials not accepted readily along the digestive tract are not accepted by its mouth. Perhaps the animal accepts undesirable material only to avoid extreme hunger or death.

Many grazing animals have little ability to search for food beyond routes learned as juveniles. They usually spend most of their lives in a restricted territory even when the food supply in that area diminishes.

Grazing herbivores differ markedly in their food habits; each animal species shows preferences for certain plant species, individual plants, parts of plants, plants in certain growth stages, areas of previous use, successional stages, range sites, and range types. Animals often continue to graze these preferred elements although their availability becomes low and associated but less desirable elements more abundant. Animals show variation in food preferences among locations, among parts of the year, over a period of a few days, within the same day, and among individuals (Van Dyne and Heady, 1965).

Food habits are not exhaustively cataloged here, but reference is made to a few of them (Table 3-2). In Chapter 9, further reference is made to diets in conjunction with the management of mixed animal species.

Environmental Influences

Climate, topography, and soil affect palatability of plants and preference for foods by animals (Cook, 1959). A plant species on different sites will vary in chemical composition, succulence, proportion of leaf, and harshness of the foliage. Animals prefer different sites, and the site affects their selection of foods. Hooper (1962) found that deer browsed the same species in different degrees when it occurred on different soil types. Degree of forage use on different sites and selectivity of area for grazing correlated positively with nitrogen, phosphorus, and potassium contents in plants and soils (Vandermark et al., 1971).

Two management practices, fertilization and burning, change palatability of plants as well as feed quantity and nutritional quality. Grazing animals prefer fertilized and burned areas.

Table 3-2 Food preferences shown by several large herbivores during four seasons of the year

Animal	Season	Percentage in Diet			Location	Source
		Grasses	Forbs	Browse		
Hereford cattle	Spring	35	40	25	New Mexico	Herbel and Nelson (1966)
	Summer	71	23	6		
	Fall	50	41	9		
	Winter	50	27	23		
Santa Gertrudis cattle	Spring	58	30	12	New Mexico	Herbel and Nelson (1966)
	Summer	81	17	2		
	Fall	49	43	8		
	Winter	65	20	15		
Sheep	Spring	37	47	16	Texas	McMahan (1964)
	Summer	61	8	31		
	Fall	68	3	28		
	Winter	82	1	17		
Mule deer	Spring	2	30	58	New Mexico	Boeker et al. (1972)
	Summer	2	42	50		
	Fall	6	8	86		
	Winter	2	4	94		
White-tailed deer	Spring	34	65	1	Texas	Drawe and Box (1968)
	Summer	5	71	24		
	Fall	27	66	7		
	Winter	37	59	4		
White-tailed deer	Spring	38	18	43	Montana	Allen (1968)
	Summer	T	54	45		
	Fall	2	17	81		
	Winter	6	29	65		

Table 3-2 Food preferences shown by several large herbivores during four seasons of the year

Animal	Season	Percentage in Diet			Location	Source
		Grasses	Forbs	Browse		
Pronghorn antelope	Spring	25	57	18	Alberta	Mitchell and Smoliak (1971)
	Summer	13	62	25		
	Fall	13	37	50		
	Winter	9	47	43		
Rocky Mountain goat	Spring	70	14	14	Montana	Saunders (1955)
	Summer	72	23	3		
	Fall	76	21	1		
	Winter	58	16	25		
Roosevelt elk	Spring	62	4	34	California	Harper et al. (1967)
	Summer	58	20	22		
	Fall	56	23	21		
	Winter	76	2	22		
Angora goat	Spring	40	25	35	Texas	Malechek and Leinweber (1972)
	Summer	65	8	27		
	Fall	47	12	41		
	Winter	47	4	49		

Grazing animals change their behavior, hence their food preferences, with differences in temperature and rainfall (Castle and Halley, 1953; Corbett, 1953) and with wetness of foliage (Tayler, 1953). Areas of heavy clay soils tend to be avoided by plains game animals in Africa during wet weather; thus weather influences their selectivity of foods.

VEGETATIONAL RESPONSES TO SELECTIVE GRAZING

A large body of literature leaves no doubt that grazing animals influence the vegetation on which they feed. Logically, even under a light grazing intensity, the selected species should be completely eaten first, and others left ungrazed. Many clipping studies indicate that defoliation handicaps grazed plants and should promote their replacement by different species. Thus, given enough time, the vegetation should change to plants with low palatability.

Innumerable accounts describe increases of all preferred plants when grazing pressures were lightened (Ellison, 1960). However, few examples exist where palatable species have completely disappeared because of grazing, especially light grazing. Wild animals have grazed through recent geological time without apparent destruction of their preferred forages. This paradox suggests a number of hypotheses: that moderate intensities of grazing may be stimulatory and beneficial to the continued well-being of rangeland ecosystems, that forage species tolerate defoliation within certain limits, that grazing factors other than forage selectivity may be major causes of vegetational changes, that the subject of grazing influences is not sufficiently understood, and that the separate influences of selective grazing have not been measured.

Definitive information on selective grazing alone as a factor causing vegetational changes remains scarce. Grazing of single sheep in small, uniform pastures of *Phalaris tuberosa* and *Trifolium subterraneum* resulted in marked differences in botanical composition after five months (Arnold, 1964c). Presumably, each animal selected a different diet, but the animals also ate different amounts, and the conclusion was reached that intensity of grazing influenced pasture changes more than did selectivity. After five years of sheep grazing in southcentral Canada, *Euphorbia esula* was reduced by 95 percent and *Agropyron desertorum* increased by 32 percent because of selective grazing (Johnston and Peake, 1960). As with the previously mentioned work, clear elimination of other grazing influences was not made. Few documented observations on the influence of selectivity alone on vegetation are available; yet it is an aspect of grazing that underlies many management recommendations.

LITERATURE CITED

Allen, E. O. 1968. Range use, foods, condition and productivity of white-tailed deer in Montana. *J. Wildl. Mgmt.* 32: 130–141.

Arnold, G. W. 1964a. Some principles in the investigation of selective grazing. *Proc. Aust. Soc. Ani. Production* 5: 258–271.

———. 1964b. Factors within plant associations affecting the behaviour and performance of grazing animals. In *Grazing in terrestrial and marine environments,* pp. 133–154. Oxford: Blackwell.

———. 1964c. Effect of between animal variation in appetite on the yield and composition of pasture. *CSIRO, Div. Plant Ind. Field Sta. Record* 3: 21–28.

———. 1966. The special senses in grazing animals: I. Sight and dietary habits in sheep. *Aust. J. Agr. Res.* 17: 521–529. II. Smell, taste, and touch and dietary habits in sheep. *Aust. J. Agr. Res.* 17: 531–542.

Bayless, S. R. 1969. Winter food habits, range use and home range of antelope in Montana. *J. Wildl. Mgmt.* 33: 538–551.

Bjugstad, A. J., H. S. Crawford, and D. L. Neal. 1970. Determining forage consumption by direct observation of domestic grazing animals. *U.S. Dept. Agr. Misc. Pub.* 1147: 101–104.

Blaser, R. E., R. C. Hames, Jr., H. T. Bryant, W. A. Hardison, J. P. Fontenot, and R. W. Engel. 1960. The effect of selective grazing on animal output. In *Proceedings of the 8th International Grassland Congress,* pp. 601–606.

Boecker, E. L., V. E. Scott, H. G. Reynolds, and B. A. Donaldson. 1972. Seasonal food habits of mule deer in southwestern New Mexico. *J. Wildl. Mgmt.* 36: 56–63.

Castle, M. E., and R. J. Halley. 1953. The grazing behaviour of dairy cattle of the National Institute for Research in Dairying. *Br. J. Ani. Behav.* 1:139–143.

Cook, C. W. 1959. The effect of site on the palatability and nutritive content of seeded wheatgrasses. *J. Range Mgmt.* 12:289–292.

———. 1962. An evaluation of some common factors affecting utilization of desert range species. *J. Range Mgmt.* 15: 333–338.

———, and L. E. Harris. 1950. The nutritive value of range forage as affected by vegetation type, site, and stage of maturity. *Utah Agr. Expt. Sta. Bull.* 344.

———, L. A. Stoddart, and L. E. Harris. 1956. Comparative nutritive value and palatability of some introduced and native forage plants for spring and summer grazing. *Utah Agr. Expt. Sta. Bull.* 385.

Corbett, J. L. 1953. Grazing behaviour in New Zealand. *Br. J. Ani. Behav.* 1: 67–71.

Cowlishaw, S. J., and F. E. Alder. 1960. The grazing preferences of cattle and sheep. *J. Agr. Sci.* 54: 257–265.

Cushwa, C. T., R. L. Downing, R. F. Harlow, and D. F. Urbston. 1970. The importance of woody twig ends to deer in the southeast. *U.S. Dept. Agr. Forest Service Research Paper* SE-67.

Drawe, D. L., and T. W. Box. 1968. Forage ratings for deer and cattle on the Welder Wildlife Refuge. *J. Range Mgmt.* 21: 225–228.

Ellison, L. 1960. Influence of grazing on plant succession of rangelands. *Bot. Rev.* 26:1–78.

Greenhalgh, J.F.D., and G. W. Reid. 1967. Separating the effects of digestibility and palatability on food intake in ruminant digestion. *Nature* 214: 744.

Hanks, D. L., J. R. Brunner, D. R. Christensen, and A. P. Plummer. 1971. Paper chromatography for determining palatability differences in various strains of big sagebrush. *U.S. Dept. Agr. Forest Service Research Paper INT-101.*

Hardison, W. A., J. T. Reid, C. M. Martin, and P. G. Woolfolk. 1954. Degree of herbage selection by grazing cattle. *J. Dairy Sci.* 37: 89–102.

Harper, J. A., J. H. Harn, W. W. Bentley, and C. F. Yocom. 1967. The status and ecology of the Roosevelt elk in California. *Wildl. Monog.* 16.

Heady, H. F. 1964. Palatability of herbage and animal preference. *J. Range Mgmt.* 17:76–82.

———, and D. T. Torell. 1959. Forage preference exhibited by sheep with esophageal fistulas. *J. Range Mgmt.* 12: 28–34.

Herbel, C. R., and A. B. Nelson. 1966. Species preference of Hereford and Santa Gertrudis cattle on a southern New Mexico range. *J. Range Mgmt.* 19: 177–181.

Hooper, J. F. 1962. Influence of soils and deer browsing on vegetation following logging redwood–Douglas fir near Korbel, Humboldt County. M.S. thesis. Univ. of California, Berkeley.

Hurd, R. M., and F. W. Pond. 1958. Relative preference and productivity of species on summer cattle ranges, Bighorn Mountains, Wyoming. *J. Range Mgmt.* 11: 109–114.

Johnston, A., and R. W. Peake. 1960. Effect of selective grazing by sheep on the control of leafy spurge *(Euphorbia esula L.)*. *J. Range Mgmt.* 13: 192–195.

Klebenow, D. A., and G. M. Gray. 1968. Food habits of juvenile sage grouse. *J. Range Mgmt.* 21: 80–83.

Leigh, J. H. 1961. The relative palatability of various varieties of weeping lovegrass *(Eragrostis curvula* (Schrad.) Nees). *J. Br. Grassland Soc.* 16: 135–140.

Longhurst, W. M., H. K. Oh, M. B. Jones, and R. E. Kepner. 1968. A basis for the palatability of deer forage plants. *Trans. N. Am. Wildl. and Nat. Resources Conf.* 33: 181–192.

Malechek, J. C., and C. L. Leinweber. 1972. Forage selectivity by goats on lightly and heavily grazed ranges. *J. Range Mgmt.* 25: 105–111.

Martin. D. J. 1964. Analysis of sheep diet utilizing plant epidermal fragments in faeces samples. In *Grazing in terrestrial and marine environments*, ed. D. J. Crisp, pp. 173–188. Oxford: Blackwell.

McIlvanie, S. K. 1942. Carbohydrate and nitrogen trends in bluebunch wheatgrass, *Agropyron spicatum,* with special reference to grazing influences. *Plant Physiol.* 17: 540–557.

McMahan, C. A. 1964. Comparative food habits of deer and three classes of livestock. *J. Wildl. Mgmt.* 28: 798–808.

Mitchell, G. J., and S. Smoliak. 1971. Pronghorn antelope, range characteristics and food habits in Alberta. *J. Wildl. Mgmt.* 35: 238–250.

Mitchell, H. L., and N. W. Hosley. 1936. Differential browsing by deer on plots variously fertilized. *Black Rock Forest Papers* 1: 24–27.

Nagy, J. G., H. W. Steinhoff, and G. M. Ward. 1964. Effects of essential oils of sagebrush on deer rumen microbial function. *J. Wildl. Mgmt.* 28: 785–790.

Nichol, A. A. 1938. Experimental feeding of deer. *Ariz. Agr. Expt. Sta. Tech. Bull.* 75.

Oh, H. K., M. B. Jones, and W. M. Longhurst. 1968. Comparison of rumen microbial inhibition resulting from various essential oils isolated from relatively unpalatable plant species. *Appl. Microbiol.* 16: 39–44.

———, T. Sakai, M. B. Jones, and W. M. Longhurst. 1967. Effects of various essential oils isolated from Douglas fir needles upon sheep and deer rumen microbial activity. *Appl. Microbiol.* 15: 777–784.

Oldemeyer, J. L., W. T. Barome, and D. L. Gilbert. 1971. Winter ecology of bighorn sheep in Yellowstone National Park. *J. Wildl. Mgmt.* 35: 257–269.

Pigden, W. J. 1953. The relation of lignin, cellulose, protein, starch and ether extract to the "curing" of range grasses. *Can. J. Agr. Sci.* 33: 364–378.

Plice, M. J. 1952. Sugar versus the intuitive choice of foods by livestock. *J. Range Mgmt.* 5: 69–75.

Range Term Glossary Committee. 1964. *A glossary of terms used in range management.* Denver: American Society of Range Management.

Reichert, D. W. 1972. Rearing and training deer for food habits studies. *U.S. Dept. Agr. Forest Service Research Note* RM-208.

Saunders, J. K., Jr. 1955. Food habits and range use of the Rocky Mountain goat in the Crazy Mountains, Montana. *J. Wildl. Mgmt.* 19: 429–437.

Smith, J. G., and O. Julander. 1953. Deer and sheep competition in Utah. *J. Wildl. Mgmt.* 17: 101–112.

Springfield, H. W., and H. G. Reynolds. 1951. Grazing preferences of cattle for certain reseeding grasses. *J. Range Mgmt.* 4: 83–87.

Tayler, J. C. 1953. The grazing behaviour of bullocks under two methods of management. *Br. J. Ani. Behav.* 1: 72–77.

Tomanek, G. W., E. P. Martin, and F. W. Albertson, 1958. Grazing preference comparisons of six native grasses in the mixed prairie. *J. Range Mgmt.* 11: 191–193.

Torell, D. T. 1954. An esophageal fistula for animal nutrition studies. *J. Ani. Sci.* 13: 878–884.

Ueckert, D. H., and R. M. Hansen. 1972. Diet of walkingsticks on sandhill rangeland in Colorado. *J. Range Mgmt.* 25: 111–113.

Vandermark, J. L., E. M. Schmutz, and P. R. Ogden. 1971. Effects of soils on forage utilization in the desert grassland. *J. Range Mgmt.* 24: 431–434.

Van Dyne, G. M., and H. F. Heady. 1965. Botanical composition of sheep and cattle diets on a mature annual range. *Hilgardia* 36:465–492.

———, and D. T. Torell. 1964. Development and use of the esophageal fistula: A review. *J. Range Mgmt.* 17: 7–19.

Wagnon, K. A., and H. Goss. 1961. The use of molasses to increase the utilization of rank, dry forage and molasses—urea as a supplement for weaner calves. *J. Range Mgmt.* 14: 5–9.

Wallmo, O. C., and D. J. Neff. 1970. Direct observations of tamed deer to measure their consumption of natural forage. *U.S. Dept. Agr. Misc. Pub.* 1147: 105–110.

Weir, W. C., and D. T. Torell. 1959. Selective grazing by sheep as shown by a comparison of the chemical composition of range and pasture forage obtained by hand clipping and that collected by esophageal-fistulated sheep. *J. Ani. Sci.* 18: 641–649.

Young, P. T. 1948. Appetite, palatability and feeding habit: a critical review. *Psychol. Bull.* 45: 289–320.

Zyznar, E., and P. J. Urness. 1969. Qualitative identification of forage remnants in deer feces. *J. Wildl. Mgmt.* 33:506–510.

Chapter 4

Physical Effects
of Grazing Animals

Whenever large grazing animals move, the exerted force affects soil, vegetation, and other animals. Major impacts on the land include eating action, which pulls plants from the soil; trampling or treading, which bruises and cuts plants; soil compaction; and covering of vegetation with soil and dung. Other, less well understood, effects occur. The mechanics, magnitude, and control of soil compaction, as results of grazing and as indirect influences on herbage production, have received most attention. This emphasis stems from the fact that soil compaction increases in direct proportion to increasing intensity of rangeland use by animals.

One of the first recommended range practices was to eliminate trampling damage by avoiding repeated use of the same bed-ground by bands of sheep grazing summer ranges (Sampson and Weyl, 1918). Large areas around each place of animal concentration, whether it was a bed-ground, watering point, gate, holding pen, or campground, had become bare of vegetation (Fig. 4-1). Designated livestock trails or stock routes throughout the world receive so much animal traffic that, typically, they are bare of vegetation and eroded. The range manager

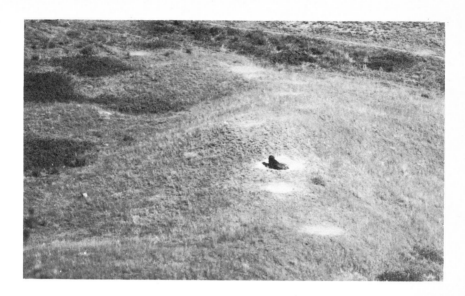

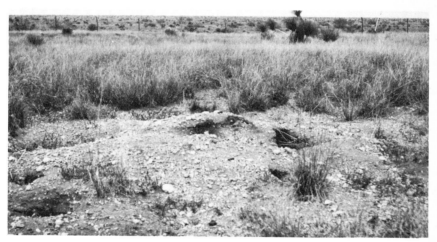

Figure 4-1 Buffalo wallows on the National Bison Range in Western Montana (upper photo) and a rodent den in *Bouteloua eriopoda* grassland, southern New Mexico (lower photo), change soil and vegetation.

seeks to understand and to control the physical effects of animals, especially those of trampling. Defoliation is a physical effect. In fact, all the grazing factors can be considered physical effects. However, this chapter centers on the impact of animal movements upon the habitats of the animals.

ANIMAL MOVEMENTS

Each species of animal, and to a lesser degree each individual, moves in its own repetitive behavioral pattern. These habits relate directly to the resultant physical effects on the land. For example, a highly selective grazing animal travels further in mixed grassland to obtain its daily ration than does a less selective individual. Burrowing activities of rodents, wallowing by bison, dusting by birds, and mixing of soil by invertebrates are other types of innate behavior which result in physical effects on rangelands.

Behavioral patterns of cattle and sheep vary according to type, breed, and age of animal; climate; season; available feed; topography; and other factors. Extensive reviews show the following characteristics for cattle and sheep on a daily basis (Hafez and Schein, 1962; Hafez and Scott, 1962):

	Cattle	Sheep
Grazing time, hr	4–9	9–11
Distance traveled during grazing, km	3–5	5–13
Rumination time, hr	4–9	8–10
Number of grazing periods	4–5	4–7

Sheep spend more time grazing and traveling than do cattle. As the available forage decreases in quantity, both animals travel further and spend more time grazing, as suggested by the maximum figures given above. Great variation in behavior exists among individual animals of the same species and in the same individual in different study conditions.

DIRECT EFFECTS ON PLANTS

Animals exert direct physical impacts on rangeland by pulling and discarding plants and plant parts, wounding bark on trees and shrubs, covering vegetation with soil and dung, and cutting plants and soil with their hooves.

Discarding of Herbage

Animals frequently pull plants from the soil, tear developing grass stems from their sheaths, and sever pieces of plants which they do not eat. *Poa ampla* appears especially susceptible to pulling from the soil (Hyder and Sneva, 1963). Plants differ seasonally in their resistance to pulling; for example, grazing cattle uprooted *Calamovilfa longifolia* and *Stipa comata* most in July but *Bouteloua gracilis* most in September (Quinn and Hervey, 1970).

Pulled and discarded plants may be found after grazing on nearly all range types. Klemmedson and Smith (1964) described such damage to *Bromus tectorum* by cattle. Horses and burros are known for their habit of pulling grasses and consuming only parts of them (McKnight, 1958). Grasshoppers cut blades of grass but eat only parts. Rabbits and rodents have been observed to nip pieces from grasses and shrubs and waste most of the material (Fitch and Bentley, 1949; Koford, 1958; Currie and Goodwin, 1966). More than likely, these actions constitute efforts by the animal to obtain preferred foods and desirable nesting materials. However, the resultant effects go beyond the influence of removing the material actually eaten.

Bark Wounding

Animal damage to the bark of woody plants may cause material above the wound to die. Bark wounding and ring-barking result from rubbing, as by mule deer removing velvet from their antlers; bears and cats sharpening their claws; rabbits, rodents, bears, beavers, and Australian opossums feeding on the inner bark; birds feeding on the sap of trees; and insects depositing their eggs in or under the bark. Many more examples may be given. Perhaps African elephants destroy woody plants more spectacularly than do any other animals (Fig. 4-2). They eliminate forests by breaking limbs for browse and by pushing down trees or tearing them apart seemingly in fun. However, other situations may be striking. Ring-barking by voles killed as much as 84 percent of the *Artemisia tridentata* in some Montana stands (Mueggler, 1967).

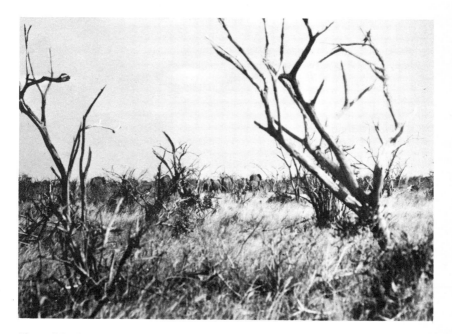

Figure 4-2 Elephants have broken the trees and fire has consumed the debris, converting woodland to grassland in Tsavo National Park, Kenya.

Covering of Live Plants

Larger animals may cover vegetation with dung. Smaller, ground-dwelling animals may dig new burrows, depositing soil on surrounding vegetation. Dung patches killed 75 percent of the grasses and legumes under them in a dairy pasture during a 15-day period (MacDiarmid and Watkin, 1971). Organic materials under the patches decomposed quickly but the affected areas produced little regrowth for a year. Dung patches averaged 0.07 square meter and were deposited at the rate of 13.9 per day (MacDiarmid and Watkin, 1972). This calculates to a coverage of approximately 0.97 square meter per day or 354 square meters per year per cow. While many factors alter these calculations for field application, the conclusion must be accepted that coverage with dung constitutes an important physical effect of grazing animals. A high stocking rate concentrates that effect into a small area. Mineral quantities in soil and vegetation changed by the dung are discussed in Chapter 5.

Mound building by soil-dwelling animals buries live vegetation and alters the habitat for establishment of new plants. Pocket gophers disturbed as much as 25 percent of the soil surface in southwestern Oregon and reduced survival of *Pinus ponderosa* seedlings from 87 percent to 12 percent (Hooven, 1971). Turner (1969) determined that pocket gopher control permitted some plant species to increase, but others decreased. Gopher impact was from both burial of plant and foraging. Ellison (1946) found an average of about 11,000 kilograms of oven-dry soil per hectare per year in the casts of pocket gophers on subalpine range in Utah. This material covered 3.5 percent of the land surface. Julander, Low, and Morris (1969) reported 4,000 to 4,500 pocket gopher mounds per hectare in the Cache National Forest, Utah, which is a higher population density than the one studied by Ellison. Prairie dogs and ground squirrels may move as much soil as to pocket gophers (Koford, 1958).

Whether or not burrowing, mound building, and other activities of ground dwellers result in benefits to range forage production remains unclear. A drier habitat results where pocket gophers burrow than where they are absent; erosion may be increased with the freshly turned soil; and the new mounds provide sites on which germination and establishment of plants are difficult (Laycock, 1958; Julander et al., 1969). Conversely, burrowing counteracts soil compaction; mixes soil and organic matter; covers erosion pavement; and increases water infiltration, soil porosity, soil aeration, and rate of soil formation (Ellison and Aldous, 1952). Species of early successional stages often occur on abandoned two- and three-year-old mounds. There seems little question that rodents in peak numbers consume large quantities of forage and permanently reduce seeded and planted stands of grasses and trees by their physical activities. However, small populations may be more beneficial than harmful to range ecosystems.

Trampling of Plants

Trampling affects plants directly, as animals cut, bruise, and break them during walking and running. This damage or effect on vegetation has been recognized in many instances but has not often been quantatively separated from indirect effects resulting from soil changes. Direct losses of herbage by trampling have been reported as 1 to 5 percent in the short-grass type in Colorado (Quinn and Hervey, 1970), 23 percent of the standing crop on sheep ranges in the mountains of Utah (Laycock et al., 1972), and 68 percent of the lichen component (six *Claydonia* spp. and two *Cretraria* spp.) dislodged by reindeer during a year of grazing (Pegau, 1970). Pegau found that one crossing by reindeer in a loose herd in the dry season dislodged 15 percent of the lichens. Fitch and Bentley (1949) claimed that herbage elimination in the California annual grassland amounted to 25 percent of the annual crop by pocket gophers, 35 percent by ground squirrels, and 16 percent by kangaroo rats; but that the animals ate less than 10 percent of the plant material that they eliminated. Artificial trampling and lodging of *Mertensia arizonica* var. *leonardi* during early growth increased production but decreased production if it occured during flowering and fruiting (Laycock and Conrad, 1969).

Physical damage to plants by trampling changes with the plants' moisture content, elevation of growing points, physical strength of leaves, and flexibility of plant parts (Edmond, 1966). Dry plant materials tend to break rather than bend under the hoof, so late seasonal effects often exceed growing-season damage for many species. The breakage may be desirable if it lays dead grass materials on the soil surface, where decomposition occurs rapidly, or it may be undesirable if it results in loss of soil protection. Rhizomatous grasses as a group resist trampling more than do bunchgrasses.

EFFECTS ON SOIL

Large animals walking on the ground exert physical pressure on the soil by their weight and move soil particles about the land surface with their feet. Soil compaction may result from the first but the second often causes soil loosening and erosion. Small animals cause the same effects as do large animals; the only difference is in degree. Soil-dwelling animals may loosen the soil more than they compact it, thereby countering influences of large animals; for example, the eastern mound-building ant reduced bulk density of the soil by constructing channels and chambers and by depositing subsoil within and on the soil surface (Salem and Hole, 1968). Many species of termites in arid and semiarid regions cement soil particles in their nest building. Those nests below ground form a cap that prevents water infiltration and seedling establishment for many years, but mounds favorable to plant growth are produced by some species of termites (Lee and Wood, 1971). A wide variety of soil-dwelling animals select, transport, rearrange, mix in organic matter, and cement soil particles. Plants respond to changes in soil, so perhaps the positive affects of animals on soil and vegetation outweigh the immediate negative physical effects of animals on plants.

Soil Compaction

Soil compaction is defined as *the packing together of soil particles by forces exerted at the soil surface, which result in an increase in specific gravity by decreasing the pore space* (Lull, 1959). Untold combinations of soil-forming factors exist from place to place and from time to time, so studies of soil compaction show varied results.

The principal soil characteristics determining susceptibility to compaction include texture, structure, porosity, and moisture content. These combine to give each soil condition a capacity to hold or support a load or to resist deformation. Examples selected from Lull (1959) show the approximate deformation point of several soil materials as follows:

	kg/cm^2
Organic soils	0.21
Dry sand	2.0
Wet sand and dry clay	4.0
Packed gravel	8.0

Static loads exerted when rangeland vehicles and animals remain stationary approximate the following pressures on the soil. Values encompass a wide variation in load weights and track sizes or bearing surfaces for vehicles (Lull, 1959).

	kg/cm^2
Crawler tractor	0.32–0.63
Sheep	0.65
Wheel tractor	1.4–2.1
Horse and cow	1.7
Truck	3.5–7.0

These relationships suggest that stationary pressures on many soils do not exceed the supporting capacity of the soils. As animals walk, their weights fall on restricted areas of their hooves, whereby weight per unit area does exceed the soil strength. The result may be chipping of dry soil surfaces, compaction of moist soils, or deformation of wet soils. Supporting capacity of soils varies with moisture content and so does susceptibility to compaction. Maximum compaction occurs at soil moistures about midway between wilting and field capacity. Wetter soils give way or re-form with less compaction than do those with intermediate moisture content. Puddling, or loss of structure, and compaction may occur with repeated traffic on heavy soils.

With constant pressures and soil moisture, soils with high porosity and a wide range of particle sizes are more susceptible to compaction than are other soils. When compaction occurs, small particles replace air spaces between the large pieces. Soils composed of particles mostly of one size usually do not compact unless a well-developed structure has given them large pore spaces. Structureless sands compact very little (Fig. 4-3).

Compaction readily alters or reduces structure and pore volume, thereby increasing soil density, and increased soil density in turn reduces infiltration capacity, permeability to water, water storage capacity, aeration, root penetration, and activities of soil animals and results in less top growth of plants (Lutz and Chandler, 1946). Any of these related factors may be measured to indicate soil compaction, but the one most commonly employed is bulk density or specific gravity.

Changes in Bulk Density

Numerous, but not all, experiments that included measurements of physical effects of animals on soil have shown that grazing increases bulk density or decreases porosity of soil. Those indicating an increase include Duvall and Linnartz (1967) in longleaf pine-bluestem range of the southern United States, true prairie in

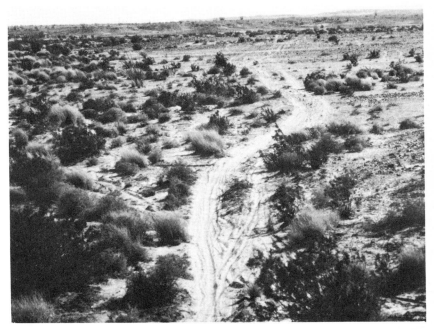

Figure 4-3 Vegetation destroyed and desert pavement altered by motorcycles in southeastern California.

Missouri (Kucera, 1958), sandy soils in Oklahoma (Rhodes et al., 1964), silt loam soils in New Zealand (Edmond, 1958), and numerous other pasture and forest situations as reviewed by Reynolds and Packer (1963). Studies in the short-grass region of the United States have generally found that bulk density increases directly as intensity of grazing becomes more severe (Brown and Schuster, 1969; Knoll and Hopkins, 1959; Rauzi and Hanson, 1966; Read, 1957; and Reed and Peterson, 1961).

In contrast, Canadian workers reported lowered pH and changed carbon content of soils, but little effect on moisture tension, bulk density, total available phosphorus, and total nitrogen. One report was on fescue grassland (Johnston et al., 1971) and the other on the short-grass type after 19 years of heavy grazing at Manyberries Station in southern Alberta (Smoliak et al., 1972). Earlier, Lodge (1954) in southern Canada and Orr (1960) in the Black Hills of South Dakota found increased bulk density in some grazed soils but not in others. Bunchgrass ranges in southeastern Washington (Daubenmire and Colwell, 1942) and subalpine grasslands in Utah (Meeuwig, 1965; Laycock and Conrad, 1967) showed no change in bulk density with heavy grazing.

Packer (1963) maintained that winter grazing by elk reduced plant cover and increased soil bulk density in the *Artemisia-Agropyron* areas north of Yellowstone Park. He suggested that ground cover should not be allowed to diminish below 70 percent and bulk density to increase above 1.04 grams per cubic centimeter. Standards have not been suggested for other soils. Work with tractors on forest soils showed that the most compaction for any trip occurs during the first trip and the maximum compaction occurs between the fourth and tenth trips (Steinbrenner, 1955). If this principle can be extended to grazing, it would suggest that soil compaction by livestock has a maximum value for each set of soil conditions. Ideal and maximum possible bulk density values should be determined for major types of rangeland soils.

Interpretation of changes in bulk density requires care. Soil density changes with moisture content, as it did when soils were compared during early and late growing season (Laycock and Conrad, 1967). Removal of mulch from the soil surface resulted in changes in botanical composition and significant increases in soil bulk density, without trampling by animals (Heady, 1965). These results suggest that altering animal impact on the vegetation itself, and thus changing species composition and soil water content, has an influence on soil density which is separate from the influence of compaction by trampling. Thus, soil compaction may not be caused entirely by animal trampling.

Increased bulk density correlated with decreased soil porosity (Read, 1957; Kucera, 1958; Reed and Peterson, 1961). Grazing of farm woodlots reduced water infiltration (Alderfer and Merkle, 1941; Steinbrenner, 1951; Johnson, 1952), which justified recommendation that they not be grazed. Trampling with an artificial hoof increased overland flow of water in the *Agropyron spicatum– Bromus tectorum* type in southern Idaho (Packer, 1953).

Depth of soil compaction due to grazing seldom reaches 15 centimeters, frequently is limited to the surface 5 centimeters, and probably recovers in five to ten years after heavy grazing is reduced (Reynolds and Packer, 1963). Lusby (1970) reported soil recovery in three years after removal of cattle from the salt-desert-shrub type in Colorado. These conclusions were based on an insufficient number of reports and are likely to change with additional studies in more soil types. Alternating swelling and shrinking, as with freezing-thawing and wetting-drying, reduced the persistence of soil compaction in the studies described above. More than likely, freezing-thawing and wetting-drying together with the activities of animals begin to reduce soil compaction as soon as it occurs.

Desirable Trampling Effects

Although trampling usually implies damage to vegetation and compaction of soil, a number of benefits result from the physical impact of animals. Without disturbance, the surface few millimeters of soil may become sealed and capped with algae and mosses, and intake of water and establishment of new seedlings may be reduced thereby. The mosses and algae often given the surface a dark appearance during dry conditions, as may be observed in long-term livestock exclosures. The trampling action of livestock breaks the cap, moves soil, and helps to cover seeds (Davies, 1938).

Trampling action lays standing dead material onto the soil surface, where decomposition increases and the minerals return to the soil. In addition, trampling reduces large accumulations of mulch and litter by breaking it and may actually stir plant materials into the mineral soil. Like many other factors in moderation, a small amount of treading may be beneficial or show no detrimental effects (Campbell, 1966).

Livestock have been used to trample broadcasted seed into the soil in order to increase chances for successful seedling establishment (Tanganyika Agriculture Corporation, 1961). Rolling or compaction of seedbeds on light soils tends to increase moisture retention and moisture per unit volume of soil and improve several factors for plant survival (Hyder and Sneva, 1956).

Effects of Soil Compaction on Vegetation

Compaction of the soil has been shown to reduce root growth of sunflowers (Veihmeyer and Hendrickson, 1948), development of sugarbeet roots (Pendleton, 1950), root growth of several tree species (Forristall and Gessel, 1955), and penetration into soil of mustard and wheat roots (Fountaine and Payne, 1952). Soil compaction reduced yields of ryegrass—white clover pastures in New Zealand (Edmond, 1963; 1966), alfalfa-brome mixtures in Wisconsin (Federer et al., 1961), bluegrass pastures (Bryant et al., 1972), and sugar maple in grazed woodlands (Dambach, 1944). Artificial trampling reduced ground cover and production of *Agropyron spicatum* and *Bromus tectorum* in southern Idaho

(Packer, 1953). Similar results were reported as a result of use by elk on their winter range in southwestern Montana (Packer, 1963). Compaction of soil below the plowed zone reduced emergence and first-year yields of seeded range grasses (Barton et al., 1966). Roots of *Bouteloua curtipendula,* cv Premier, did not penetrate a compacted layer in old fields during the first year after seeding (Fryrear and McCully, 1972).

Although most of these results confound grazing and trampling, they suggest that soil compaction reduces growth of roots and thereby lowers yield of tops. Extension of these principles to dry rangelands seems reasonable, but results there may be less severe than those from moist soils. Apparently, dry soils do not compact easily. Extensive range grazing, much of it during the dry season, may have little effect on soil compaction and herbage yield.

Animals often walk the same paths again and again as they move across slopes or to and from water. Lange (1969) showed that a network of radial trails developed around water in relatively flat desert-shrub vegetation in Australia. Herbaceous vegetation at the path sides tended to be different from herbaceous vegetation between the paths. In moist regions with long growing season, the paths may be bare in the center and support annual grasses and weedy species or even tall grasses along the edges. Somewhat shorter grasses dominate between the paths (Bates, 1938; Thomas, 1959). Probably, treading exerts major influence in the paths and grazing exerts major influence away from them. Tall growth at the path edge may result from increased soil water beneath the bare paths with less competition for it. These strips of different vegetational compositions in both dry rangelands and moist pastures suggest successional stages that result from various degrees of animal use.

MEASUREMENT OF PHYSICAL EFFECTS

Separation of the physical effects of animals from changes due to defoliation presents difficult problems; these results have been confounded in nearly all grazing studies. Two techniques have been used to determine trampling effects by livestock: One requires herding of muzzled animals along narrow fenced pathways (Edmond, 1958) or across plots for a certain number of trips (Bryant et al., 1972). Another uses a type of cage that allows grazing inside but prevents animals from walking in it (Smith et al., 1971). In the second technique, the investigator beats or strikes vegetation and soil with a weighted device that approximates the size and pressure of a hoof. It may approach the vertical pressure from hooves but is unlikely to duplicate walking. Experimental control of other physical effects, such as direct damage to plants and burrowing of rodents, has been reported less frequently.

Measurements of the effects of trampling on vegetation include those commonly used to sample for changes in botanical composition and biomass of the vegetation. Measurements of changes in the internal geometry of soil include specific gravity or bulk density, porosity, pore size distribution, conductivity of air and water, and infiltration. Changes in the pressures needed to displace soil particles and the load that a soil will hold without failure can indicate trampling effects. These techniques have been defined and evaluated for soil compaction studies (ASAE/SSSA Soil Compaction Committee, 1958).

EVALUATION OF PHYSICAL EFFECTS

Relating vegetational changes to the causes of those changes remains a difficult problem of separation of multiple interrelationships. For example, disappearance of plant materials in grazed-ungrazed treatments may be due to foraging by insects, birds, and other animals; to trampling; to pulling or breakage of plants; to falling of mature plant parts such as flowers, lower leaves, and fruits; and to the shattering action of wind, rain, hail, and windblown materials. Obscuring of these losses by regrowth may further complicate measurement and interpretation. Martin (1970) called the losses *invisible utilization* because difference in and out of cages or before and after grazing confused all changes in biomass due to physical impacts with those due to actual eating of forage by the excluded animals.

Physical effects of animals are as ageless as the animal species themselves. England and De Vos (1969) reported the presence of fossil trails and wallows made by bison on the Canadian prairies. Burrowing animals have pushed more soil materials downhill than uphill for as long as these animals have existed. Ground birds have changed soil characteristics by their scratching and dusting; all animals have exerted pressure by walking; and many more physical effects have occurred during geological time. Therefore, trampling and other physical effects of animals are unavoidably parts of the grazing process.

As one evaluates these related effects, compensations or counterinfluences become increasingly obvious and the concept that physical effects mean damage becomes less important. It is true that livestock compact the soil and break plants by their trampling, but, immediately, other animals and the physical environment tend to reduce the compaction. Breaking of plants may stimulate them to new growth. Bare soil quickly becomes occupied with new plants. Populations of plants and animals succeed as their physical requirements become available, and they diminish as their surroundings become more favorable for other species. Thus, the physical effects of animals may be either desirable or harmful depending upon the context of evaluation.

Permanent changes in rangeland ecosystems can result from excessive physical effects of animals, but usually compensations quickly cover one physical effect with another. The vigor of rangeland systems likely depends as much on favorable physical conditions for the dominant plant species as upon adequate quantities of nutrients and energy. Unfortunately the physical state of rangeland systems has received little attention.

LITERATURE CITED

Alderfer, R. B., and F. G. Merkle. 1941. Structural stability and permeability of native forest soils compared with cultivated areas of the same soil type. *Proc. Soil Sci. Soc. Am.* 6: 98–103.

ASAE/SSSA Soil Compaction Committee. 1958. Concepts, terms, definitions and methods of measurements for soil compaction. *Agri. Engin.* 39: 173–176.

Barton, H., W. G. McCully, H. M. Taylor, and J. E. Box. 1966. Influence of soil compaction on emergence and first-year growth of seeded grasses. *J. Range Mgmt.* 19: 118–121.

Bates, G. H. 1938. Life forms of pasture plants in relation to treading. *J. Ecol.* 26: 452–454.

Brown, J. W., and J. L. Schuster. 1969. Effects of grazing on a hardland site in the southern high plains. *J. Range Mgmt.* 22: 418–423.

Bryant, H. T., R. E. Blaser, and J. R. Peterson. 1972. Effect of trampling by cattle on bluegrass yield and soil compaction of a Meadowville Loam. *Agron. J.* 64: 331–334.

Campbell, A. G. 1966. Effects of treading by dairy cows on pasture production and botanical structure, on a Te Kowhai soil. *N. Z. J. Agr. Res.* 9: 1009–1024.

Currie, P. O., and D. L. Goodwin. 1966. Consumption of forage by black-tailed jackrabbits on salt desert ranges of Utah. *J. Wildl. Mgmt.* 30: 304–311.

Dambach, C. A. 1944. Comparative productiveness of adjacent grazed and ungrazed sugar-maple woods. *J. For.* 42: 164–168.

Daubenmire, R. F., and W. E. Colwell. 1942. Some edaphic changes due to overgrazing in *Agropyron-Poa* prairie of southeastern Washington. *Ecol.* 23: 32–40.

Davies, W. 1938. Vegetation of grass verges and other excessively trodden habitats. *J. Ecol.* 26: 38–49.

Duvall, V. L., and N. E. Linnartz. 1967. Influences of grazing and fire on vegetation and soil of longleaf pine-bluestem range. *J. Range Mgmt.* 20: 241–247.

Edmond, D. B. 1958. Some effects of soil physical conditions on ryegrass growth. *N. Z. J. Agr. Res.* 1: 652–659.

———. 1963. Effects of treading perennial ryegrass (*Lolium perenne* L.) and white clover (*Trifolium repens* L.) pastures in winter and summer at two soil moisture levels. *N. Z. J. Agr. Res.* 6: 265–276.

———. 1966. Influence of animal treading on pasture growth. *Proceedings of the 10th International Grassland Congress,* pp. 453–458.

Ellison, L. 1946. The pocket gopher in relation to soil erosion on mountain range. *Ecology* 27: 101–114.

———, and C. M. Aldous. 1952. Influence of pocket gophers on vegetation of subalpine grassland in central Utah. *Ecology* 33: 177–186.

England, R. E., and A. De Vos. 1969. Influence of animals on pristine conditions on the Canadian grasslands. *J. Range Mgmt.* 22: 87–94.

Federer, C. A., G. H. Tenpas, D. R. Schmidt, and C. B. Tanner. 1961. Pasture and soil compaction by animal traffic. *Agron. J.* 53: 53–54.

Fitch, H. S., and J. R. Bentley. 1949. Use of California annual-plant forage by range rodents. *Ecology* 30: 306–321.

Forristall, F. F., and S. P. Gessel. 1955. Soil properties related to forest cover type and productivity on the Lee Forest, Snohomish County, Washington. *Proc. Soil Sci. Soc. Am.* 19: 384–389.

Fountaine, E. R., and P. C. J. Payne. 1952. *The effect on tractors on volume weight and other soil properties.* Wrest Park, England-National Institute of Agricultural Engineering.

Fryrear, D. W., and W. G. McCully. 1972. Development of grass root systems as influenced by soil compaction. *J. Range Mgmt.* 25: 254–257.

Hafez, E. S. E., and M. W. Schein. 1962. The behaviour of cattle. In *The behaviour of domestic animals,* pp. 247–296. Baltimore: Williams and Wilkins.

————, and J. P. Scott. 1962. The behaviour of sheep and goats. In *The behaviour of domestic animals,* pp. 297–333. Baltimore: Williams and Wilkins.

Heady, H. F. 1965. The influence of mulch on herbage production in an annual grassland. *Proceedings of the 9th International Grassland Congress,* pp. 391–394.

Hooven, E. F. 1971. Pocket gopher damage on ponderosa pine plantations in southwestern Oregon. *J. Wildl. Mgmt.* 35: 346–356.

Hyder, D. N., and F. A. Sneva. 1956. Seed- and plant-soil relations as affected by seedbed firmness on a sand loam range land soil. *Proc. Soil Sci. Soc. Am.* 20: 416–419.

————, and ————. 1963. Studies of six grasses seeded on sagebrush-bunchgrass range. *Ore. Agr. Expt. Sta. Tech. Bull. 71.*

Johnson, E. A. 1952. Effect of farm woodland grazing on watershed values in the Southern Appalachian Mountains. *J. For.* 50: 109–113.

Johnston, A., J. F. Dormaar, and S. Smoliak. 1971. Long-term grazing effects on fescue grassland soil. *J. Range Mgmt.* 24: 185–188.

Julander, O., J. B. Low, and O. W. Morris. 1969. Pocket gophers on seeded Utah mountain range. *J. Range Mgmt.* 22: 325–329.

Klemmedson, J. O., and J. G. Smith. 1964. Cheatgrass *(Bromus tectorum* L.). *Bot. Rev.* 30: 226–262.

Knoll, G., and H. H. Hopkins. 1959. The effects of grazing and trampling upon certain soil properties. *Trans. Kan. Acad. Sci.* 62: 221–231.

Koford, C. B. 1958. Prairie dogs, whitefaces, and blue grama. *Wildl. Monog.* 3: 1–79.

Kucera, C. L. 1958. Some changes in the soil environment of a grazed prairie community in central Missouri. *Ecology* 39: 538–540.

Lange, R. T. 1969. The piosphere: sheep track and dung patterns. *J. Range Mgmt.* 22: 396–400.

Laycock, W. A. 1958. The initial pattern of revegetation of pocket gopher mounds. *Ecology* 39: 346–351.

————, H. Buchanan, and W. C. Krueger. 1972. Three methods for determining diet, utilization, and trampling damage on sheep ranges. *J. Range Mgmt.* 25: 252–256.

————, and P. W. Conrad. 1967. Effect of grazing on soil compaction as measured by bulk density on a high elevation cattle range. *J. Range Mgmt.* 20: 136–140.

————, and ————. 1969. How time and intensity of clipping affect tall bluebell. *J. Range Mgmt.* 22: 299–303.

Lee, K. E., and T. G. Wood. 1971. *Termites and soils.* New York: Academic Press.

Lodge, R. W. 1954. Effects of grazing on the soil and forage of mixed prairie in southwestern Saskatchewan. *J. Range Mgmt.* 7: 166–170.

Lull, H. W. 1959. Soil compaction on forest and rangelands. *U.S. Dept. Agr. Misc. Pub.* 768.

Lusby, G. C. 1970. Hydrologic and biotic effects of grazing vs. non-grazing near Grand Junction, Colorado. *J. Range Mgmt.* 23: 256–260.

Lutz, H. J., and R. F. Chandler, Jr. 1946. *Forest soils.* New York: Wiley.

MacDiarmid, B. N., and B. R. Watkin. 1971. The cattle dung patch: 1. Effect of dung patches on yield and botanical composition of surrounding and underlying pasture. *J. Br. Grassland Soc.* 26: 239–245.

———, and ———. 1972. The cattle dung patch: 3. Distribution and rate of decay of dung patches and their influence on grazing behavior. *J. Br. Grassland Soc.* 27:48–54.

Martin, S. C. 1970. Relating vegetation measurements to forage consumption by animals. *U.S. Dept. Agr. Misc. Pub.* 1147: 93–100.

McKnight, T. L. 1958. The feral burro in the United States: distribution and problems. *J. Wildl. Mgmt.* 22: 163–179.

Meeuwig, R. O. 1965. Effects of seeding and grazing on infiltration capacity and soil stability of a subalpine range in central Utah. *J. Range Mgmt.* 18: 173–180.

Mueggler, W. F. 1967. Voles damage big sagebrush in southwestern Montana. *J. Range Mgmt.* 20: 88–91.

Orr, H. K. 1960. Soil porosity and bulk density on grazed and protected Kentucky bluegrass range in the Black Hills. *J. Range Mgmt.* 13: 80–86.

Packer, P. E. 1953. Effects of trampling disturbance on watershed conditions, runoff, and erosion. *J. For.* 51: 28–31.

———. 1963. Soil stability requirements for the Gallatin elk winter range. *J. Wildl. Mgmt.* 27: 401–410.

Pegau, R. E. 1970. Effect of reindeer trampling and grazing on lichens. *J. Range Mgmt.* 23: 95–97.

Pendleton, R. A. 1950. Soil compaction and tilling operation effects on sugar beet root distribution and seed yields. *Proceedings of the American Society of Sugar Beet Technology,* pp. 278–285. Fort Collins, Colo.: The Beet Sugar Development Foundation.

Quinn, J. A., and D. F. Hervey. 1970. Trampling losses and travel by cattle on sandhills range. *J. Range Mgmt.* 23: 50–55.

Rauzi, F., and C. L. Hanson. 1966. Water intake and runoff as affected by intensity of grazing. *J. Range Mgmt.* 19: 351–356.

Read, R. A. 1957. Effect of livestock concentration on surface-soil porosity with shelterbelts. *J. For.* 55: 529–530.

Reed, M. J., and R. A. Peterson. 1961. Vegetation, soil, and cattle response to grazing on northern Great Plains range. *U.S. Dept. Agr. Tech. Bull.* 1252.

Reynolds, H. G., and P. E. Packer. 1963. Effects of trampling on soil and vegetation. *U.S. Dept. Agr. Misc. Pub.* 940: 116–122.

Rhodes, E. D., L. F. Locke, H. M. Taylor, and E. H. McIlvain. 1964. Water intake on a sandy range as affected by 20 years of differential cattle stocking rates. *J. Range Mgmt.* 17: 185–190.

Salem, M. Z., and F. D. Hole. 1968. Ant *(Formica exsectoides)* pedoturbation in a forest soil. *Proc. Soil Sci. Soc. of Am.* 32: 563–567.

Sampson, A. W., and L. H. Weyl. 1918. Range preservation and its relation to erosion control on western grazing lands. *U.S. Dept. Agr. Bull.* 675.

Smith, A., R. A. Arnott, and J. M. Peacock. 1971. A comparison of the growth of a cut sward with that of grazed swards, using a technique to eliminate fouling and treading. *J. Br. Grassland Soc.* 26: 157–162.

Smoliak, S., J. F. Dormaar, and A. Johnston. 1972. Long-term grazing effects on *Stipa-Bouteloua* prairie soils. *J. Range Mgmt.* 25: 246–250.

Steinbrenner, E. C. 1951. Effect of grazing on floristic composition and soil properties of farm woodlands in southern Wisconsin. *J. For.* 49: 906–910.

———. 1955. The effect of repeated tractor trips on the physical properties of forest soils. *Northwest Sci.* 29: 155–159.

Tanganyika Agriculture Corporation. 1961. The influence of cattle trampling on the establishment of perennial grasses. *Herb. Abst.* 31: 265, Abst. No. 1500.

Thomas, A. S. 1959. Sheep paths. *J. Br. Grassland Soc.* 14: 157–164.

Turner, G. T. 1969. Responses of mountain grassland vegetation to gopher control, reduced grazing, and herbicide. *J. Range Mgmt.* 22: 377–383.

Veihmeyer, F. J., and A. H. Hendrickson. 1948. Soil density and root penetration. *Soil Sci.* 65: 487–493.

Chapter 5

Energy Flow and Nutrient Cycling

The mass of live and dead organic materials in any rangeland system exists within a potential energy level determined by the inherent capabilities of organisms and by the energy sources of the site. Assessment of the magnitude of the many pathways of energy flow has characterized much recent ecological work. Studies of arid and semiarid rangeland ecosystems usually concern energy use by grazing mammals, but the uses of energy and minerals by other animals need to be emphasized.

The energy transformations actually achieved in the primary production of photosynthates and the secondary production of biomass in other tropic levels—herbivores, predators, and decomposers—depend upon minerals as well as upon energy. The cyclic flow of nitrogen and the essential minerals, especially phosphorus, calcium, magnesium, sodium, potassium, chlorine, and sulfur, closely associates with energy transfer. At each trophic level, energy is partitioned and minerals altered by assimilation, respiration, excretion, defecation, and production. These transfers of energy through biological systems and the cycling of minerals from soil through plants and back to the soil constantly change in rate and magnitude. An objective in range management is to increase the efficiency of energy and nutrient cycles.

ENERGY FLOW

Primary productivity transforms radiant energy from the sun into chemical energy by photosynthesis. *Gross primary production* includes energy stored by the plant and used in its own respiration. The more useful concept, *net primary production,* excludes the energy used in respiration and is the accumulated plant biomass.

Williams (1966) estimated that his range plots in the San Joaquin Valley, California, received 1,600,000 kilocalories per square meter of solar energy of which 700,000 or 44 percent were in the wavelengths usable by plants. Net primary production amounted to 3,275 kilograms per hectare or 1,410 kilocalories per square meter. This was 0.09 percent of the total energy received at the site. Steers, one type of secondary producer on those plots, had a net productivity of 69 kilocalories per square meter for an efficiency of 0.004 percent relative to the total energy income.

Although studies in other ecosystems have shown different proportions of energy converted from plants to animals, all are in broad agreement that a small fraction of the total energy becomes net primary production and that a still smaller part becomes net secondary production (Williams, 1964). For example, Buechner and Golley (1967) reported in a review that the meadow mouse produced 17.5 kilocalories per square meter a year, the African elephant 23.3, the white-tailed deer 43.1, and the Uganda kob 62.4 kilocalories per square meter a year.

Energy passes through biological systems with tremendous unrecoverable losses at each transfer. Because energy is not recycled, increased efficiency of energy use depends upon prevention of losses.

Macfadyen (1963) estimated that metabolic activity in kilocalories per square meter per year was 186 for herbivorous and decomposer organisms including molluscs, arthropods, and earthworms in an oak woodland in Holland. Biomass and mean annual respiration of harvester termites in tropical regions may be of the same order of magnitude as that of mixed populations of mammalian herbivores in Africa and much greater than that of the marsupial fauna in northern Australia (Lee and Wood, 1971). Macfadyen (1964) maintained that energy respired by a temperate meadow was proportioned about one-seventh by plants, two-sevenths by herbivores, and four-sevenths by decomposers. Apparently poikilothermic animals transfer energy more efficiently than homiotherms do because most of the former have an extremely efficient digestive system and use the energy efficiently (McNeill and Lawton, 1970; Petrusewicz and Macfadyen, 1970). Small animals process more energy relative to their weight than do larger animals. Clearly, small soil-dwelling animals have a little known but significant influence on energy flow.

Cook (1970) suggested that energy transfer presents a new approach to calculating biological efficiency of range ecosystem for domestic animals. On the assumption that 40 to 50 percent range utilization expresses forage consumption, between 18 and 25 percent of the herbage produced becomes metabolizable energy in cattle and sheep. Cook allocated that amount of energy among the various physiological functions such as reproduction, growth, heat, and travel. This information and body weight changes of grazing animals permitted him to calculate energy productivity on rangeland. Different classes of animals had different energy requirements. For example, a yearling steer required energy equivalent to 0.85 of a nonlactating cow unit and about 0.67 of a cow-calf unit. A ewe and lamb rated 0.21 of a cow-calf unit.

Energy transformation and animal responses can be used to establish standards for measuring range livestock production. Cook (1970) showed that summer mountain ranges in Utah produced about three times more energy than did desert winter ranges, and that steers converted dietary energy to meat about 45 percent more efficiently than did cows.

Partitioning of energy draws attention to points of energy dissipation where ecosystem modifications to increase efficiency of energy use may be effective (Fig. 5-1). The energy budget shows the relative impact of different organisms. Because different kinds of animals use energy at different rates, biomass comparisons between such diverse species as grasshoppers, mice, and livestock have much less value than do comparisons of energy transfer. The aboveground species account for a small proportion of the secondary production. Macfadyen (1961, 1968) maintains that microorganisms in the soil produce as much as 90 percent of the secondary production because of their large numbers and rapid metabolic rates. Apparently, far more energy is liberated through soil-dwelling organisms than through aboveground herbivores. If this is so, the decomposers may limit range ecosystems, and increasing range productivity can depend upon speeding their

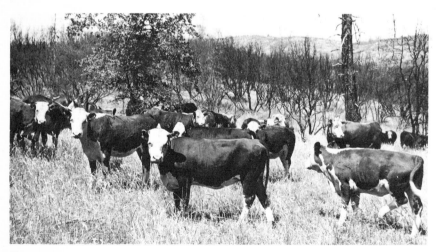

Figure 5-1 Conversion of brushlands to grasslands increases those energy pathways needed to produce range livestock. *(Photo by Lineer Studio.)*

activities. Proper assessment of the importance of cattle, sheep, and other large herbivores as energy transfer agents within the total range ecosystem requires knowledge of energy flow rather than of biomass.

NUTRIENT CYCLING

Herbivores divert portions of plant nutrients into animal food chains. Unlike energy, which leaves the system when released from chemical bonds, nutrients return to the soil. They may be circulated from soil to plants to animals to soil numerous times. Each nutritive element follows its own particular pathway because each serves separate functions and is held by different chemical bonds. Grazing animals alter these pathways, change the rates of nutrient release by decomposition, reposition nutrients in the pasture, and may even remove significant amounts of nutrients from the area. Without herbivory, nutrients in vegetation leach directly to the soil or return to the soil via decomposition or organic material.

Generalized Nutrient Cycling

A generalized diagram of nutrient cycling is shown in Figure 5-2. The boxes represent nutrient accumulations, and the arrows show pathways of transfer from one sink to another. Descriptions abound of quantities of minerals in the various pools such as the soil and the litter. A common type of study partitions or budgets the total quantity of minerals among all the compartments.

Detailed analysis of mineral reserves describes the system organization and provides a base for the study of mineral flow through the system, the system physiology. Such an analysis depends upon estimates of the sizes of the various nutrient pools and the transport of minerals from one pool to another. Transfers occur in both space and time. The annual cycle of plant biomass accumulation and litter decomposition has received much attention. Comprehensive reviews of this information are available (Rodin and Basilevich, 1965; Charley, 1972; Pieper, 1974).

Without herbivores, minerals cycle from soil to plants, to litter, and back to soil. Grazing adds many more routes because minerals pass through the animals and are deposited as dung or urine, which decompose at rates different from those of the uneaten plant litter. The herbivores may die, may be eaten by carnivores, or may be removed from the area by man; thus many more pathways for the flow of minerals are added (Fig. 5-2). Lemming cycles have been correlated with cycling of nitrogen, phosphorus, potassium, and calcium. Schultz (1964, 1969) speculated that primary production in the arctic grassland declines and the lemming populations crash when vegetation is overgrazed and a high proportion of the nutrients become unavailable in plant and animal detritus. As decomposition releases the nutrients, primary production increases and the lemmings soon increase.

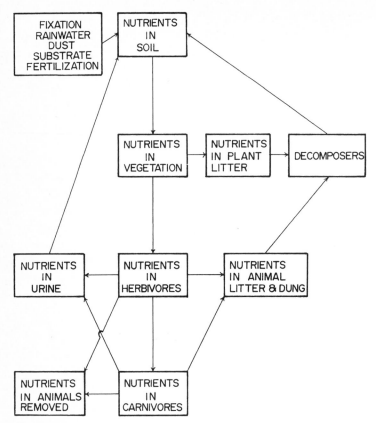

Figure 5-2 Generalized nutrient cycles in range ecosystems. *(Redrawn from Pieper, 1973).*

The pattern of accumulation and decomposition of dead herbage on rangeland is closely related to productivity. Early recognition of this point is evidenced in stipulations that proper utilization was removal of 50 to 80 percent of the herbage crop. Mulch—litter or plant residue—in terms either of amounts per unit area or of percent of soil cover, has been used to evaluate range conditions and trend. Generally, litter cover correlates directly with production, but an excess may decrease herbage growth.

Recent studies suggest that dead herbage is an important but neglected constituent of pasture and range systems. Beginning at the low point of plant residue accumulations, near the end of the rapid-growth season, amounts accumulate rapidly as current growth dies. Decomposition, consumption by invertebrates, and grazing by vertebrates gradually reduce the amount of residue until the next yearly increment is added. However, that addition does not occur as a single large amount at one time. Growth and decomposition are overlapping in time; for example, flowers and lower leaves in herbaceous vegetation begin to die almost as soon as they begin to grow. The living and dead materials are tangled in space. Both the time-related and space-related variables are subject to modification by grazing and the physical environment. Dead herbage must be included or used to modify conventional range production and utilization parameters if vegetational changes and the nutritional environment of the grazing animal are to be understood.

Man adds minerals to any system by fertilization and supplemental feeding of livestock, which in effect borrow from some other system. Natural additions of minerals include those in rainwater, dust, fixation by microorganisms, and continual decomposition of soil parent material.

After analysis of data in several papers, Pieper (1974) constructed an approximate budget of nutrient cycling in the desert grassland of southern New Mexico (Table 5-1). This table shows that domestic livestock at moderate stocking rates altered the routing of only a small quantity of minerals as they cycled and that rodents were unimportant in the area. Commonly, soil reserves constitute many times the amounts of cycled minerals (Charley, 1972).

Elements Returned to the Soil

Grazing animals return a large proportion of the consumed plant nutrients to the soil. Petersen et al. (1956) have determined that a mature cow produces 25 kilograms of dung and 9 kilograms of urine daily. Chemical composition on a percentage net weight basis of the excreted materials was as follows:

	Nitrogen	P_2O_5	K_2O
In feces	0.38	0.18	0.22
In urine	1.1	0.01	1.15

Most of the voided phosphorus occurred in the dung whereas the urine was rich in nitrogen and potassium.

Table 5-1 Annual compartmental budget, in kilogram per hectare, for quantities of five elements on a desert grassland range in southern New Mexico (*Pieper, 1974*)

Transfer or compartment	Nitrogen	Phosphorus	Potassium	Calcium	Magnesium
Taken up by vegetation	6.6	0.3	4.5	1.4	2.1
Average wt. in herbage	4.4	0.2	3.0	1.0	1.4
Average wt. in litter	4.5	0.5	2.6	1.4	0.3
Transferred from litter to soil	4.5	0.5	2.6	1.4	0.3
Consumed by cattle	4.6	0.2	3.1	1.0	1.4
Consumed by rodents	0.19	0.01	0.13	0.04	0.06
Returned in feces	0.5	0.10	0.2	0.65	1.1
Returned in urine	3.8	0.03	2.9	0.25	0.2
Removed by sale of calves	0.26	0.07	0.02	0.10	0.003

Hutton et al. (1965, 1967) found that dairy cattle voided most of the minerals consumed, excreted from 5 to 26 percent in milk, and retained less than 10 percent of any element. The elements were distributed in the following percentages:

	In feces	In urine	In milk	Retained
Nitrogen	26	53	17	4
Potassium	11	81	5	3
Phosphorus	66	0	26	8
Sodium	30	56	8	6
Calcium	77	3	11	9

These values vary according to the nutrient content of the forage, condition of the animal, and physiological state of the animal. However, direct relationships were found for nitrogen in dung and in forage (Raymond, 1966) and between nitrogen, phosphorus, and potassium in forage and in soil (Vandermark et al., 1971). Although exact estimates vary, it is accepted that 80 to 95 percent of all ingested nutrients are returned to the soil in the excreta of domestic animals.

Elements from Outside Sources

Rainfall, dust, and microorganisms that fix materials from the atmosphere continuously increase the reserves of nitrogen and several of the major minerals in the soil (Henzell and Norris, 1962). Rock decomposition may be the only significant source of additional phosphorus for range soils. Decomposition of soil parent material adds other minerals to the available supply.

Fried and Broeshart (1967) and Allison (1965) showed that rainwater adds about 9 kilograms (range 2 to 45) of nitrogen to each hectare per year as a worldwide average. Sulfur additions in rainwater may be over 112 kilograms per hectare per year near industrial plants that burn large amounts of fossil fuel. Extensive rangelands receive less, perhaps as little as 100 grams per hectare per year. In Great Britain, Robertson and Davies (1965) showed that minerals added to the soil in rainwater each year were calcium, 7 kilograms per hectare; magnesium, 4 kilograms per hectare; potassium, 3 kilograms per hectare; and essentially no phosphorus. Arid and semiarid regions with more dust than Great Britain likely have greater quantities of minerals in rainwater. Relatively high contents of ammonia, nitrate, and sulfate in rainwater occurred in the industrial regions and central part of North America. Chlorine and sodium were concentrated near the oceans, potassium occurred uniformly across the continent, and calcium concentrated in dry regions (Junge, 1958; Junge and Werby, 1958).

Numerous studies reported nitrogen fixation by *Rhizobia* on planted pasture legumes to be between 56 and 670 kilograms per hectare per year (Fried and Broeshart, 1967; Sears et al., 1965). Most native legumes contribute nitrogen to range ecosystems. Becking reported in 1968 that about one-third of the 330 species in 13 genera of nonleguminous seed plants were known to fix nitrogen. The genera are as follows: *Alnus, Casuarina, Ceanothus, Cercocarpus, Coriaria, Discaria, Dryas, Elaeagnus, Gale, Hippophae, Myrica, Purshia,* and *Shepherdia.* Numerous species of bacteria, actinomyces, fungi, yeasts, and blue-green algae are known to be nonsymbiotic fixers of nitrogen from the air (McKee, 1962). Nonsymbiotic nitrogen fixation is difficult to measure, but it is likely to be 22 to 56 kilograms per hectare per year on unfertilized pastures (Whitehead, 1970).

Elements Lost from an Area

The bovine body contains about 20 percent ash and 80 percent protein on a fat-free and water-free basis (Reid et al., 1955). Both water and fat contents vary tremendously but have little influence on the amounts of protein and ash. A 450-kilogram animal contains about 15.9 kilograms of nitrogen, 5.9 of calcium, 3.2 of phosphorus, 0.9 of potassium, 0.7 of sodium and sulfur, 0.5 of chlorine, and 0.2 kilograms of magnesium (Maynard and Loosli, 1969). If that animal were two years old and required the forage from 4 hectares, it would remove 2 kilograms per hectare per year of nitrogen, 0.7 of calcium, 0.4 of phosphorus, and less than 0.1 of the other elements. A dry sheep on the Australian pastures which ingests 450 kilograms of feed in a year might fix half a kilogram or so of nitrogen in its body each year (Barrow and Lambourne, 1962). Annual transport of nutrients by sheep from heather lands in England amounted to 1 kilogram per hectare of calcium and phosphorus and 2 kilograms per hectare of nitrogen (Robertson and Davies, 1965). Domestic animals that are sold or removed from the land take elements with them, but not large amounts. In contrast, grain crops may remove 67 to 78 kilograms per hectare of nitrogen, 11 to 17 of phosphorus, and 67 to 78 of potassium (Fried and Broeshart, 1967).

Recoveries of fertilizer nitrogen in forages seldom reach 50 percent. Many attempts have been made to account for the losses (Martin and Skyring, 1962). Nutrients are eroded and leached from an area in runoff and ground water. Likens et al. (1967) found that forested watersheds had losses of calcium, magnesium, and sodium but the losses were balanced with release from rocks through weathering. Domestic animals removed from rangeland take minor amounts of nutrients with them.

DOMESTIC ANIMALS AND NUTRIENT CYCLING

Although they remove few nutrients, large grazing animals have a small but probably significant effect on the overall mineral cycles on rangeland. Hannon (1958) in Australia suggested that less than 0.1 percent of the total nitrogen in the soil actually cycles. Williams (1964), working with improved pastures, accounted for 7 percent of the total nitrogen that annually cycled through plants and animals. Nitrogen fixed in the yearly crop of California annual grassland averaged less than 22 kilograms per hectare and accounted for less than 0.5 percent of the total nitrogen in the soil-plant system. Phosphorus in the herbage amounted to approximately 0.2 percent of the total (Heady, 1965). Microorganisms have been shown to use most of the net primary energy (Macfadyen, 1968), so they probably cycle more nutrients than domestic animals do.

The preceding conclusion and others about nutrient cycling lean heavily on work with pastures grown under humid and irrigated conditions. However, energy transfer and nutrient cycling on dry rangeland are likely to differ from those situations more in degree than in principle. Research underway in several range areas will shed light on these relationships.

THE NITROGEN CYCLE

Nitrogen, which is the largest component of air and tends to return to its relatively inert gaseous state in the atmosphere, is an ideal indicator of nutrient cycling. Unlike energy, which moves through an ecosystem once and is lost, nitrogen cycles continuously from the atmospheric and soil reservoirs to primary producers, to consumers, and back to the reservoirs. None is lost from the system, although time may need to be reckoned on a geological basis for completion of the longest cycles. Pathways that nitrogen may follow are numerous and complicated (Doak, 1952; Allison, 1965).

Figure 5-3 depicts a generalized nitrogen cycle for rangeland. It indicates that losses and gains occur continuously as nitrogen moves from place to place and alters in chemical form. Figure 5-3 should be considered a flow chart of possibilities, not a closed cycle nor a steady state of nitrogen movements. Nitrogen was selected to illustrate cycling because of the key role it plays in range production, the large body of available information about it, and the emphasis on urinary nitrogen describing animal influences.

Urinary nitrogen from cattle and sheep was found to be 76 percent or more in urea form, 12 percent in amino acids, 1 percent ammonia, and the remainder in numerous other nitrogenous compounds (Doak, 1952). Most of the amino form of nitrogen is glycine (Bathurst, 1952). Depending upon temperatures and soil moisture, urinary nitrogen moves rapidly through the various pathways in the nitrogen cycle (Fig. 5-3), and its effects on plants may disappear in a few weeks.

Nitrogen deposited on the leaves may be absorbed or returned to the atmosphere. Most of it, however, is added to the soil reservoir, where it changes to ammonia, to nitrite, and finally to nitrate. At each step, nitrogen may be absorbed by plants, lost by leaching, or returned to the atmosphere. Volatilization results when ammonia is formed from chemical decomposition of nitrogen oxides and by enzymatic reduction of nitrogen oxides (Woldendorp, 1968).

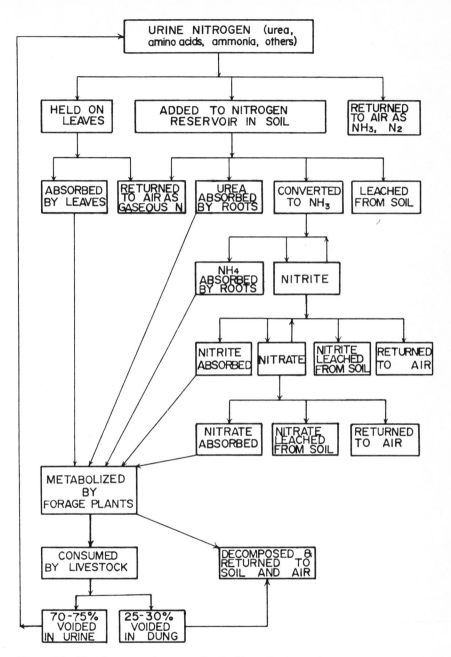

Figure 5-3 The nitrogen cycle on rangeland, with emphasis on urinary nitrogen.

Simpson and Freney (1967) found that nitrogen reactions were most rapid in soils with low quantities of nitrogen. However, Power (1972) claimed that fertilizer nitrogen may become immobilized in any part of the cycle and suggested a three to four-year cycle for complete nitrogen turnover in the northern Great Plains. Apparently the rate of nitrogen release from urine is much faster and from dung slower than from decomposing plant litter (Barrow, 1961). On balance, turnover of nitrogen is accelerated by passage through animals but, like other nutrients, it may go into reserves anywhere in the cycle.

THE SULFUR CYCLE

Sulfur, like nitrogen, is cycled from soil through plant and animal and back to the soil (Blair, 1971). The sulfate ion ($SO_4 =$) is the principal form of sulfur used by plants. The sulfur cycle begins with the oxidation of rock sulfides and elemental sulfur into sulfates. These may be leached from the soil, precipitated as sulfate salts, absorbed on the surface of clay particles, absorbed by organisms, or reduced to sulfides. Sulfur is added in fertilizers, introduced into the cycle in rainwater, and absorbed as SO_2 from the atmosphere.

The sulfur that becomes bound in organic matter is unavailable to plants and must be converted to sulfate form, largely by microbial action, before it can be used again.

The ultimate source of sulfur, unlike that of nitrogen, is the soil parent material, which releases sulfates during weathering. High atmospheric sulfur contents are primarily due to burning of fossil fuels. Much of the sulfur in range ecosystems is associated with plants, animals, and organic detritus. Till and May

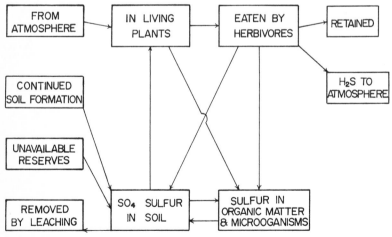

Figure 5-4   The sulfur cycle in a rangeland context. *(After Till and May, 1970.)*

(1970a, 1970b), in Australia, found about 200 kilograms per hectare total sulfur of which 14 kilograms per hectare were available to plants and 100 in the cycling pools (Fig. 5-4). Undoubtedly other grazing situations would show different amounts. These authors maintained that the sulfur cycle formed a highly complex closed system with few losses and net additions essentially from fertilization (Till and May, 1971). Reductions of the total pool were due to cropping, which takes about 4.5 kilograms of sulfur in 2,700 kilograms of grass hay and 11.3 kilograms in alfalfa hay (Whitehead, 1964). A 450-kilogram steer has about 0.7 kilograms of sulfur retained in its body. A cow probably consumes 9 kilograms of sulfur in a year, nearly all of which is returned to the soil. Voided sulfur is about 30 percent in dung and 70 percent in urine (Frame, 1970; Walker, 1957).

OTHER ELEMENTS

Animals influence rates and amounts of other cycling elements as well as those of nitrogen and sulfur. Voided phosphorus occurs almost completely in the dung, where it apparently is more concentrated than in the original feed. It leaches slowly from dung, especially that of sheep and other animals that produce pellets. Approximately 20 percent is inorganic and readily available to plants (Bromfield, 1961; Bromfield and Jones, 1970). Organic phosphorus in dung becomes slowly available to plants as the dung decomposes (Doak, 1952; Petersen et al., 1956; Williams, 1962; Floate, 1971).

Complexity of mineral cycling is further illustrated by phosphrous turnover within the ruminant animal (Tomas et al., 1967). Saliva constitutes the principal source of phosphorus for rumen organisms. It determines the inorganic phosphorus level in the rumen fluid. The cycle is from gut to blood to saliva to rumen.

Potassium, mostly in the urine, is readily taken in by plants (Sears, 1956); hence its effectiveness disappears in a few months. Wolton (1963) found potassium in the urine of grazing animals to be the key to favorable response to fertilization with nitrogen and phosphorus. This illustrates the fact that nutrients in animal excreta have interacting influences. If one is in short supply in the pasture system, increases in the others have little effect.

MANAGEMENT BASED UPON MINERAL CYCLING

Living matter is likened to a chemical engine that transforms the energy of biomass to usable form. Minerals are important to that transformation. Availability to plants of all minerals except phosphorus appears to be enhanced by passage of herbage through grazing animals. Animals increase the rate of cycling, especially of those ions, such as chorides and nitrates, which move easily in soil solution. Evidence supporting this contention appears in the relationships of animals to pasture productivity. Frame (1970) showed that dung patches have the equivalent of over 112 kilograms per hectare of phosphorus and 224 kilograms per hectare of potassium. Urine spots have fertilizer rates of nitrogen above 336 kilograms per hectare and potassium rates above 560 kilograms per hectare. Urine spots from a single cow may cover a combined area of 1 or more square meters each day. Even though part of the deposited nutrients is lost, more than 50 to 60 percent becomes effective in forage production in which the nutrients constitute an important factor (Herriott et al., 1959). Grazing may increase the need for supplements of the mobile nutrients but is likely to have little effect on the supply of phosphorus (Barrow, 1967).

Working in a pasture situation in New Zealand, Sears (1953) found that dung and urine increased the grass component of pastures and decreased the *Trifoliums*. Other investigations repeated this general conclusion (Wheeler, 1958; Norman and Green, 1958; Green and Cowling, 1960; Mundy, 1961). Brockman et al., (1971) maintained that mineral cycling due to grazing increases the efficiency of fertilizer use over cutting. For example, dry-matter pasture yield increased from 10,000 to 12,000 kilograms per hectare for grazing over cutting and removal with the same rates of fertilization (Brockman, 1971). Apparently, rate of nitrogen circulation increases directly as grazing intensity becomes severe and nitrogen status in the soil improves. Nitrogen recirculation by grazing animals permits maintenance of pasture production with fewer inputs than with forage harvesting.

While these results were found on pastures with high stocking rates, it would seem logical that they should apply, in principle, to rangelands. Low rainfall and low stocking rates should change only the speed of cycling and the amounts of nutrients in the cycle. Wight and Black (1972) found that unfertilized range systems in the northern Great Plains cycled about 67 kilograms per hectare per year of nitrogen but that two to three times more biomass production occurred when cycling nitrogen amounted to 112 to 185 kilograms per hectare per year.

Rates of dung decomposition depends upon coprophagous insects in many regions of the world. Their activities incorporate dung into the soil, reduce infective stages of parasitic worms, reduce breeding areas for flies, and increase rate of mineral cycling (Fig. 5-5). Dung-feeding insects have been shown to vary in kinds and numbers in different adjacent vegetational types (White, 1960). Australia has introduced dung beetles from Africa to improve organic matter decomposition and soil fertility in their tropical pastures (Bornemissza, 1960; Gillard, 1967).

The bottleneck in mineral cycling likely rests in the slow decomposition of organic accumulations. Management to increase the rate of mineral turnover includes trampling and laying of standing dead materials so that contact with moisture and soil organisms is increased, addition of nutrients to reduce imbalances, and spreading of unnecessarily large accumulations of litter.

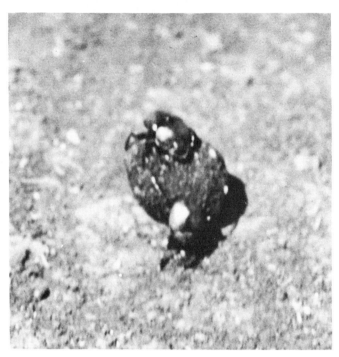

Figure 5-5 Dung beetles rolling a ball of dung that will be buried and will serve as the larval food supply.

LITERATURE CITED

Allison, F. E. 1965. Evaluation of incoming and outgoing processes that affect soil nitrogen. In Soil nitrogen, eds. W. V. Bartholomew and F. E. Clark. *Am. Soc. Agron. Monog.* 10:573–606.

Barrow, N. J. 1961. Mineralization of nitrogen and sulphur from sheep faeces. *Aust. J. Agri. Res.* 12:644–650.

———. 1967. Some aspects of the effects of grazing on the nutrition of pastures. *J. Aust. Inst. Agr. Sci.* 33:254–262.

———, and L. J. Lambourne. 1962. Partition of excreted nitrogen, sulphur, and phosphorus between the faeces and urine of sheep being fed pasture. *Aust. J. Agr. Res.* 13:461–471.

Bathurst, N. O. 1952. The amino-acids of sheep and cow urine. *J. Agr. Sci.* 42:476–478.

Becking, J. H. 1968. Nitrogen fixation by non-leguminous plants. *Stikstof* 12:47–74.

Blair, G. T. 1971. The sulphur cycle. *J. Aust. Inst. Agr. Sci.* 37:113–121.

Bornemissza, G. F. 1960. Could dung eating insects improve our pastures? *J. Aust. Inst. Agr. Sci.* 26:54–56.

Brockman, J. S. 1971. The difference in yield between cut and grazed swards. *J. Br. Grassland Soc.* 26:192.

————, C. M. Rope, and M. T. Stevens. 1971. The effect of the grazing animal on the N status of grass swards. *J. Br. Grassland Soc.* 26:209–212.

Bromfield, S. M. 1961. Sheep faeces in relation to the phosphorus cycle. *Aust. J. Agr. Res.* 12:111–123.

————, and O. L. Jones. 1970. The effect of sheep on the recycling of phosphorus in hayed-off pastures. *Aust. J. Agr. Res.* 21:699–711.

Buechner, H. K., and F. B. Golley. 1967. Preliminary estimation of energy flow in Uganda Kob *(Adenota kob thomasi* Newmann). In *Secondary productivity of terrestrial ecosystems (principles and methods),* ed. K. Petrusewicz, pp. 243–254. Warsaw: Polish Academy of Sciences.

Charley, J. L. 1972. The role of shrubs in nutrient cycling. In Wildland shrubs—their biology and utilization. *U.S. Dept. Agr. Forest Service General Tech. Rep.* INT-1, pp. 182–203.

Cook, C. W. 1970. Energy budget of the range and range livestock. *Colo. State Univ. Expt. Sta. Bull.* TB 109.

Doak, B. W. 1952. Some chemical changes in the nitrogenous constituents of urine when voided on pasture. *J. Agr. Sci.* 42:162–171.

Floate, M. J. S. 1971. Plant nutrient cycling in hill land. *Fifth Report of the Hill Farming Research Organization,* 1967-1970, Edinburgh, pp. 15–34.

Frame, J. 1970. Fundamentals of grassland management. Part 10: The grazing animal. *Scottish Agr.* 50:28–44.

Fried, M., and H. Broeshart. 1967. *The soil-plant system in relation to inorganic nutrition.* New York: Academic Press.

Gillard, P. 1967. Coprophagous beetles in pasture ecosystems. *J. Aust. Inst. Agr. Sci.* 33:30–34.

Green, J. O., and D. W. Cowling. 1960. The nitrogen nutrition of grassland. *Proceedings of the 8th International Grassland Congress,* pp. 126–129.

Hannon, Nola J. 1958. The status of nitrogen in the Hawkesburg sandstone soils and their plant communities in the Sydney district. 11. The distribution and circulation of nitrogen. *Proceedings Linnean Soc. New S. Wales* 83:65–85.

Heady, H. F. 1965. The influence of mulch on herbage production in an annual grassland. *Proceedings of the 9th International Grassland Congress,* pp. 391–394.

Henzell, E. F., and D. O. Norris. 1962. Processes by which nitrogen is added to the soil/plant system. In A review of nitrogen in the tropics with particular reference to pastures. *Commonwealth Bureau of Pastures and Field Crops Bull.* 46:1–18.

Herriott, J. B. D., O. A. Wells, and J. Dilnot. 1959. The grazing animal and sward productivity. *J. Br. Grassland Soc.* 14:191–198.

Hutton, J. B., K. E. Jury, and E. B. Davies. 1965. Studies of the nutritive value of New Zealand dairy pastures. 4. The intake and utilization of magnesium in pasture herbage of lactating dairy cattle. *N. Z. J. Agr. Res.* 8:479–496.

————, ————, and ————. 1967. Studies of the nutritive value of New Zealand dairy pastures. 5. The intake and utilization of potassium, sodium, calcium, phosphorus,and nitrogen in pasture herbage by lactating dairy cattle. *N. Z. J. Agr. Res.* 10:367–388.

Junge, C. E. 1958. The distribution of ammonia and nitrate in rainwater over the United States. *Trans. Am. Geophys. Union* 39:241–248.

————, and R. T. Werby. 1958. The concentration of chloride, sodium, potassium, calcium, and sulphate in rainwater over the United States. *J. Meteorology* 15:417–425.

Lee, K. L., and T. G. Wood. 1971. *Termites and soils.* London: Academic Press.

Likens, G. E., F. H. Bormann, N. M. Johnson, and R. S. Pierce. 1967. The calcium, magnesium, potassium, and sodium budgets for a small forested ecosystem. *Ecology* 48:772–785.

Macfadyen, A. 1961. Metabolism of soil invertebrates in relation to soil fertility. *Ann. Appl. Biol.* 49:215–218.

————. 1963. The contribution of the microfauna to total soil metabolism. In *Soil organisms,* eds. J. Doeksen, and J. van der Drift, pp. 3–16. Amsterdam: North-Holland.

————. 1964. Energy flow in ecosystems and its exploitation by grazing. In *Grazing in terrestrial and marine environments,* ed. D. J. Crisp, pp. 3–20. Oxford: Blackwell.

————. 1968. The animal habitat of soil bacteria. In *The ecology of soil bacteria,* eds. T. R. G. Gray and D. Parkinson, pp. 66–76. Toronto: Univ. of Toronto Press.

Martin, A. E., and G. W. Skyring. 1962. Losses of nitrogen from the soil/plant system. In A review of nitrogen in the tropics with particular reference to pastures. *Commonwealth Bureau of Pastures and Field Crops Bull.* 46:19–34.

Maynard, L. A., and J. K. Loosli. 1969. *Animal nutrition.* New York: McGraw-Hill.

McKee, H. S. 1962. *Nitrogen metabolism in plants.* Oxford: Clarendon Press.

McNeill, S., and J. H. Lawton. 1970. Annual production and respiration in animal populations. *Nature* 225:472–474.

Mundy, E. J. 1961. The effect of urine and its components on the botanical composition and production of a grass/clover sward. *J. Br. Grassland Soc.* 16:100–105.

Norman, J. J. T., and J. O. Green. 1958. The local influence of cattle dung and urine upon the yield and botanical composition of permanent pasture *J. Br. Grassland Soc.* 13:39–45.

Petersen, R. G., H. L. Lucas, and W. W. Woodhouse. 1956. The distribution of excreta by freely grazing cattle and its effect on pasture fertility. 1. Excretal distribution. *Agron. J.* 48:440–444. 11. Effects of returned excreta on the residual concentrations of some fertilizer elements. *Agron. J.* 48:444–449.

Petrusewicz, K., and A. Macfadyen. 1970. Productivity of terrestrial animals: Principles and methods. *IBP Handbook No. 13.* London: Blackwell.

Pieper, R. D. 1974. Effects of herbivores on nutrient cycling and distribution. *Proceedings of the 2nd U.S.-Australia Range Workshop.*

Power, J. F. 1972. Fate of fertilizer nitrogen applied to a northern great plains rangeland ecosystem. *J. Range Mgmt.* 25:367–371.

Raymond, W. F. 1966. The nutritive value of herbage. In *Recent advances in animal nutrition,* ed. J. T. Abrams, pp. 81–116. London: Churchill.

Reid, J. T., G. H. Wellington, and H. O. Dunn. 1955. Some relationships among the major chemical components of the bovine body and their application to nutritional investigations. *J. Dairy Sci.* 38:1344–1359.

Robertson, R. A., and G. E. Davies. 1965. Quantities of plant nutrients in heather ecosystems. *J. Appl. Ecol.* 2:211–219.

Rodin, L. E., and N. I. Basilevich. 1965. *Production and mineral cycling in terrestrial vegetation,* Transl. Scripta Technica Ltd. London: Oliver and Boyd.

Schultz, A. M. 1964. The nutrient-recovery hypothesis for arctic microtine cycles. 11. Ecosystem variables in relation to arctic microtine cycles. In *Grazing in terrestrial and marine environments,* ed. D. J. Crisp, pp. 57–68. Oxford: Blackwell.

———. 1969. A study of an ecosystem: the arctic tundra. In *The ecosystem concept in natural resource management,* ed. G. Van Dyne, pp. 77–93. New York: Academic Press.

Sears, P. D. 1953. Pasture growth and soil fertility. VII. General discussion of the experimental results, and of their application to farming practice in New Zealand, *N. Z. J. Sci. Tech.* 35:221–236.

———. 1956. The effect of the grazing animal on pasture. *Proceedings of the 7th International Grassland Congress,* pp. 92–103.

———, V. C. Goodall, R. H. Jackman, and G. S. Robinson. 1965. Pasture growth and soil fertility. VIII. The influence of grasses, white clover, fertilizers and the return of herbage clippings on pasture production of an impoverished soil. *N. Z. J. Agr. Res.* 8:270–283.

Simpson, J. R., and J. R. Freney. 1967. The fate of labelled mineral nitrogen after addition to three pasture soils of different organic matter contents. *Aust. J. Agr. Res.* 18:613–623.

Till, A. R., and P. F. May. 1970a. Nutrient cycling in grazed pastures. II. Further observations with (^{35}S) gypsum. *Aust. J. Agr. Res.* 21:253–260.

———, and ———. 1970b. Nutrient cycling in grazed pastures. III. Studies of labelling of the grazed pasture system by solid (^{35}S) gypsum and acqueous mg ^{35}SO$_4$. *Aust. J. Agr. Res.* 21:455–463.

———, and ———. 1971. Nutrient cycling in grazed pastures. IV. The fate of sulphur-35 following its application to a small area in a grazed pasture. *Aust. J. Agr. Res.* 22:391–400.

Tomas, F. M., R. J. Moir, and M. Somers. 1967. Phosphorus turnover in sheep. *Aust. J. Agr. Res.* 18:635–645.

Vandermark, J. L., E. M. Schmutz, and P. R. Ogden. 1971. Effects of soils on forage utilization in the desert grassland. *J. Range Mgmt.* 24:431–434.

Walker, T. W. 1957. The sulphur cycle in grassland soils. *J. Br. Grassland Soc.* 12:10–18.

Wheeler, J. L. 1958. The effect of sheep excreta and nitrogenous fertilizer on the botanical composition and production of a ley. *J. Br. Grassland Soc.* 13:196–202.

White, E. 1960. The distribution and subsequent disappearance of sheep dung on Pennine moorland. *J. Ani. Ecol.* 29:243–250.

Whitehead, D. C. 1964. Soil and plant-nutrition aspects of the sulphur cycle. *Soils and Fertilizers* 27:1–8.

———. 1970. The role of nitrogen in grassland productivity. A review of information from temperate regions. *Commonwealth Bureau of Pasture and Field Crops Bull.* 48.

Wight, J. R., and A. L. Black. 1972. Energy fixation and precipitation-use efficiency in a fertilized rangeland ecosystem of the northern Great Plains. *J. Range Mgmt.* 25:376–380.

Williams, C. H. 1962. Changes in the nutrient availability in Australian soils as a result of biological activity. *J. Aust. Inst. Agr. Sci.* 28:196–205.

Williams, O. B. 1964. Energy flow and nutrient cycling in ecosystems. *Proc. Aust. Soc. Ani. Prod.* 5:291–300.

Williams, W. A. 1966. Range improvement as related to net productivity, energy flow, and foilage configuration. *J. Range Mgmt.* 19:29–34.

Woldendorp, J. W. 1968. Losses of soil nitrogen. *Stikstof* 12:32–46.

Wolten, K. M. 1963. An investigation into the simulation of nutrient returns by the grazing animal in grassland experimentation. *J. Br. Grassland Soc.* 18:213–219.

Chapter 6

Redistribution
of Minerals

At any location, the supply of nutrients in the ecosystem constantly changes. Increased and improved nutrient availability results from weathering of rocks, deposit of erosion products, precipitation and fixation from the atmosphere, immigration of organisms, and fertilizer applications. This chapter describes the redistribution of minerals attributable to the presence of plants and actions of animals. Displacements in quantities of minerals occur vertically and horizontally. An influx one place means an outflux from another. Although nitrogen is a gas, many references to nitrogenous compounds are made in this chapter.

REDISTRIBUTION BY PLANTS

Minerals absorbed throughout the root zone become a part of the aboveground plant biomass or fall back to the soil in leaves, flower parts, bark, and other plant parts. Eventually the woody structure dies and its stored minerals return to the soil reserve or are removed from the system. Roots gather minerals from a wider area than that receiving most of the litter; thus localized concentrations of minerals and organic matter under the woody plant canopy result. This movement of minerals has been examined in many ways: as a vertical and horizontal mosaic of minerals, environmental conditions, and organisms; as an annual cycle of production, deposit, and decomposition of litter; as to variations among regions due to climate and vegetational types; in relation to plant succession and changing species composition; and as the cause for changing mineral status of soil.

Gradients of minerals, organisms, and microenvironments occur because plants are discrete and live sufficiently long for striking patterns to develop. Open canopies foster mosaics, which may be highly regular or random in their distribution. Once formed the pattern may remain, as shown by gradients of nitrogen around stumps of the legume *Acacia aneura* and chlorides of sodium and potassium around *Atriplex vesicaria* (Charley, 1972). Perennial herbaceous plants and even annuals contribute to the mosaic, but less is known about their influence than about that of woody plants. Vegetational mosaics are patterns of foods and cover for animals (Fig. 6-1). They may be altered in their development by grazing animals.

Trees

The transfer of various chemical elements between trees and soil follows a number of routes and occurs at different rates according to the species of plant and the kind of chemical. Studies have shown that radioactive elements introduced into roots

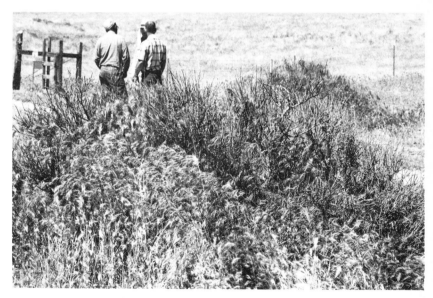

Figure 6-1 *Bromus rigidus,* an annual grass, has reached exceptional height within a plant of *Atriplex polycarpa.*

and stems rapidly pass into other plant parts, from which they may be leached by rain, fall in litter, and be released from the roots. Rain leached approximately 15 percent of cesium-134 from innoculated *Quercus alba* trees before leaf fall (Witherspoon, 1964). Potassium reacts much like cesium. Calcium apparently leaches at a slower rate than does potassium and falls in the litter. Rainfall under *Pseudotsuga menziesii* contained as much phosphorus and twice the potassium as that dropped in litter fall (Will, 1959). Potassium, calcium, magnesium, and sodium occurred as leachates in rainwater that dripped through tree canopies and ground flora and flowed down the stems (Carlisle et al., 1967). *Cornus florida* functioned through uptake and subsequent leaching to keep more calcium in circulation and to increase exchangeable calcium in the soil of a *Pinus taeda* plantation over that in a pure pine stand (Thomas, 1969). These results show that part of the nutrients complete a cycle from plant to soil and return to plants without intervening leaf fall and decay.

Accumulations of wood and litter contain large amounts of mineral nutrients in unavailable form. After rapid initial leaching of soluble nutrients, further release occurs slowly by decomposition, which may be the limiting factor on rate of nutrient cycling in forests (Olson and Crossley, 1963). Of the aboveground material in a *Pinus taeda* plantation, Switzer and Nelson (1972) estimated that 18 percent cycled during the twentieth year after planting. This percentage varied from 7 percent of the calcium to 28 percent of the potassium.

Soil contained more phosphates under both pines and oaks than under grass in a transect from the central valley of California (elevation 225 meters) to the mixed conifer type in the Sierra Nevada Mountains at 1,250 meters (Johannesson, 1958). Botanical composition of the herbaceous vegetation differs under tree canopy from that in open areas, plant development may be somewhat later under the trees, and differences in selectivity of forages occur between shaded and unshaded sites. These differences may be due in part to the combined redistribution of nutrients by both plants and animals. Soil phosphates and other accumulations could decrease to the grassland levels if the woody plants were removed. Cycling of one item influences another; hence mosaic development of organisms as well as nutrients occurs.

Shrubs

Nutrient and organic matter gradients become sharper with increasing aridity, especially where individual shrubs are separated by unoccupied soil, as in most shrub steppes. Closed canopies often show little pattern in the distribution of nutrients (Charley, 1972). Distribution of nitrogen under a bush of *Atriplex vesicaria* (Fig. 6-2) illustrates concentration near the soil surface and somewhat to one side of the central stem due to wind action and gravity. Oxygen uptake and nitrification under *Atriplex* bushes averaged about twice that in the interbush area. The shrubs may be cycling nitrogen, speeding the nitrification process, or doing

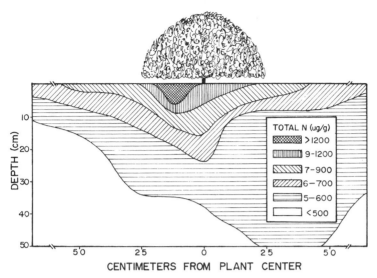

Figure 6-2 Distribution of nitrogen in the soil beneath a single bush of *Atriplex vesicaria (Charley, 1972).*

both (Rixon, 1971). Nitrogen in soils under *Acacia gregii, Cassia armata,* and *Larrea divaricata* decreased significantly as a function of distance from the center of the shrub canopy (Garcia-Moya and McKell, 1970). Beaty and Tan (1972) described a situation in which 23 percent more nitrogen occurred under pensacola bahiagrass *(Paspalum notatum)* than in fallow soil after three years without harvests or fertilization of the grass.

Distributions of other nutrients, as well as nitrogen, correlate with shrub presence. Five species of *Atriplex* concentrated salts of sodium, potassium, calcium, and magnesium in their leaves and fruiting bracts (Beadle, 1952). These minerals tended to reach constant concentrations in the materials, regardless of soil content (Beadle et al., 1957; Ashby and Beadle, 1957). The five desert-shrub species varied in their ability to concentrate minerals in the soil beneath them. In another situation, *Grayia spinosa* concentrated potassium in the leaves and soil beneath the plants and *Sarcobatus vermiculatus* accumulated sodium. *Bromus tectorum* reflected the concentration with higher sodium content when growing under *Sarcobatus* shrubs than between them (Rickard, 1965).

REDISTRIBUTION BY LARGE HERBIVORES

Large herbivorous animals tend to concentrate near water, salt, feeding areas, bed-grounds, and shade. These are focal points to which animals move in more or less regular daily or seasonal migratory patterns. By consuming forages away from these focal points and depositing excreta near them, animals cause a redistribution of minerals. Hilder (1966) found that sheep deposited about a third of their excreta on only 5 to 7 percent of the total area of pastures 40 hectares in size. About 30 percent of the pasture became enriched and 70 percent impoverished. Earlier in the same study, Hilder and Mottershead (1963) showed that sheep bed-grounds, in comparison with areas 128 meters away, had twice the total nitrogen and exchangeable calcium, 5 times the magnesium, 14 times the available phosphorus, and a 130-fold increase in potassium.

Weir (1971) described a situation in Wankie National Park, Rhodesia, in which herds of about ten wild species of game gathered around water during drought. Accumulation of minerals occurred within a kilometer of water and depletion occurred from 3 to 5.5 kilometers away from water. Losses of minerals were likely in the area along the edges between grassland and woodland, a favorite grazing habitat for several species.

A number of workers showed that excreta was not distributed uniformly in dairy and other intensively used pastures, especially if the grazing period was more than a few days (Petersen et al., 1956a, 1956b; Hilder, 1966). Cattle droppings appeared more random than those of sheep. Not only do animals redistribute nutrients that they consume, but also they remove nutrients disproportionately because of their selectivity for certain feeds (Van Dyne and Heady, 1965).

Defecation rates for cattle vary between 10 and 16 times per day (MacLusky, 1960). After review and experimentation with two kinds of dairy cows, MacDiarmid and Watkin (1972) showed that the average defecation rate was 14 times per day and the dung covered an area of approximately a square meter. Dung affects vegetation on an area three to six times larger than the area covered or three to six square meters on a daily basis, if no overlap occurs. Castle and MacDaid (1972) suggested an average affected area of 4 square meters per cow day. Urination rates per day vary from 8 to 12 times, but each urination patch affects an area larger than the dung patch (MacLusky, 1960; Lotero et al., 1966). According to these approximations, cattle apparently influence about 8 square meters per day by deposit of dung and urine. This is 7 to 8 percent of the total grazed area in a year if the stocking rate is one cow per 4 hectares per year.

Many factors alter these influences. Effects of urine decrease in a linear manner from the center outward (Lotero et al., 1966). The greatest impact of dung on vegetation occurs under the deposit and at its edge (MacDiarmid and Watkin, 1971). Rapid losses of moisture and ammonia immediately follow deposition of both dung and urine. After initial decomposition of fine materials, disappearance of dung occurred at a slow rate and from the bottom upward. If the upper surface of a dung pat dries, it tends to shed rainwater and remain for a year or two before disappearing (Lotero et al., 1966). Both the magnitude of effect and rate of dissipation directly relate to precipitation and temperature, to rate of plant growth, and to actions of coprophagus insects (Davies et al., 1962).

Estimates have varied as to the importance of dung and urine in pasture management. Sears (1956), Weeda (1967), Watkin (1954), Wheeler (1958), and

Wolton (1963) maintained that return of dung and urine to pastures increased production of forage and altered botanical composition. Norman and Green (1958) found effects from urine to last no longer than two pasture rotations and effects from dung, about four rotations. Herriott and Wells (1963), Lotero et al., (1966), and Marsh and Campling (1970) suggested that little fertility is contributed to the pasture as a whole but concentration of nutrients has considerable local influence. However, concentration leads to losses of nutrients by leaching and evaporation (Watson and Lapins, 1969). Except where animals congregate and enrich the soil with large accumulations of dung and urine, effects may be minor. Effects of dung and urine on rangeland remain poorly understood.

Forage production on ranges and pastures depends upon grazing intensity, selectivity by animals, trampling, and many other influences that have not been separated from the redistribution of nutrients by animals. Little wonder that contrasting results accrue from different studies. Still, abundant observations have established that congregations of grazing animals alter soil and vegetation.

REDISTRIBUTION BY OTHER ANIMALS

Other animals in addition to the large herbivores consume foods in one place and concentrate their waste at a central point in their territories. Termiteria in Africa are richer in nutrients than is the surrounding soil because of the gathering of plant materials by termites. The mounds are high in organic material because termites use salivary or fecal materials to cement the soil (Goodland, 1965). Lee and Wood (1971) found two- to ten-fold increases of nitrogen, phosphorus, calcium, and potassium in a mound of *Nasutitermes triodiae* in northern Australia. These authors cited other studies that illustrate nutrient gathering by several soil animals as follows:

	In termite galleries	In anthills	In earthworm casts	In soil
Nitrogen, %	0.102	0.126	0.192	0.087
Phosphorus, %	1.20	0.058	0.061	0.041
Potassium, %	0.61	0.37	0.89	0.48

The conclusion that all animals alter the distribution of nutrients seems reasonable, although the influence of many species on their habitats has not been determined.

MINERAL CONCENTRATIONS DUE TO LIVESTOCK FEEDING

Confinement and feeding of animals in a small space concentrates waste materials and results in mineral concentrations in soil and water. The element of greatest concern is nitrogen because it may reach concentrations in drainage water which exceed health standards (45 ppm NO_3 or 10 ppm $NO_3 - N$) (U.S. Public Health

Service, 1962). Examples in which these standards have been exceeded include areas with numerous dairy herds in southern California (Adriano et al., 1971) and the livestock feedlot area along the North Platte River Valley in Colorado (Stewart et al., 1967).

Nitrate standards mentioned previously are based on dangers of methemoglobinemia, which may occur when the body converts nitrates to nitrites. Excessive concentrations of nitrates in feed and water endanger both livestock and humans.

Minerals concentrated in corrals or in home and community sewage systems often find their way into streams and lakes. This fertilization of the water may increase algae and other aquatic plants, eventually resulting in large amounts of decaying organic matter that reduces oxygen content of the water, kills fish, and causes unpleasant odors. Other sources of leachable minerals include fertilizers used on cropland; decomposing crop residues; industrial discharges; and natural sources such as erosion, fixation from the atmosphere, rainwater, and rock decomposition. Evaluation of the relative contributions to mineral pollution in both surface and ground water remains difficult. Nitrogen undergoes rapid and complex transformations as it moves in and out of soil reservoirs, making the evaluation of nitrate as a water pollutant difficult. Allison (1966) described the principal soil losses of nitrogen as leaching of nitrates, denitrification, and volatilization of ammonia. Stewart et al. (1967) found about 100 kilograms per hectare of nitrate in a natural grassland in the North Platte River Valley and 16 times that amount under corrals. Shallow wells and surface water generally have much more nitrate than do deep wells, according to Smith (1967), who believes that most nitrate in water comes from natural sources and that little comes from fertilizer nitrogen. The most common minerals in underground water are calcium, sodium, potassium, magnesium, and ammonium. Usually, abundance of these and other minerals relates directly to composition of local soil and rocks. However, excessive concentrations of nitrate in water do occur in relation to livestock concentration and to crop fertilization.

High concentrations in water of phosphorus and other elements that rapidly become fixed on soil colloids result from direct discharges of sewage and industrial wastes. Eroded soil material from runoff plots in Wisconsin contained 3 times the available phosphorus and 19 times the exchangeable potassium found in the soil proper (Massey and Jackson, 1952). Radioactive phosphorus, potassium, and calcium moved more rapidly into a forest soil as a result of colloidal particle transport and faunal activity than by leaching (Riekerk, 1971). Normally, water filtered through soil does not contain large amounts of readily fixed elements until saturation has been exceeded.

MANAGEMENT BASED ON MINERAL DISTRIBUTIONS

Movements and redistributions of minerals are important to rangeland management, especially when the whole range is considered (Fig. 6-3). Corrals need to be

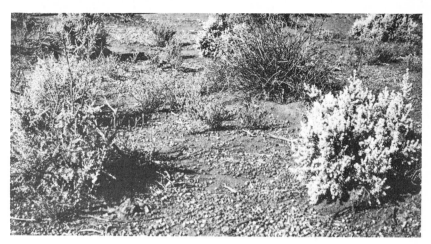

Figure 6-3 *A flash flood accumulated these sheep and kangaroo pellets in the saltbush type, South Australia.*

below the domestic water supply to lessen danger of pollution. Winter feeding of livestock should be located in a different area each year to lessen concentration of nutrients that increase danger of discharges into surface water and shallow wells. Domestic water supplies should be sealed and wells adequately cased to prevent contamination from corrals, septic-tank drain fields, and fertilization of crops and gardens. Each ranch presents its peculiar problems in positioning of water supply, homestead, and livestock.

Nitrate leaching and cycling appear to be related to depth of moisture penetration (White and Moore, 1972). Even where annual precipitation is too low to leach minerals beyond the root zone, an occasional flood or unusual weather even may cause pollution of water supplies if care has not been taken in positioning the various ranch functions.

Grazing management obviously plays an important role in nutrient cycling and redistribution. Proper grazing protects the soil resource from accelerated erosion that carries away valuable elements. Control of animal distribution minimizes nutrient redistribution by preventing local overgrazing and livestock concentration.

Recognition that patterns of minerals and organisms occur naturally and that animals contribute to them provides the land manager with a better understanding of his landscape. The mineral pattern formed in one vegetational type continues when another vegetation is established. The effect may be seen as varied results of plot treatments, varied success in seeding, patterned response to fetilization, and areas selected by animals for grazing. The "tracks" of previous plant and animal communities may disappear slowly. Reestablishment of original assemblages usually follows the earlier pattern.

People on small acreages in Africa and other parts of the world have used redistribution and management of minerals to increase total production and kinds of products from their farms. The central and new effort is to stall feed a cow or two and perhaps a steer with forages hand cut and carried to them. The droppings from a few caged chickens may be added to the chopped feed to increase the amount of nitrogen. Manure from the stall goes to the cropland as each new crop is established. Commercial fertilizers may be given to either food or pasture crops.

Normal expectations from establishment of this system would include (1) as much crop productivity from less land than before because of improved soil mineral status and physical conditions; (2) improved nutrition for the family because of better-quality crops, proteins from the stall-fed animals, and more eggs from the chickens; (3) less soil erosion because forage crops are rotated with food crops; (4) more cash flow to the small farmer; (5) reduced livestock trespassing on crops; and (6) relief to overgrazed rangeland surrounding the farms. Professional range managers find that range improvement may come more easily with an indirect attack, as illustrated by this example, rather than with a frontal attack on the range problem alone. Control of mineral redistribution in its broadest sense helps the range manager to put his problems and their solutions into the total ecosystem.

LITERATURE CITED

Adriano, D. C., P. F. Pratt, S. E. Bishop, W. Brock, J. Oliver, and W. Fairbank. 1971. Nitrogen load of soil in ground water from dairy manure. *Calif. Agr.* 25 (12):12–14.

Allison, F. E. 1966. The fate of nitrogen applied to soils. *Adv. Agron.* 18:219–258.

Ashby, W. C., and N. C. W. Beadle. 1957. Studies in halophytes III. Salinity factors in the growth of Australian saltbushes. *Ecology* 38:344–352.

Beadle, N. C. W. 1952. Studies in halophytes I. The germination of the seed and establishment of the seedlings of five species of *Atriplex* in Australia. *Ecology* 33:49–62.

———, R. D. B. Whalley, and J. B. Gibson. 1957. Studies in halophytes II. Analytical data on the mineral constituents of three species of *Atriplex* and their accompanying soils in Australia. *Ecology* 38:340–344.

Beaty, E. R., and K. H. Tan. 1972. Organic matter, N, and base accumulation under Pensacola bahiagrass. *J. Range Mgmt.* 25:38–40.

Carlisle, A., A. H. F. Brown, and E. J. White. 1967. The nutrient content of tree stem flow and ground flora litter and leachates in a sessile oak *(Quercus petraea)* woodland. *J. Ecol.* 55:615–627.

Castle, M. E., and E. MacDaid. 1972. The decomposition of cattle dung and its effect on pasture. *J. Br. Grassland Soc.* 27:133–137.

Charley, J. L. 1972. The role of shrubs in nutrient cycling. In Wildland shrubs—their biology and utilization. *U.S. Dept. Agr. Forest Service General Tech. Rep.* INT-1, pp. 182–203.

Davies, E. B., D. E. Hogg, and H. G. Hopewell. 1962. Extent of return of nutrient elements by dairy cattle: possible leaching losses. *Transactions of the Joint Meeting of Commissions IV and V,* International Society of Soil Science, New Zealand, pp. 715–720.

Garcia-Moya, E., and C. M. McKell. 1970. Contribution of shrubs to the nitrogen economy of a desert-wash plant community. *Ecology* 51:81–88.

Goodland, R. J. A. 1965. On termitaria in a savanna ecosystem. *Can. J. Zoo.* 43:641–650.

Herriott, J. B. D., and D. A. Wells. 1963. The grazing animal and sward productivity. *J. Agr. Sci.* 61:89–99.

Hilder, E. J. 1966. Distribution of excreta by sheep at pasture. *Proceedings of the 10th International Grassland Congress,* pp. 977–981.

———, and B. R. Mottershead. 1963. The redistribution of plant nutrients through free-grazing sheep. *Aust. J. Sci.* 26:88–89.

Johannesson, C. 1958. Higher phosphate values in soils under trees than in soil under grass. *Ecology* 39:373–374. ·

Lee, K. E., and T. Wood. 1971. *Termites and soil.* London: Academic Press.

Lotero, J., W. W. Woodhouse, Jr., and R. G. Petersen. 1966. Local effect on fertility of urine voided by grazing cattle. *Agron J.* 58:262–265.

MacDiarmid, B. N., and B. R. Watkin. 1971. The cattle dung patch. 1. Effect of dung patches on yield and botanical composition of surrounding and underlying pasture. *J. Br. Grassland Soc.* 26:239–245.

———, and ———. 1972. The cattle dung patch. 2. Effect of a dung patch on the chemical status of the soil, and ammonia nitrogen losses from the patch. 3. Distribution and rate of decay of dung patches and their influence on grazing behavior. *J. Br. Grassland Soc.* 27:43–54.

MacLusky, D. S. 1960. Some estimates of the areas of pasture fouled by the excreta of dairy cows. *J. Br. Grassland Soc.* 15:181–188.

Marsh, R., and R. C. Campling. 1970. Fouling of pastures by dung. *Herb. Abst.* 40:123–130.

Massey, H. F., and M. L. Jackson. 1952. Selective erosion of soil fertility constituents. *Soil Sci. Soc. Am. Proc.* 16:353–356.

Norman, M. J. T., and J. O. Green. 1958. The local influence of cattle dung and urine upon the yield and botanical composition of permanent pasture. *J. Br. Grassland Soc.* 13:39–45.

Olson, J. S., and D. A. Crossley, Jr. 1963. Tracer studies of the breakdown of forest litter. In *Radioecology,* eds. V. Schultz and A. W. Klement, Jr., pp. 411–416. New York: Reinhold.

Petersen, R. G., H. L. Lucas, and W. W. Woodhouse, Jr. 1956a. The distribution of excreta by freely grazing cattle and its effect on pasture fertility: I. Excretal distribution. *Agron. J.* 48:440–444.

———, W. W. Woodhouse, Jr., and H. L. Lucas. 1956b. The distribution of excreta by freely grazing cattle and its effect on pasture fertility: II. Effect of returned excreta on the residual concentration of some fertilizer elements. *Agron. J.* 48:444–449.

Rickard, W. H. 1965. Sodium and potassium accumulation by greasewood and hopsage leaves. *Bot. Gaz.* 126:116–119.

Riekerk, H. 1971. The mobility of phosphorus, potassium and calcium in a forest soil. *Soil. Sci. Soc. Amer. Proc.* 35:350–356.

Rixon, A. J. 1971. Oxygen uptake and nitrification by soil within a grazed *Atriplex vesicaria* community in semiarid rangeland. *J. Range Mgmt.* 24:435–439.

Sears, P. D. 1956. The effect of the grazing animal on pasture. *Proceedings of the 7th International Grassland Congress,* pp. 92–103.

Smith, G. E. 1967. Are fertilizers creating pollution problems? *Soil Cons. Soc. Amer. Proc.* 22:108–114.

Stewart, B. A., F. G. Viets, Jr., and G. L. Hutchinson. 1967. Effect of agriculture on nitrate pollution of groundwater. *Soil. Cons. Soc. Amer. Proc.* 22:115–118.

Switzer, G. L., and L. E. Nelson. 1972. Nutrient accumulation and cycling in Loblolly pine *(Pinus taeda,* L.) plantation ecosystems: the first twenty years. *Soil Sci. Soc. Am. Proc.* 36:143–147.

Thomas, W. A. 1969. Accumulation and cycling of calcium by dogwood trees. *Ecol. Monog.* 39:101–120.

U.S. Public Health Service. 1962. Drinking water standards. *U.S. Public Health Service Pub.* 956, 47–52.

Van Dyne, G. M., and H. F. Heady. 1965. Dietary chemical composition of cattle and sheep grazing in common on a dry annual range. *J. Range Mgmt.* 18:78–86.

Watkin, B. R. 1954. The animal factor and levels of nitrogen. *J. Br. Grassland Soc.* 9:35–46.

Watson, E. R., and P. Lapins. 1969. Losses of nitrogen from urine on soils from southwestern Australia. *Aust. J. Exp. Agr. Anim. Husb.* 9:85–91.

Weeda, W. C. 1967. The effect of cattle dung patches on pasture growth, botanical composition, and pasture utilization. *N. Z. J. Agr. Res.* 10:150–159.

Weir, J. S. 1971. The effect of creating additional water supplies in a Central African National Park. In *The scientific management of animal and plant communities for conservation, British Ecological Society 11th Symposium,* eds. E. Duffey and A. S. Watt, pp. 367–385.

Wheeler, J. L. 1958. The effect of sheep excreta and nitrogenous fertilizer on the botanical composition and production of a ley. *J. Br. Grassland Soc.* 13:196–202.

White, E. M., and D. G. Moore. 1972. Nitrates in South Dakota range soils. *J. Range Mgmt.* 25:27–29.

Will, G. M. 1959. Nutrient return in litter and rainfall under some exotic conifer stands in New Zealand. *N. Z. J. Agr. Res.* 2:719–734.

Witherspoon, J. P., Jr. 1964. Cycling of cesium-134 in white oak trees. *Ecol. Monog.* 34:403–420.

Wolton, K. M. 1963. An investigation into the simulation of nutrient returns by the grazing animal in grassland experimentation. *J. Br. Grassland Soc.* 18:213–219.

Chapter 7

Redistribution
of Plants

The fact that a plant grows on a spot of soil indicates that somehow a seed or other bit of germ plasm arrived there and became established. This chapter concerns the dispersal of plants by herbivorous animals. No attempt is made to review dispersal of organisms in general, as that was done by Ridley (1930), Good (1964), Carlquist (1965), and van der Pijl (1972).

In 1971, Stebbins claimed that animal dispersal of seed plants was the most effective means by which those plants moved. He based that conclusion on the large number of plant species which have adopted animal dispersal mechanisms. Apparently, every animal that is large enough to move seeds does so. At least no evidence was found to the contrary. Animals actively transport disseminules to nests and caches. They egest unharmed at least a few seeds of most, but not all, ingested species, and they passively carry disseminules that adhere to fur, feathers, and feet. The materials moved may be seeds, fruits, living pieces of plants, and whole plants. *Distribution of plants by animals* is considered here to mean *movement of disseminules beyond the territory where they normally would occur without animal influence.*

ACTIVE TRANSPORT

Among small mammals, birds, termites, and ants, numerous species gather and store plant disseminules in their nests and in other hiding places, usually small excavations in the soil. More material is collected than consumed, some caches may not be found, and mortality of the caching animals results in some of the hidden material not being eaten. Clusters of *Oxalis cernua* occur where mole rats have cached the bulbs (Galil, 1967). Birds are perhaps the most effective transporters. For example, the jay in England actively buries acorns, one per hole, for about two months each autumn in a radius of about 1 kilometer from the source (Chettleburgh, 1952). Active transport may be the principal dispersal mechanism for large fruited species such as oaks, walnuts, and hazelnuts. Obviously this activity, as well as other types of dispersal, peaks at the time of seed maturity. Caching of *Purshia tridentata* seeds in small soil pits by rodents has occurred as far as 300 meters from any seed source (Nord, 1965). Clusters of perhaps a dozen seedlings may appear if the seeds are not eaten. The kangaroo rat and Great Basin pocket mouse in Nevada cache seeds of *Bromus tectorum, Agropyron intermedium, Agropyron cristatum, Chrysothammus* spp., and many other species in soil pits about 5 centimeters deep and 3 centimeters wide. One pit contained 65 plants and 155 seeds of *Bromus tectorum*. Heteromyid rodents generally recover few cached seeds, leaving many planted. La Tourrette, Young, and Evans (1971) believed that this activity influences the dynamics of plant populations by enhancing plant establishment. Other species of kangaroo rats and pocket mice in Arizona cached and favored establishment of *Prosopis, Opuntia,* and large-seeded grasses (Reynolds, 1950).

Harvester termites collect leaves, stems, and seeds that are stored in their nests and may be exposed and planted by termite-eating mammals that destroy the nests. Bare soil and vegetation of low density around termite mounds often become colonized with *Cynodon* spp. in subtropical grasslands. Ridley (1930) suggested that collection of the seeds plays a part in the establishment of the particular vegetation found on these mounds.

Accumulations of seed and chaff from consumed seed around ant mounds indicate that harvesters occupy the burrows. Transport of seeds by harvester ants is not for great distances, but the diffusion of plants in the locality is altered and planted seed may be eliminated. Working in the Sonoran Desert of southern California, Tevis (1958) found that the ant *Veromessor pergandei* selected and gathered 8 percent of the seed crop of three plant species. He concluded that *Veromessor* had no significant influence on the native seed supply.

INGESTION AND SPREAD OF FRUITS

Animals spread plants by ingesting seeds at one location and egesting them at another place. In reviewing 94 papers on the dispersal of viable seeds by birds, McAtee (1947) found that crow droppings contained more than two viable seeds per gram and that some 50 avian species ate and voided the seeds of *Juniperus virginiana*. Predators that feed on seed eaters secondarily disperse seeds. The killdeer and mallard duck egested seeds of many aquatic and semiaquatic plants in viable condition. Many hydrophytes have small, hard seeds; thus they can pass unharmed through the gizzard and are resistant to digestive acids (DeVlaming and Proctor, 1968). Ringnecked pheasants and bobwhite quail destroyed beyond recognition the seeds of 3 common fencerow plant species and voided at least a few seeds of 16 species (Krefting and Roe, 1949; Swank, 1944). *Bromus mollis* seeds, which easily imbibe water, were completely digested by four different bird species (Krach, 1959). Olson and Blum (1968) found viable seeds in all parts of the digestive tracts of the tropical birds they examined.

Fruit bats disperse seeds by anal discharge or expectoration anywhere between the place of consumption and the roost (van der Pijl, 1957). Riegel (1941, 1942) recovered viable seeds of several grasses and *Opuntia* sp. from pellets of cottontails and California jackrabbits. Ten herbaceous species germinated from deer fecal pellets placed on sterile sand in the glasshouse (Heady, 1954).

Apparently ruminant animals will pass a few seeds of nearly every species that they consume. Burton and Andrews (1948) recovered the following proportions of seeds fed to dairy cows: one-half *Paspalum notatum* and *Cynodon dactylon,* one-third *Axonopus affinis* and *Sorghum halepense,* one-fourth *Paspalum dilatatum,* and one-eighth *Lespedeza striata.* Seeds of six common farm weeds were recovered at average rates of 11 to 24 percent when fed to calves, horses, sheep, and hogs, but few survived digestion by chickens (Harmon and Keim, 1934). McCully (1951) recovered half the *Rosa bracteata* seeds fed to mature cows, and 90 percent of the seed showed no damage. Kern (1921) found 45 seedlings of *Berberis vulgaris* in a single cow dropping. He attributed spread of the barberry from fencerows to pasture to dispersal by cattle. Thirty percent of hard seed but only 3 percent of scarified seed of *Trifolium repens* passed through sheep (Suckling, 1952). Sheep grazing rangeland in California voided 15 species as determined by germination tests with seeds in fecal pellets (Heady, 1954). Based on germination tests of seed in dung, Dore and Raymond (1942) claimed that in a grazing season a single cow on pasture redistributed 36 species totaling over 900,000 viable seeds.

Seeds that pass through digestive tracts unharmed include desirable pasture grasses and legumes, undesirable range species, and weeds of cultivated crops. Fecal pellets of sheep and jackrabbits collected where animals had been grazing areas heavily infested with *Halogeton glomeratus* contained 14 and 18 viable seeds, respectively, per 500 grams of material. This quantity is sufficient for sheep to have spread *Halogeton* over its wide area of distribution in a few years (Cook and Stoddart, 1953).

Studies to determine the reasons for *Prosopis* invasion into semiarid grassland of the southwestern United States implicate livestock, deer, peccary, cottontail rabbits, jackrabbits, coyotes, rodents, and Gambel's quail for their roles in seed dispersal (Reynolds, 1954). Between 12 and 45 percent of the hard *Prosopis* seeds passed through livestock (Reynolds and Glendening, 1949). Twenty-seven percent of the total seeds fed to sheep germinated after egestion (Glendening and Paulsen, 1950). Many rodent caches remained unopened and produced *Prosopis* seedlings, sometimes several years after the cache was deposited (Reynolds, 1958). Rodents, most of which have small home ranges, may not carry the seed more than 100 meters and would seem to be less important distributors of seeds than are the larger animals. Livestock trailed at the rate of 15 kilometers per day might transport *Prosopis* seeds in their digestive tracts more than 100 kilometers.

The seeds show improved germination following passage through a digestive tract. Passed *Rosa bracteata* seed germinated at a 50 percent rate in dung (Fig. 7-1) whereas the controls and stratified seed failed to germinate (McCully, 1951). *Opuntia* seed germination increased 50 percent after passage through jackrabbits (Timmons, 1942). Consumption of the wild tomato *(Lycopersicon esculentum* var. *minor)* by the giant tortoise on the Galapagos Islands broke dormancy of the seed and increased germination from 0 to 80 percent (Rick and Bowman, 1961). Seeds of farm weeds recovered from farm animals germinated at a higher percentage than did uneaten controls but less than did uneaten acid-treated seed (Harmon and Keim, 1934).

The seeds of different species germinate differently in response to passage through the digestive tract. About half the species fed to pheasants and quail showed no change in percentage germination (Krefting and Roe, 1949; Swank, 1944). *Cynodon dactylon* was the only one among seven southern forage species which increased in germination rate after passage through cattle. The other species decreased (Burton and Andrews, 1948). *Atriplex confertifolia* was the only one among seven common species of the sagebrush-grass type in southern Idaho which

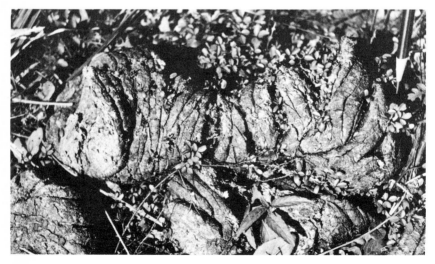

Figure 7-1 Germinating seeds of *Rosa bracteata* after they passed through cattle.

showed increased germination by passage through sheep. *Bromus tectorum, Elymus caput-medusae,* and *Agropyron cristatum* exhibited > 90 percent germination before and < 2.4 percent after consumption by sheep, but jackrabbits reduced germination of these three species to less than 0.6 percent (Lehrer and Tisdale, 1956).

PASSIVE TRANSPORT

Adaptations of seeds and other plant parts which facilitate their dispersal by animals include burrs; hooks; barbs; mucilaginous coverings; and retrorse arrangements of hairs, spines, spikelet parts, etc. Large accumulations of *Xanthium* burrs in the tails of livestock, *Stipa* and *Erodium* fruits under the skin of sheep, and cactus joints hanging on the faces of cattle illustrate obvious dispersal mechanisms. Many are more subtle, as abundantly cataloged by Ridley (1930). The magnitude of seed dispersal by animals may be greater than commonly realized. Almost half of 369 hares *(Lepus capensis)* collected in Kenya had disseminules in their fur which totaled 810 and included 17 plant species (Agnew and Flux, 1970). Since these hares groom themselves daily, the number of seeds they carry in a season must be considerable.

Sharp, Hironaka, and Tisdale (1957) commented that seeds of *Elymus caput-medusae* were carried and spread by men and machinery as well as by animals. Few studies have been made of this hitchhiking kind of plant dispersal by man. Clifford (1956), working in England, listed 43 species that he found in dried mud on footwear; the maximum disseminule number in one sample was 176. In a later Nigerian study (1959), he found over 40 species in samples of mud taken from automobiles. This material averaged one to two seeds per 10 grams of mud. Clearly, man and his equipment are agents of plant dispersal. Robbins (1940) listed 526 alien species growing without cultivation in California and stated that the invasion began in 1769 with the first permanent settlement at San Diego. Very likely, alien plants arrived to stay in California before 1769. Discarded packing materials and livestock debris from sailing vessels along the California coast no doubt contained seed. Animals and men put ashore for short trips inland. The first European settlers into Mexico and the eastern United States arrived long before 1769, and plants brought by them could have been spread by migrating birds and mammals. In fact, once man brings an alien plant species onto a new continent, it has potential to spread and occupy suitable habitats throughout that continent without further dispersal by him.

MANAGEMENT IMPLICATIONS

Dispersal of plants by animals and man has a number of implications for management of rangelands. Obviously, clean shoes, trouser cuffs, truckbeds, feeds, and seed reduce chances of invasion by undesirables.

Duration of Seed Retention in Digestive Tracts

Apparently cattle retain a few seeds in their digestive tracts for seven to ten days (McCully, 1951; Burton and Andrews, 1948). After feeding known quantities of *Trifolium repens* seed in gelatin capsules to sheep, Suckling (1952) found the first seed in the dung 24 hours later, the maximum number on the second day, and decreasing amounts through the sixth day. One autopsied sheep had 1,559 seeds in the digestive tract, mostly in folds of the omasum, six days after feeding. Sheep in Idaho were found to retain viable seeds for nine days, and New Zealand rabbits still had seeds after four days (Lehrer and Tisdale, 1956). Trailing and hauling of animals spreads the retained viable seed along stock routes.

Other animal species may retain seed for various intervals; for example, the maximum seed retention time was five days for killdeer and four days for mallards (DeVlaming and Proctor, 1968). Different seed species pass through a single animal at different rates. Details are largely unknown, but small, hard seeds are likely to be retained longer and with less reduction in germination than are large seeds and those that rapidly imbibe water. Cud chewing, grinding in gizzards, and contact with digestive acids do not destroy all seeds.

Longevity of Seeds in Dung

Harmon and Keim (1934) found that seeds of six common weeds lost their viability within four months of burial in fermenting manure, but *Trifolium repens* showed 16 percent germination after burial in dung for five months. Manures used for fertilizer may contain viable seed of undesirable species. Although return of manures to rangeland may not be a common practice and seeds may not survive long storage in manure, alien plants may become established in a corral area where shipped livestock are unloaded.

The Use of Animals to Spread Seed

Animals can be used to spread desirable forage plants. Burton and Andrews (1948) mentioned cattle as a factor in the spread of *Axonopus affinis* in the South and suggested this method as an aid to reseeding in the piney woods. At least one rancher in Lake County, California, fed *Medicago hispida* to sheep in order to spread it over his rangeland. Jones and Carroll in California (1953) found that *Oryzopsis miliacea* and, in a few cases, *Trifolium hirtum* were established by feeding seed to cattle. *Phalaris tuberosa, Lolium* spp., and *Melilotus indica* failed to establish themselves in the same experiment. The practicality of this method of seeding rangelands is yet to be determined.

Feeding hay with considerable seed attached results in subsequent seed dispersal by animals. Feeding on rangeland should be rotated from place to place to spread seed and reduce undesirable effects of concentrated animals.

In rough country, such as cutover timberland, planting of forage species often can be done only in irregular patches or strips. Animals will spread the seeded plants when grazing occurs at the time of seed maturity.

Seed Collection

Squirrel caches yield seeds of coniferous species. Many rodents pile grass seeds around or in their burrows. Farmers have raided these caches to obtain seeds of wild plants for commercial purposes. Hawbecker (1944) described stocks of *Bromus rubens* seed gathered by giant kangaroo rats (Fig. 7-2). Ridley (1930) gave many examples of animal caching habits being used to advantage for seed collections. Hard seeds that pass through the digestive tract become concentrated in the dung, which may be collected more easily than seeds gathered directly from plants. Improved germination may give a double advantage to the use of these seeds.

Effective Dispersal Distance

Duration and rate of travel by animals determine dispersal distances. For example, a migrating mallard flying at 75 kilometers per hour could easily carry seeds for distances of 1000 or more kilometers before they were voided. DeVlaming and Proctor (1968) believed that the characteristic widespread distribution of many aquatic and semiaquatic plants is due to migration of aquatic and shore birds.

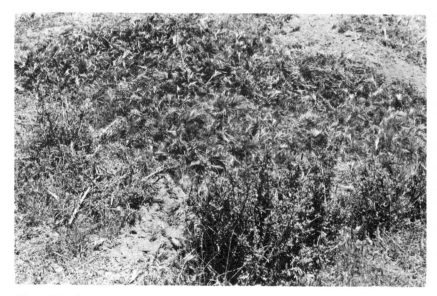

Figure 7-2 Kangaroo rats collected this cache of *Bromus rubens* seed.

Table 7-1　Number of flowering plant species with different dispersal mechanisms on three islands at different distances from Java *(From Ridley, 1930)*

	Distance from Java, km	Age of island	Seaborne	Windborne	Carried internally by birds	Adhesive to birds	Carried in mud on birds
Krakatau	30	36 yr	60	34	34	9	3
Christmas	225	Eocene	44	9	36	15	0
Cocos-Keeling	1,125	Unknown	17	0	0	5	0

The classic study (Ridley, 1930) of revegetation on the island of Krakatau after all organisms on it had been destroyed by volcanic eruption in 1883 gave a rough estimate of dispersal rates. This island lies in the path of prevailing sea and air currents from Java, 30 kilometers away. Thirty-six years after the eruption, many plants had reached Krakatau. Many were not present on similar islands further from Java (Table 7-1). These data and Ridley's interpretations suggest that distance is a factor in dispersal, that seaborne dispersal is highly effective, and that birds carry disseminules for greater distances than does wind.

EFFECTIVENESS OF PLANT DISPERSAL BY ANIMALS

On a small scale, say one or two square kilometers, animals probably serve to keep plant populations thoroughly mixed. They bring disseminules to each point of ground in such numbers and variety that every species growing nearby has potential to become established on each new bare area. This vicinity effect from neighboring stands functions directly with distance. Dansereau and Lems (1957) claimed that dispersal rates as a function of distance alter the pace of vegetational change but that little is know concerning magnitudes of these effects. An example of plant-animal interaction was given by Janzen (1972). Seeds falling from *Sterculia apetala* trees were eaten immediately by the insect *Dysdercus fasciatus*. Squirrels and monkeys carried seeds and lost or discarded a few in nearby grasslands where the insects did not occur. There appeared to be no survival of this species within the forest, and only a few plants were able to become established in the grassland habitat. The results are a scattered population, characteristic of many tropical-forest trees. This interaction between dispersal and herbivory, which involves more than one animal species, illustrates complexities of animal influences on vegetation. Although the example came from a tropical forest, the hypothesis is presented here that many such interactions are likely between domestic animals and range vegetation.

Hawbecker (1944) considered the giant kangaroo rat as beneficial on California rangelands because it increased *Erodium cicutarium* and *Bromus rubens* and it contributed to soil formation. Sheep preferentially grazed the burrow precincts. Although 12 rodent species consumed 14 kilograms of vegetation and 7 kilograms of insects and stored about 11 kilograms of plant materials per hectare as well as denuding 10 percent of the land area with their dens in the desert grassland of New Mexico, several beneficial effects occurred (Wood, 1969). Part of the cached seed escaped consumption, it germinated, and plants became established. Rodent consumption of herbivorous insects reduced grazing pressures on seeds and plants. Magnitudes of animal effects depend upon many factors, especially upon the niche and behaviorial characteristics of each animal species and upon the numbers of animals. Food-habit information alone does little to reveal dispersal of plants by animals or animal impacts on rangelands.

Animals consume seeds and fruits of many plants in amounts varying with individual preferences and seasonal availability. A portion of the seeds consumed passes through the animals in viable condition, that portion being dependent both on the nature of the seed and on characteristics of the animal. These and other actions contribute to the dispersal of plants and to the vegetational composition on rangeland. The magnitude of animal influences and effective management of plant dispersal by animals are still largely matters of speculation, needing further exploration.

LITERATURE CITED

Agnew, A. D. W., and J. E. C. Flux. 1970. Plant dispersal by hares *(Lepus capensis* L.) in Kenya. *Ecology* 51:735–737.

Burton, G. W., and J. S. Andrews. 1948. Recovery and viability of seeds of certain southern grasses and lespedeza passed through the bovine digestive tract. *J. Agr. Res.* 76:95–103.

Carlquist, S. 1965. *Island life.* New York: American Museum of Natural History.

Chettleburg, M. R. 1952. Observations on the collection and burial of acorns by jays in Hainault Forest. *Brit. Birds* 45:359–364.

Clifford, H. T. 1956. Seed dispersal on footwear. *Proc. Bot. Soc. Brit. Isles.* 2:129–131.

———. 1959. Seed dispersal by motor vehicles. *J. Ecol.* 47:311–315.

Cook, C. W., and L. A. Stoddart. 1953. The halogeton problem in Utah. *Utah Agr. Expt. Sta. Bull* 364.

Dansereau, P., and K. Lems. 1957. The grading of dispersal types in plant communities and their ecological significance. *Contributions de l' Institut Botanique de l' Université de Montréal* 71.

DeVlaming, V., and V. W. Proctor. 1968. Dispersal of aquatic organisms: Viability of seeds recovered from the droppings of captive killdeer and mallard ducks. *Am. J. Bot.* 55:20–26.

Dore, W. G., and L. C. Raymond. 1942. Viable seeds in pasture soil and manure. *Sci. Agric.* 23:69–79.

Galil, J. 1967. On the dispersal of bulbs of *Oxalis cernua* Thunb. by molerats *(Spalax ehrenbergi* Nehring). *J. Ecol.* 55:787–792.

Glendening, G. E., and H. A. Paulsen. 1950. Recovery and viability of mesquite seeds fed to sheep receiving 2, 4-D in drinking water. *Bot. Gaz.* 111:486–491.

Good, R. V. 1964. *The geography of the flowering plants,* 3rd ed. New York: Wiley.

Harmon, G. W., and F. D. Keim. 1934. The percentage and viability of weed seeds recovered in the feces of farm animals and their longevity when buried in manure. *J. Am. Soc. Agron.* 26:762–767.

Hawbecker, A. C. 1944. The giant kangaroo rat and sheep forage. *J. Wildl. Mgmt.* 8:161–165.

Heady, H. F. 1954. Viable seed recovered from fecal pellets of sheep and deer. *J. Range Mgmt.* 7:259–261.

Janzen, D. H. 1972. Escape in space by *Sterculia apetala* seeds from the bug *Dysdercus fasciatus* in a Costa Rican deciduous forest. *Ecology* 53:350–361.

Jones, R. G., and F. D. Carroll. 1953. Spread of range forage plants. *Calif. Agric.* 7(12):4, 12.

Kern, F. D. 1921. Observations of the dissemination of the barberry. *Ecology* 2:211–214.

Krach, K. E. 1959. Untersuchungen über die Ausscheidung unverdauter Klee-, Gras- und Unkrautsamen durch Vögel und die Beeinflussung ihrer Keimwerte durch die Magen- und Darm-passage. *Z. Acker-u. PflBau.* 107(4):405–434.

Krefting, L. W., and E. I. Roe. 1949. The role of some birds and mammals in seed germination. *Ecol. Monog.* 19:269–286.

LaTourrette, J. E., J. A. Young, and R. A. Evans. 1971. Seed dispersal in relation to rodent activites in seral big sagebrush communities. *J. Range Mgmt.* 24:118–120.

Lehrer, W. P., Jr., and E. W. Tisdale. 1956. Effect of sheep and rabbit digestion on the viability of some range plant seeds. *J. Range Mgmt.* 9:118–123.

McAtee, W. L. 1947. Distribution of seeds by birds. *Am. Midl. Nat.* 38:214–223.

McCully, W. G. 1951. Recovery and viability of Macartney rose seeds fed to cattle. *J. Range Mgmt.* 4:101–106.

Nord, E. C. 1965. Autecology of bitterbrush in California. *Ecol. Monog.* 35:307–334.

Olson, S. L. and K. E. Blum. 1968. Avian dispersal of plants in Panama. *Ecology* 49:565–566.

Reigel, D. A. 1941. Some coactions of rabbits and rodents with cactus. *Trans. Kan. Acad. Sci.* 44:96–103.

———. 1942. Some observations of the food coactions of rabbits in western Kansas during periods of stress. *Trans. Kan. Acad. Sci.* 45:369–375.

Reynolds, H. G. 1950. Relation of Merriam kangaroo rats to range vegetation in southern Arizona. *Ecology* 31:456–463.

———. 1954. Some interrelations of the Merriam kangaroo rat to velvet mesquite. *J. Range Mgmt.* 7:176–180.

———. 1958. The ecology of the Merriam kangaroo rat (*Dipodomys Merriami* Mearns) on the grazing lands of southern Arizona. *Ecol. Monog.* 28:111–127.

———, and G. E. Glendening. 1949. Merriam kangaroo rat a factor in mesquite propagation on southern Arizona range lands. *J. Range Mgmt.* 2:193–197.

Rick, C. M., and R. I. Bowman. 1961. Galapagos tomatoes and tortoises. *Evolution* 15:407–417.

Ridley, H. N. 1930. *The dispersal of plants throughout the world.* Ashford, England: L. Reeve.

Robbins, W. W. 1940. Alien plants growing without cultivation in California. *Calif. Agr. Expt. Sta. Bull.* 637.

Sharp, L. A., M. Hironaka, and E. W. Tisdale. 1957. Viability of medusa-head *(Elymus caput-medusae L.)* seed collected in Idaho. *J. Range Mgmt.* 10:123–126.

Stebbins, G. L. 1971. Adaptive radiation of reproductive characteristics in Angrosperms. II: Seeds and seedlings. *Annual Rev. Ecol. and Systematics* 2:237–260.

Suckling, F. E. T. 1952. Dissemination of white clover *(Trifolium repens)* by sheep. *N.Z. J. Sci. Tech.* 33 (Section A) (5):64–77.

Swank, W. G. 1944. Germination of seeds after ingestion by ring-necked pheasants. *J. Wildl. Mgmt.* 8:223–231.

Tevis, L., Jr. 1958. Interrelations between the harvester ant *Veromessor pergandei* Mayr and some desert ephemerals. *Ecology* 39:695–704.

Timmons, F. L. 1942. The dissemination of prickly pear seed by jackrabbits. *J. Am. Soc. Agron.* 34:513–520.

van der Pijl, L. 1957. The dispersal of plants by bats. *Acta. Bot. Neerl.* 6:291–315.

———. 1972. *Principles of dispersal in higher plants.* New York: Springer-Verlag.

Wood, J. E. 1969. Rodent populations and their impact on desert rangelands. *N. Mex. Agr. Expt. Sta. Bull.* 555.

Part Two

Management of Grazing Animals

Chapter 8

Numbers of Animals

As each animal grazes, it reduces available herbage both in quantity and in quality, thereby changing the habitat for itself and altering its future response. Control of animal numbers is the most important single tool available to the rangeland manager. Grazing pressure is the principal force—other than, perhaps, fire and cultivation—controlling species composition and forage production which the manager can manipulate. However, without stipulation of kind of animal, grazing distribution, and season of use, stocking rate has little meaning.

In areas of natural vegetation, regeneration of desirable plants maintains good range condition. However, grazing by too many animals or too heavy use by a few animals result in overuse, loss of vigor, and ultimately disappearance of the desirable plants (Fig. 8-1). Deterioration of the range begins when less valuable forage species replace the desirable plants. Diminished land values, lowered income, and soil instability eventually result.

Replacement of destroyed vegetation by seeding remains expensive. Furthermore, animal numbers must be strictly controlled if new seedlings are to become established. Other range-improvement practices also require relief from

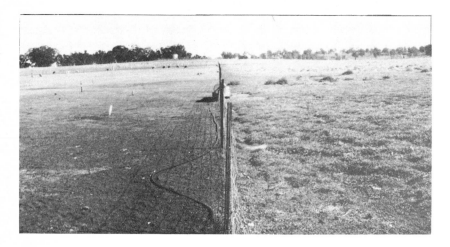

Figure 8-1 An extreme stocking rate (37 sheep per hectare) (left pasture) destroyed a stand of *Phalaris* and *Trifolium* near Armidale, Australia. At 2.5 sheep per hectare (right pasture), damage occurred near water.

heavy grazing. If range resources are to be perpetuated at the highest productivity levels, the range must be properly stocked and utilized. Excessive forage utilization by either livestock or game reduces weight gains, growth rates, and profit. Coordination of forage utilization with forage growth through control of animal numbers usually determines the success or failure of other range practices and the economic stability of the operation. This principle can hardly be overemphasized. It is the result of many stocking rate experiments, for example, Woolfolk (1949), Hurtt (1951), Launchbaugh (1957), Klipple and Costello (1960), Reed and Peterson (1961), Beetle, et al. (1961), and Merrill and Miller (1961), which have shown that moderate and conservative stocking rates give greater returns than does a heavy stocking rate because with those stocking rates there are higher selling prices, improved animal condition, more wool, greater percentage calf crops, higher weaning weights, fatter cull animals, less death loss, and need for less supplementary feed.

CONCEPTS AND DEFINITIONS

Range management literature lists many terms related to numbers of animals. *Grazing capacity* refers to *the number of animals over a long time period,* and *stocking rate* means *the number of animals in a pasture for a stated time period.* Other terms describe the degree of forage utilization at a given time in the current year and the effects of utilization over a longer time period. Measurement concepts such as *animal unit* and *sheep day* are employed in attempts to quantify the grazing pressure. The following sections group and define related terms applicable to grazing influences, grazing products, and other values of wildlands.

Carrying Capacity and Grazing Capacity

Range resources are supplies of commodities and services originating from rangelands with certain capacities. The relative utility of these resources is a result of physical environmental factors, effects of organisms upon the resources, available technology concerning their use, and their current or potential value to the society of man. Recent. extensive changes in the use of all wildlands, including grazing land, stem from changes in the types of goods and services demanded in the marketplace. Carrying capacity is defined in terms of products, generally, useful ones. Managerial inputs that combine personal ability and available technology alter production strategies and carrying capacities.

Rangeland resources result from more than the physical characteristics of the site. Individual resources increase or decrease in importance and new ones are created as a result of demands by society and inputs by management (Lime and Stankey, 1971). The concept of rangeland resources signifies a synthesis of physical environment, plants, and animals as enhanced by the manager and produced for society.

Rangeland carrying capacity results from the productivity levels of the several rangeland resources. Therefore, as many carrying capacities can be defined as there are management objectives. If inputs and management objectives did not change over time, carrying capacity would have an unchanging maximum value or combination of values that could be maintained. But inputs and objectives do change; thus the notion of carrying capacity as a biological constant becomes untenable, as does the concept of sustained yield when applied to a single unchanging product.

The Range Term Glossary Committee (1964) defined *carrying capacity* as *"the maximum number of individual animals that can survive the greatest period of stress each year on a given land area."* Sharkey (1970) defined *carrying capacity* as *"the total weight of animals that can be supported permanently."* These definitions should be rejected because they do not encompass the capability of rangeland to produce several different products. *Carrying capacity* includes more than maximum numbers of animals that can survive and that do no damage. It expresses the greatest return of combined products without damage to the physical resources. It should not be confused with grazing capacity.

Grazing capacity is *the number of animals that produces the greatest return without damage to the physical resources and in concert with other values received from the land.* Optimum carrying capacity expresses the most profitable levels of all products and services. Optimum grazing capacity suggests the most profitable stocking rate (Cowlishaw, 1969; Hart, 1972).

Many factors determine grazing capacity. For both livestock and game, the principal limits on grazing capacity are quantity and seasonal availability of feed. Winter snow, which lowers food availability, limits populations that, at other times of the year, do not completely use available forage. High-quality summer forage promotes large individual size and general good health that enhances winter survival and reproductive success. Thus, the desirable herd size of any animal population on a summer range may be considerably different from that of the same herd on a winter basis. Alternating wet and dry seasons have effects similar to those of alternating winter and summer seasons. During a year, range livestock operations combine feeds from native forages, seeded ranges, seeded pastures, crop aftermath, hay, and concentrates. No two ranches produce or purchase the same proportions of feed types. Efforts to increase grazing capacity center on increasing the feed supply at the time of greatest stress.

Where both feed supply and livestock numbers cycle, three types of calculations have been used in quantifying basic herd size for yearlong operations. One method requires identifying the feed supply and number of animals supportable during the months of least available homegrown forages. A second method determines a yearlong herd size on the basis of average monthly feed supply; usually this method gives high estimates of animal numbers that can be maintained. A third method arrives at the basic herd size by comparing month-by-month estimates of feed supplies and requirements by animals of all ages (Workman and MacPherson, 1973).

Merely increasing the feed supply cannot increase grazing capacity where overriding behavioral mechanisms control numbers. The populations of Uganda kob are limited by territoriality (Buechner, 1963). Interaction between predators and prey can result in relatively stable numbers of both, as in the wolf-moose relationship on Isle Royale (Mech, 1966).

Grazing capacity is more difficult to define in populations that ''explode'' or cycle than in those that tend to be stable, such as the numbers of livestock on a ranch. Examples of exploding populations are those of species introduced onto islands; some examples are the reindeer, which rapidly increased, then crashed, on St. Matthew Island in 1963–1964 (Klein, 1968), and the moose on Isle Royale in Lake Superior (Mech, 1966). In these instances, the limiting factor seemed to be only one—the food supply. Control or crash was both sudden and severe. The common sequence of events is a geometric population increase beginning with a few animals, summer food in short supply, and animals entering the winter in poor condition. Extreme weather conditions result in a heavy die-off.

In a catastrophic decline, the numbers of reindeer on St. Matthew Island crashed from 6,000 to less than 50 during one winter. When a second limiting factor, predation, was introduced onto Isle Royale, the numbers of moose fluctuated much less severely than they did with only changing food supply.

These examples illustrate the difficulties in defining and interpreting the concepts of carrying capacity and grazing capacity. To avoid misunderstanding, one should use them sparingly after defining them tersely in each given situation.

Units of Animals and Grazing

An *animal unit* (AU) is widely accepted as *a mature cow with calf, or their equivalent.* Horses, sheep, and goats commonly are converted to animal units at the rates of 1.25, 0.2, and 0.17, respectively. Young animals between weaning and maturity vary from 0.6 to 0.9 of their adult female equivalent animal units. Adult bulls are about 1.25 animal units. These conversion factors are indicators of equivalent amounts of forage needed by different kinds and classes of domestic animals with similar diets. They have little application in expressing equivalent impacts on range vegetation from animals with wide differences in food habits. *Animal unit requirement* refers to *forage needed by an AU for one year.*

An *animal unit month* (AUM) is *the amount of forage required by an animal unit for one month of grazing.* Related terms for specific instances include *band day, sheep day, cow day, cow month,* and many others that refer to different kinds of animals and time periods.

Animal unit equivalents symbolize mixed herds as groups of average animals, whether they are different kinds of mature animals that change little in feed requirements from day to day or growing animals that gradually increase their daily intake. Coordination of varying AUM requirements and forage increments in day-to-day livestock management still is a matter of judgment by the manager. Animal unit months of grazing, or a variant such as steer months, are widely used as leasing units and as a basis for pasture rental. Grazing fees on public lands and on many private pastures are attached to animal units on a yearly or monthly basis.

Grazing Pressure

The pressure of grazing at any given moment is defined as *a relationship between demand for forage by animals and a combination of daily herbage increment and standing crop of vegetation* (Fig. 8-2). This function is related only indirectly to numbers of animals and area of pasture. The standing crop of new forage available for grazing begins at 0, proceeds to a peak at plant maturity, and falls to 0 as herbage is consumed by herbivores and decomposers. In many vegetational types, the cycle of herbage produced one year overlaps part of the following cycle before it disappears. Animals, or their demand for forage, are imposed on the cycle at a more or less constant rate in most range operations. Exceptions include gradually increasing demands for feed by young animals, a sudden decrease in needs at sale time, and complete use of feed during the growing period in steer operations.

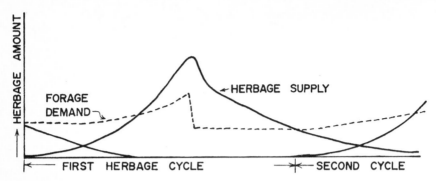

Figure 8-2 Grazing pressure expressed diagramatically. The supply of forage for one full yearly cycle, which overlaps the end of other cycles, appears as an accumulation and decay of standing forage crop (solid line). Demand for forage (dashed line) increases as young animals grow and suddenly decreases at sale time. Grazing pressure is light when daily consumption is less than the increment in forage supply.

Thus, almost all range grazing programs result in varying seasonal grazing pressures on the vegetation. Grazing pressure is light during times when the daily growth increment is greater than the daily harvest and during times of grazing on accumulated mature growth. Heavy pressure occurs when daily consumption exceeds the daily growth increment and the available forage supply is low. Yearly as well as seasonal variations alter these relationships.

Expressions and measurements of grazing pressure on rangeland have embodied the concept that the degree or percentage of forage utilization signifies the influence of grazing on the vegetation (Campbell, 1937). This relationship suggests that grazing pressure is proportional to the amount of herbage eaten during a season or a year. A better expression of grazing pressure for rangelands and pastures may be one relating numbers of animals to available forage (Hyder, 1954; Heady, 1956; Mott, 1960). Campbell (1966) expressed this concept of grazing pressure as a ratio of animal days per 1,120 kilograms of available dry matter per hectare. The influence of day-to-day changes in grazing pressure (ratio of forage demand to supply) on range condition and production needs further clarification.

Stocking Rate and Density

Stocking rate is *the actual number of animals or animal units on a specific area for a specific period of time, usually for a grazing season.* Where the grazing season is yearlong, a time period may not be stipulated, but in temperate and mountainous regions, *stocking rate* commonly defines all the grazing that occurs during a year, for example, 30 AUs per hectare for four months of grazing. It may be expressed as 120 AUMs per hectare or 1 AUM per 0.0092 hectare. This is an animal-to-land relationship fully controlled by the operator. He decides which animals will graze a pasture and in what concentration they will harvest the forage.

Stocking rate should be used to express *the animal-to-land allotment* on a ranch or on a complete unit *for the entire grazing season.* It differs from *stocking density,* which describes *the animal-to-land relationship at an instant of time* (Booysen, 1967). Stocking density is a function of herd and pasture sizes.

The distinction between stocking rate and stocking density becomes important in any rotational grazing plan. For example, 1 animal per 5 hectares could be the density of animals in each unit of a 5-pasture rotational plan, but the stocking rate for the grazing season is 1 animal per 25 hectares.

Because stocking density does not refer to degree of herbage use, the concepts of understocking and overstocking should be applied to interanimal rather than to animal-to-pasture relationships. Stress due to crowding, for example, has been shown to be density-dependent in some species of animals and is a function of stocking density.

Stocking rates have been expressed as units of area for each animal as well as animals per unit area. These expressions of stocking rate have shown differently shaped functions when plotted against a third variable such as animal gains per individual or land unit. Animal-to-area expressions are preferred because they are more directly related to grazing pressure and production per hectare than is area per animal (Shaw, 1970). However, in regions with low grazing capacity, the ideal designation may be area per animal because it avoids the use of fractional terms for animals.

PRODUCTION PER HECTARE VERSUS PER ANIMAL

Given the same length of grazing period, as numbers of animals are increased per unit of area, closer utilization, less feed, and less nutritious forage per animal result. Each animal gains less, and animals vary more in weight gain. Slow-growing animals and those with great fluctuations in weight must be fed for a longer period of time and often to a heavier weight than must animals that are rapidly grown. Stocking at rates that reduce weight gains per animal often leads to range and financial problems. If gains per animal are plotted against numbers of animals per unit area, the relationship usually is linear and the two factors negatively correlated within the range of practical stocking rates (Riewe et al., 1963; Cowlishaw, 1969; Peterson et al., 1965; Blackburn, et al., 1973). This relationship is one of animal response to nutrition rather than to stocking rate or feed availability (Harlan, 1958).

At low stocking rates, individual animals show little response to changing numbers because the food supply is beyond their capacity to use it. Individual animal potential rather than pasture productivity is defined when few animals graze abundant forage (Morley and Spedding, 1968). Occasionally in practice, low forage utilization may allow plants to become coarse and of low quality, resulting in less gain per animal than at moderate stocking rates.

At high stocking rates, gains per animal fall rapidly with relatively small change in numbers of animals (Mott, 1960). The point where the curve breaks, the *optimum* level or slightly to the right of it in Figure 8-3, has been called the peril point for management (Harlan, 1958). Above that point, range-forage availability declines and animals rapidly lose condition although livestock numbers or grazing pressure increase relatively little. Stocking below the peril point gives more leeway in management and little response to changing stocking rates.

Quantities of animal products per hectare increase directly as stocking rate increases, reach a peak, and fall rapidly at high stocking rates (Fig. 8-3). Many, but not all, studies have shown the greatest per-hectare gains in productivity with the highest stocking rates (Riewe, 1961). However, treatments in the narrow range of stocking between the highest gain and no gain per hectare are difficult to select; therefore many experiments have missed them. Furthermore, managers and experimenters alike deliberately eliminate high stocking rates in order not to damage range and livestock. Maximum gains per hectare over the long term indicate ample opportunity for animals to select nutritious feed without range damage. Animal numbers and duration of stay in a pasture normally should not exceed a degree of forage utilization that causes excessive weight loss.

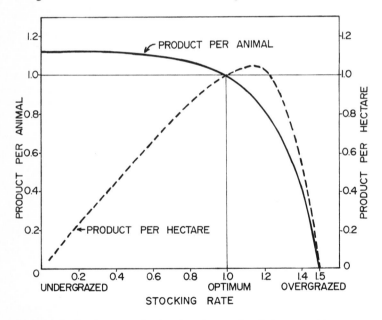

Figure 8-3 Product per animal and per hectare in relation to stocking rate. Units on all axes are ratios of actual to optimum values; therefore the value 1 indicates the situation in which actual stocking and product are optimum. Ratios permit plotting both curves on the same scale. *(Adapted from Mott, 1960.)*

After assuming equal beginning weights, grade changes, and other animal characteristics; taking no account of pasture and fixed costs; and selling steers at the same price per kilogram as the purchase price, Riewe (1961) calculated that the highest gross returns came from a stocking rate that yielded maximum gain per hectare. As selling price increased over purchase price, gross income increased at all stocking rates and remained maximum at or near the point of highest gain per hectare. If prices fell, high stocking rates tended to maximize financial loss. The least financial loss occurred with the greatest weight gain per animal at low stocking rates. Intermediate price reductions resulted in gross losses at high stocking rates and lowered returns at low stocking rates. Apparently high stocking rates produce high gross returns when price changes are favorable and produce the greatest financial losses when prices fall.

Analyses that assume changes only in prices tell little about net return or profit from changes in stocking rate or from the whole enterprise. Production per unit of labor, per kilogram of fertilizer, per centimeter of rainfall; number of game animals harvested; and other factors may be as relevant to economic analysis as is production per hectare. These input and output factors vary widely in time and place. As costs increase and prices decrease, the economically optimum stocking rate appears to decrease. Lower stocking rate does not always yield lower net returns. If rapidly gaining animals develop a price differential in their favor, the manager may need to redress stocking rate toward lower levels and less gain per hectare to maintain high rates of gain and profit.

Other factors being equal, the curve of profit against stocking rate appears to be relatively flat (Hildreth and Riewe, 1963). This relationship gives the manager considerable flexibility. He is not required to have stocking rate at a fixed point to obtain near-maximum profit. As Mott (1960) wrote, optimum stocking is a range of rates rather than a single one. The manager should strive for stocking rates that maximize net profit, as continually modified by risk and his ability to cope with changing factors.

Partially controlled game populations present stocking rate problems similar to those of livestock. For example, for deer and elk, changes in fecundity rate correlate inversely with changes in stocking density, net production per breeding animal decreases as population size increases, and the stocking density at optimum yield of young animals demands less feed than the habitat supplies (Gross, 1969). At maximum stocking density, the harvest is reduced for game as well as for livestock.

FORAGE UTILIZATION

The amount of plant material consumed by herbivores, expressed as a percentage of the current herbage crop, has been known as *range utilization, degree of use, percentage use, actual use, herbage use,* and *range use. Actual use* may be an expression of the AUMs obtained in a grazing season and thereby may be confused with *stocking rate*. In this book, *actual use* refers to *the current utilization of herbage* without stipulation of kind or numbers of animals or recommended levels of utilization. *Range use* may mean *herbage utilization on a broad scale* or *any service derived from rangeland.* Where the word *use* is a synonym for *utilization,* the context will leave the meaning clear.

The distinction is made here between stocking, which is a daily phenomenon; range forage utilization, which is seasonal; and grazing, which has a longer time reference. Thus, overstocking can be corrected in a day and overutilization (or overuse) in a growing season, but the results of overgrazing may take several years to eliminate with proper utilization each year.

Many comparative terms result from combining the prefixes *under,* and *over* and the word *proper* with *stocking, use,* and *grazing.* Definitions of these terms may be self-evident, but several are given here as follows: *Overstocking, if continued for the season, results in overuse at the end of the current grazing period, and if continued for years, will result in overgrazed or deteriorated range.* In comparison, *proper stocking results in proper use at the end of the grazing period and promotes maintenance or improvement in range condition.* Other terms modifying *utilization* and suggesting different effects include *close, destructive, extreme, full, light, local, moderate, slight,* and *severe.*

Determination of Forage Utilization

Stockmen and range technicians estimate and measure forage utilization to determine when the correct amount of grazing has occurred, to indicate the amount of forage that remains to be harvested, and to ascertain the extent of livestock distributional problems. Utilization may be expressed in percentages of the herbage weight removed, of the number of plants grazed, and of the height removed. These expressions emphasize the proportion of material that has been removed. Sixty percent utilization means that forty percent of the herbage crop remains on the ground. The 60 percent that was eaten and therefore is unmeasurable directly also is the portion that was converted into livestock products. The 40 percent that remains as organic residue can be measured directly. It is the portion that initiates future growth and indicates continued good health of the range. Quantity of material rather than proportion of the crop likely is the better indicator of grazing effects. Therefore amount of herbage ungrazed should be used increasingly to express proper utilization. Amounts of herbage on the ground after grazing can be measured directly, and standards of range utilization based on those amounts can eliminate the inaccuracies of estimating the proportion of the herbage crop that has disappeared.

Several techniques give estimates of forage weight removed by herbivores and herbage remaining on the ground. The most accurate method compares the weight of herbage before and after short periods of grazing. When herbage growth occurs during the grazing period, these estimates of forage use are inaccurate. On rangelands, the preceding method may be used for measuring utilization during short rotation periods and on both browse and grass types that are grazed during the dormant season.

Grazed and ungrazed herbage weights are widely obtained by the use of paired plots, one caged or fenced to prevent grazing and the other nearby and grazed. Measurements made include clipping and weighing of the materials or ocular estimates of the weights or differences in weights. A combination of estimates and measurements of weight is used in standardizing the ocular estimates. If grazing is light or moderate, many individual plants or plant parts are ungrazed, and a random sample of the number of ungrazed and grazed plants and the weight of each permits measurement of utilization without protection of plots. Usually the key species are measured separately.

The percentage of ungrazed plants has been used to indicate utilization of rhizomatous species such as *Agropyron smithii*. The Range Analysis Field Guide for Region 5 of the national forests suggests that, for bunchgrasses, fewer than 53 percent ungrazed plants indicates less than 35 percent utilization and fewer than 5 percent ungrazed indicates more than 75 percent use. The technician most commonly measures utilization of annual grasslands by determining the amount of unused herbage at the beginning of the growing season. This determination may be based on weights on clipped plots or on ocular comparisons between the appearance of the herbage residue and a set of standard photographs. After a technician has gained considerable experience with measurement techniques and standardization of his estimates, he may judge directly the degree of use on individual species or on the range unit as a whole. Commonly these estimates are recorded as one of five categories; slight, light, moderate, heavy, or severe utilization.

Few methods are available for measuring the utilization of browse. During the dormant season, tagged twigs may be measured for length before and after grazing and samples of grazed and ungrazed twigs of current growth may be taken for weighing. More commonly, utilization of browse is described in qualitative terms, which include hedging of key species ranked severe, moderate, or not evident, and categories that describe the browse line.

Proper Utilization

Methods of determining utilization have received more attention than has the interpretation of the accumulated measurements. Use measurements indicate effects of different intensities of grazing if adequate cause and effect relationships have been shown. Plants have a tolerance to grazing, and many are stimulated by low levels of defoliation by grazing animals. If herbage removal exceeds a certain critical point, however, most plants will lose vigor, produce less herbage, and eventually die. Proper use is that maximum point of defoliation which continues to maintain excellent range productivity or to improve poor range. Many factors cause variation in actual use and in proper use of a range, so any expression of proper utilization must be considered a general guide to be used with care.

Animals select and graze any single species in relation to other available species. On a summer cattle range in the mountains of eastern Oregon, the grassland portion was 23 percent grazed when 60 percent of the herbage produced by *Agropyron spicatum* and 55 percent of the herbage produced by *Koeleria cristata* had been removed (Pickford and Reid, 1948). Commonly no two species in a vegetational type will be grazed to the same degree, and the degree of use will not be the same for a single species in different parts of a vegetational mosaic (Table 8-1). Cattle in the Oregon study foraged on open grassland sites to a greater degree than they did on timbered range, although several of the major forage species occurred in both areas (Harris, 1954; Johnson, 1956, 1966; Smith, 1967). Other factors such as season of use, kind of animal, and distribution of animals contribute to variation in range utilization. These factors are discussed in other chapters.

If stocking rate remains approximately the same from year to year, variation in forage production in response to climatic variations will cause large yearly differences in degree of forage utilization (Table 8-1). In only one year of ten was utilization considered proper by Harris (1954); and the variations in utilization were too great to justify yearly changes in stocking. As summarized by Hedrick (1958), an average utilization of the key species over a number of years which approximates 50 percent removal is a reasonable expression of proper use for most grassland ranges.

Estimates of production and utilization of actually used plants which are based on measurement of plants not grazed at all may be inaccurate. For example, expressions of forage removed by clipping of *Agropyron desertorum* varied from 54 to 82 percent depending upon the method of calculation (Cook and Stoddart, 1953). Spring clipping resulted in 82 percent removal of mature herbage weight produced by the plant itself, but this amount was equivalent to only 54 percent

Table 8-1 Ten-year fluctuations of actual forage utilization, in percentage of growth removed by cattle on mixed grassland and timbered range, Starkey Experimental Range in eastern Oregon (*Harris, 1954*)

	Grassland, % removed		Timbered range, % removed	
	Mean	Extremes	Mean	Extremes
Agropyron spicatum	52	38–69	41	30–60
Festuca idahoensis	41	26–67	32	15–48
Koeleria cristata	38	16–55	22	18–38
Danthonia unispicata	43	18–76		
Poa secunda	15	4–34		
Carex geyeri			28	18–40
Calamagrostis rubescens			10	4–12

removal from mature plants that were not spring-clipped. In another example, allowable spring use may be heavy on *Agropyron spicatum* if it ceases early enough to permit stem growth and maturation of seeds, but grazing later should occur after food storage (Stoddart, 1946). What constitutes proper degree of herbage removal for most species at different times along the growth curve remains unclear.

Standards of utilization which are expressed as a proportion of the current herbage crop removed require reconstruction of the total crop as if it were ungrazed. Large annual variations in the total crop make reconstruction a difficult exercise. The physiological dependence of each plant on the ungrazed or remaining regenerative tissue makes reconstruction of the total crop of doubtful value in evaluating range responses. Accordingly, a number of workers have suggested that measurements of utilization and establishment of proper utilization standards should be based on herbage residue rather than on herbage removed. Among the first workers to use this concept were those concerned with Mediterranean annual-type grassland in California (Hormay and Fausett, 1942; Bentley and Talbot, 1951). Their method required matching range appearance with a set of standard photographs. Under moderate utilization, the residue is patchy, reflecting a mosaic of lightly and heavily used areas. Vegetation in swales is used to an even stubble height of approximately 2.5 centimeters. Small objects on the ground are masked from view by plant residue at 6 to 9 meters from the viewer. The landscape has the patchy, yellowish cast of varying amounts of vegetation rather than a uniform gray or brown soil color. Both under- and overutilization give more uniform appearances than does moderate utilization. Heady (1956, 1965) and Hooper and Heady (1970) showed that productivity and species composition in the California annual type are directly related to herbage residue on the ground at the beginning of the growing season. They recommended 560 kilograms of mulch per hectare when utilization is proper (Fig. 8-4). Hyder (1953) developed the residue approach for sagebrush-grass range in eastern Oregon and suggested that the proper amount is 270 kilograms per hectare.

In a summary of data from grazing trials over a 19-year period on the Central Plains Experimental Range in Colorado, Bement (1969) emphasized that the most satisfactory way to assess forage utilization was in kilograms of ungrazed herbage per hectare (Table 8-2). Analysis showed the greatest animal gains per hectare when the herbage residue was 280 kilograms per hectare, a plateau of greatest gains per animal when the residue was 390 kilograms and the highest net profit when the residue was 335 kilograms, equivalent to an average stocking rate of 1.06 hectares per heifer month. The net return column (Table 8-2) was calculated on the basis of 1964–1966 prices, interest on the purchase cost of animals for the six-month grazing period, and other costs of $1.16 per head. Proper use was recommended at 335 kilograms of plant residue per hectare. This study indicated that short-grass range is ready for grazing when the herbage supply reaches 335

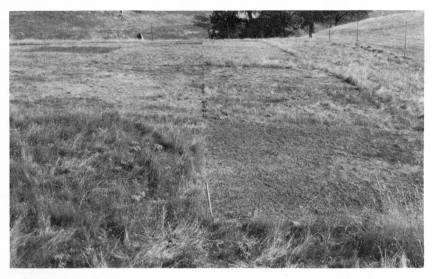

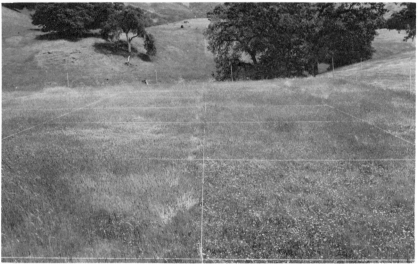

Figure 8-4 Upper photo shows mulch removal in late summer and lower photo the response the following spring in the California annual type. Absence of mulch promoted small broad-leaved plants (lower right) while abundant mulch favored grasses (lower left).

kilograms per hectare. Animals should be removed from a pasture anytime during the grazing season when the residue becomes less than that amount. This amount is an optimum standard for livestock production because the vegetation will withstand heavier use (Hyder et al., 1966).

Table 8-2 Relation of animal gains to the amount of herbage residue at the end of summer grazing on *Bouteloua gracilis* [*based on 19 years of grazing trials at the Central Plains Experimental Range (Bement, 1969)*]

Ungrazed herbage, kg/ha	Animal gains for 6 months		Net return per kg	Hectares per heifer month
	kg/ha	kg per animal		
168	14.67	57.2	$0.48	0.65
224	16.34	73.5	0.75	0.75
280	16.89	89.8	0.78	0.89
336	16.61	106.1	0.88	1.06
392	15.28	116.1	0.85	1.26
448	14.15	118.4	0.80	1.40
504	13.16	118.4	0.74	1.50
560	12.85	118.4	0.71	1.54

Considerable information on proper use factors has accumulated through experience as part of range reconnaissance surveys and other types of range inventories. Some of the plant lists that are associated with those surveys mention stubble heights of individual species when they are properly utilized. In general, these heights are estimates of the residue after grazing. The selected group of species and stubble heights for proper utilization in Table 8-3 has resulted from grazing trials and clipping studies. The stubble heights indicate that 40 to 60 percent of the herbage crop remains. Utilization of browse usually is given in percent of the current crop remaining.

Deteriorated ranges if they are to recover, require less severe utilization than those in excellent condition. Valentine (1970) recommended proper use at 50 percent removal on good *Bouteloua eriopoda* ranges and 32 percent removal on those in poorer condition.

Variability in Proper Utilization

Several types of grassland appear to be difficult to damage permanently by overgrazing. Among these are the short-grass plains of central North America and the Mitchell grass downs in Australia. Severe droughts in these types cause extensive reduction of ground cover and herbage production irrespective of grazing pressure. As has been shown in the short-grass plains, heavy grazing retards recovery in years of good rainfall. Stocking rate in these situations appears to be more important to the immediate welfare of the animal than to the health of the range vegetation.

The Northwestern bunchgrass type in the United States can be damaged easily by grazing, but the mixed prairie type of the Great Plains is difficult to damage permanently by overgrazing. Production can be maintained at a low level with

Table 8-3 Proper utilization of selected grass and browse species expressed as stubble height or percent of current growth remaining on the plant

Species	Stubble height, cm	Location	Authority
Agropyron desertorum	5	Central Colorado	Johnson (1959)
Agropyron intermedium	10	Central Colorado	Johnson (1959)
Agropyron smithii	8.5	Arizona–New Mexico	Parker and Glendening (1942)
	7.5–10	Eastern Montana	Holscher and Woolfolk (1953)
Bouteloua eriopoda	7.5–10	Arizona–New Mexico	Parker and Glendening (1942)
Bouteloua gracilis	5–7.5	Arizona–New Mexico	Parker and Glendening (1942)
	2.5–5	Eastern Montana	Holscher and Woolfolk (1953)
Bromus inermis	10	Central Colorado	Johnson (1959)
Buchloe dactyloides	3	Central Colorado	Costello and Turner (1944)
Carex filifolia	2.5–5	Eastern Montana	Holscher and Woolfolk (1953)
Deschampsia caespitosa	7.5	Oregon–Washington	Reid and Pickford (1946)
Elymus junceus	7.5	Central Colorado	Currie and Smith (1970)
Festuca viridula	7.5	Eastern Oregon	Pickford and Reid (1942)
Hilaria belangeri	4	Arizona–New Mexico	Parker and Glendening (1942)
Koeleria cristata	5	Arizona–New Mexico	Parker and Glendening (1942)
Stipa comata	5	Eastern Montana	Holscher and Woolfolk (1953)
Amelanchier alnifolia	35*	Northern Idaho	Young and Payne (1948)
Ceanothus sanguineus	40*	Northern Idaho	Young and Payne (1948)
Fraxinus americana	75*	Southeast Texas	Lay (1965)
Ilex vomitoria	50*	Southeast Texas	Lay (1965)
Purshia tridentata	40*	California	Hormay (1943)

*Proper utilization expressed as a percent of the current growth which is ungrazed.

close forage utilization. Heavy grazing pressure may be extremely damaging to range vegetation. The degree of damage depends on the characteristics of the dominant plants.

Consequences of Overutilization

The degree of herbage removed by the grazing animal has more influence on range vegetation than does any other grazing factor. Reduction in plant vigor results when too high a proportion of the photosynthetic tissue is removed. Experiments in which the treatments included a series of stocking rates, some too high and some too low, have characterized many pasture and range studies. Vegetational changes that resulted from the different stocking rates have permitted range managers to describe over-, moderately, and lightly grazed ranges for many different vegetational types.

Plants most palatable to the animals present on rangeland are selected for the first bite and perhaps selected again and again as grazing continues. Preferred species, especially where they exist in preferred areas, receive repeated defoliation. A gradual demise of plants and a gradual deterioration of the vegetation result. The individual plant responds with fewer and smaller leaves, stems, seed stalks, and roots. Energy capture and flow are interrupted, as also is the accumulation of carbohydrates. Destruction of vegetation, where plants die and their replacement falters, continues.

During the process of vegetational destruction, the soil surface becomes exposed to the beating action of raindrops and the scouring action of running water because its protection by mulch and live plants is reduced. The environment at the soil surface increases in variability, and its extremes increase in severity. The soil may be puddled by rain and by stirring as animals walk over it. Infiltration is reduced, runoff increased, and the available water for plant growth diminished. A bare and eroded landscape ultimately occurs. Desert-like vegetation appears in regions where the amount of rainfall can support less xeric species.

Many of the concepts regarding vegetational changes and plant succession have resulted from concern with destruction of vegetation by yearly overutilization. Early quantitative studies of overuse included those of Sampson (1919) in the mountain bunchgrass types of eastern Oregon and in Utah. He listed the successional types as (1) subclimax perennial grasses, (2) mixed grasses and weeds, (3) second weed stage, and (4) first weed or ruderal weed stage. Although the species of plants, rates of vegetational change, and relative importance of drought and overgrazing vary from one place to another and although many different plant successional terms have been applied, these stages may be identified and usefully employed to characterize the deterioration and improvement of ranges throughout the world (Fig. 8-5).

ADJUSTMENT OF ANIMAL NUMBERS TO FORAGE SUPPLY

Forage supply on all ranges varies from year to year in response to changes in weather. A few examples illustrate the magnitude of these fluctuations:

| Type of herbage | Location | Variation | | Source |
		kg/ha	yr	
Short grass	Southern Alberta, Canada	100– 925	1930–1953	Smoliak (1956)
Short grass	Eastern Montana	250–1,780	1927–1934	Campbell (1936)
Short grass	West Central Kansas	150–2,815	1940–1942	Weaver and Albertson (1944)
Bouteloua eriopoda	Southern New Mexico	0– 990	1926–1934	Campbell (1936)
Mixed perennial	Central Utah	505–1,425	1924–1935	Campbell (1936)
Annual	California	1,345–2,580	1935–1948	Bentley and Talbot (1951)

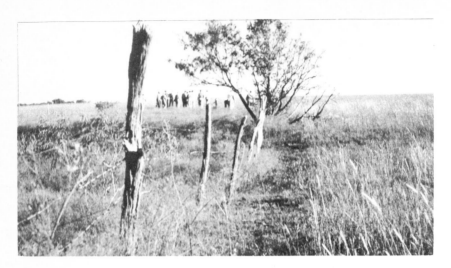

Figure 8-5 Annual broad-leaved plants within the fence on the left, a strip of short grasses where animals can reach through the fence, and tall grasses on the right constitute three successional stages due to degree of grazing in this true prairie type in Texas.

A manager may use a number of procedures to adjust stocking rate to wide variation in forage supply in order to obtain efficient forage utilization, the best possible livestock response under the circumstances imposed by the limits of each forage crop, and maintenance of range condition. One procedure stipulates stocking rates that result in proper use of the average crop, or more conservatively, that result in proper use when only 65 to 85 percent of the average crop is produced. Stocking rates may remain about the same from year to year, as, for example, permitted numbers on federal lands. Unless the grazing period is adjusted, the result can be a number of years when the range is overused and others when it is underused. The objective of the preceding plan is to balance range improvement in the years of high production against damage during the years of low production, while steady livestock numbers are maintained. Overuse is likely to occur in a quarter to a half of the years if one follows this procedure. Any strategy that maintains constant livestock numbers on rangeland results in widely varying grazing pressure and large changes in gains per animal and per hectare from one year to the next. It is an easy plan to follow for a pasture but a difficult one for a ranch. On the other hand, changes in stocking rates also are difficult in practice because they often require sale or purchase of animals in unfavorable markets.

As a managerial expediency, it probably is best to combine fixed stocking of a base herd (cows) with flexible stocking of other animals to obtain the most rapid possible improvement during the favorable years and the least damage in the poor years. The base herd should be approximately 80 percent of the average grazing capacity. Low-producing animals may be sold to reduce the herd further in very bad years. Calves may be held over, stocker animals purchased, and grazing rights leased in the good years. In this plan, a certain amount of organic residue would remain on the soil surface after grazing each year, regardless of the amount of herbage grown. In the good years, the amount would be more than in poor years, but at no time would herbage utilization be excessive.

Invariably, this plan requires yearly or, sometimes, more frequent adjustments in numbers of animals, length of grazing period, or both. As a strategist, the manager knows that these are the most important factors available for manipulation. As a tactician, he needs to arrange skillfully the numbers of animals that are put into pastures, the time when they begin grazing, the time when they are moved, and the place where they go next. The key to these animal movements is the degree of forage utilization. If future feed supplies are not available, certain animals should be sold so that those not sold will have sufficient feed. In times of surplus feed, young animals may be grown to a larger size, additional animals purchased, and forages conserved as dry hay. Ranches often need alternative feed supplies developed through irrigation, seeding, and fertilization, primarily to counter the variability of range forage.

A successful method for predicting range forage production could result in near-perfect forage utilization each year. However, success has escaped those searching for techniques that predict weather and forage in a manner useful for day-to-day management decisions. Clawson (1947) showed that consecutive years tend to be either below or above normal in precipitation in the northern Great Plains and Rocky Mountains. In the southwestern United States, the distribution is more random. Even at best, the prediction of forage production based on prediction of weather has no better chance than three years in four of being correct.

Sneva and Hyder (1962) reviewed and agreed with a common belief that winter-spring precipitation correlates closely with subsequent herbage yields of bunchgrass in the intermountain region. By the time spring rainfall is known, the time to make effective changes in animal numbers is past. A decision on the number of animals to winter often determines the number of animals on spring range. An attempt at determining number of cattle to winter by applying Sneva and Hyder's procedures shows that half the calves should be sold in late fall if below-normal July through October precipitation occurs and all the calves should be kept until they are yearlings if rainfall is above normal (Rogers and Peacock, 1968). This procedure needs more testing before it can be recommended, as do all methods that use weather as a determinant for adjusting stocking rates.

LITERATURE CITED

Beetle, A. A., W. M. Johnson, and R. L. Lang. 1961. Effect of grazing intensity on cattle weights and vegetation of the Bighorn Experimental Pastures. *Wyo. Agr. Expt. Sta. Bull.* 376.

Bement, R. E. 1969. A stocking-rate guide for beef production on blue-grama range. *J. Range Mgmt.* 22: 83–86.

Bentley, J. R., and M. W. Talbot. 1951. Efficient use of annual plants on cattle ranges in the California foothills. *U.S. Dept. Agr. Cir.* 870.

Blackburn, A. G., M. V. Frew, and P. D. Mullaney. 1973. Estimating optimum economic stocking rates for wethers. *J. Aust. Inst. Agr. Sci.* 39: 13–23.

Booysen, P. de V. 1967. Grazing and grazing management terminology in southern Africa. *Proceedings Grassland Soc. S. Afr.* 2:45–57.

Buechner, H. K. 1963. Territoriality as a behavioral adaptation to environment in Uganda kob. *Proceedings 16th Internatl. Cong. Zool.* 3:59–63.

Campbell, A. G. 1966. The dynamics of grazed mesophytic pastures. *Proceedings of the 10th International Grassland Congress,* pp. 458–463.

Campbell, R. S. 1936. Climatic fluctuations. *The western range,* Senate Document 199, pp. 135–150.

———. 1937. Problems of measuring forage utilization on western ranges. *Ecology* 18:528–532.

Clawson, M. 1947. Sequence in variation of annual precipitation in the western United States. *J. Land and Public Utility Econ. 23: 271*–287.

Cook, C. W., and L. A. Stoddart. 1953. The quandry of utilization and preference. *J. Range Mgmt.* 6: 329–335.

Costello, D. F., and G. T. Turner. 1944. Judging condition and utilization of short-grass ranges on the central Great Plains. *U.S. Dept. Agr. Farmers' Bull.* 1949.

Cowlishaw, S. J. 1969. The carrying capacity of pastures. *J. Br. Grassland Soc.* 24: 207–214.

Currie, P. O., and D. R. Smith. 1970. Response of seeded ranges to different grazing intensities. *U.S. Dept. Agr. Forest Service Prod. Res. Dept.* 112.

Gross, J.E. 1969. Optimum yield in deer and elk populations. *Trans. N. Am. Wildl. and Nat. Res. Conf.* 34:372–387.

Harlan, J. R. 1958. Generalized curves for gain per head and gain per acre in rates of grazing studies. *J. Range Mgmt.* 11: 140–147.

Harris, R. W. 1954. Fluctuations in forage utilization on ponderosa pine ranges in eastern Oregon. *J. Range Mgmt.* 7: 250–255.

Hart, R. H. 1972. Forage yield, stocking rate, and beef gains on pasture. *Herb. Abst.* 42: 345–353.

Heady, H. F. 1956. Changes in a California annual plant community induced by manipulation of natural mulch. *Ecology* 37: 798–812.

———. 1965. The influence of mulch on herbage production in an annual grassland. *Proceedings of the 9th International Grassland Congress,* pp. 391–394.

Hedrick, D. W. 1958. Proper utilization—A problem in evaluating the physiological response of plants to grazing use: A review. *J. Range Mgmt.* 11: 34–43.

Hildreth, R. J., and M. E. Riewe. 1963. Grazing production curves. II. Determining the economic optimum stocking rate. *Agron. J. 55:* 370–372.

Holscher, C. E., and E. J. Woolfolk. 1953. Forage utilization by cattle on northern Great Plains ranges. *U.S. Dept. Agr. Cir.* 918.

Hooper, J. F., and H. F. Heady. 1970. An economic analysis of optimum rates of grazing in the California annual-type grassland. *J. Range Mgmt.* 23: 307–311.

Hormay, A. L. 1943. A method of estimating grazing use of bitterbrush. *Calif. Forest and Range Expt. Sta. Research Note 35.*

————, and A. Fausett. 1942. Standards for judging the degree of forage utilization on California annual-type ranges. *Calif. Forest and Range Expt. Sta. Tech. Note* 21.

Hurtt, L. C. 1951. Managing northern Great Plains cattle ranges to minimize effects of drought. *U.S. Dept. Agr. Cir.* 865.

Hyder, D. N. 1953. Grazing capacity as related to range condition. *J. For.* 51: 206.

————. 1954. Forage utilization. *J. For.* 52:603–604.

————, R. E. Bement, E. E. Remmenga, and C. Terwilliger, Jr. 1966. Vegetation-soils and vegetation-grazing relations from frequency data. *J. Range Mgmt.* 19: 11–17.

Johnson, W. M. 1956. The effect of grazing intensity on plant composition, vigor, and growth of pine-bunchgrass ranges in Colorado. *Ecology* 37: 790–798.

————. 1959. Grazing intensity trials on seeded ranges in the ponderosa pine zone of Colorado. *J. Range Mgmt.* 12: 1–7.

————. 1966. Effects of stocking rates and utilization on herbage production and animal response on natural grasslands. *Proceedings of the 10th International Grassland Congress,* pp. 944–947.

Klein, D. R. 1968. The introduction, increase, and crash of reindeer on St. Matthew Island. *J. Wildl. Mgmt.* 32: 350–367.

Klipple, G. E., and D. F. Costello. 1960. Vegetation and cattle responses to different intensities of grazing on short-grass ranges on the central Great Plains. *U.S. Dept. Agr. Tech. Bull.* 1216.

Launchbaugh, J. L. 1957. The effect of stocking rate on cattle gains and on native shortgrass vegetation in west-central Kansas. *Kan. Agr. Expt. Sta. Bull.* 394.

Lay, D. W. 1965. Effects of periodic clipping on yield of some common browse species. *J. Range Mgmt.* 18: 181–184.

Lime, D. W., and G. H. Stankey. 1971. Carrying capacity: Maintaining outdoor recreation quality. *Proceedings of the Recreation Symposium, U.S. Dept. Agr. Forest Service,* pp. 174–184.

Mech, L. D. 1966. The wolves of Isle Royale. *Fauna of the National Parks of the U.S. Fauna Series 7.*

Merrill, L. B., and J. E. Miller. 1961. Economic analysis of year-long grazing rate studies on Substation No. 14, near Sonora. *Texas Agr. Expt. Sta.* MP-484.

Morley, F.H.W., and C.R.W. Spedding. 1968. Agricultural systems and grazing experiments. *Herb. Abst.* 38: 279–287.

Mott, G. O. 1960. Grazing pressure and measurement of pasture production. *Proceedings of the 8th International Grassland Congress,* pp. 606–611.

Parker, K. W., and G. E. Glendening. 1942. General guide to satisfactory utilization of the principal southwestern range grasses. *S. W. Forest and Range Expt. Sta. Research Note* 104.

Peterson, R. G., H. L. Lucas, and G. O. Mott. 1965. Relationship between rate of stocking and per animal and per acre performance on pasture. *Agron. J.* 57: 27–30.

Pickford, G. D., and E. H. Reid. 1942. Basis for judging subalpine grassland ranges of Oregon and Washington. *U.S. Dept. Agr. Cir.* 655.

————, and ————. 1948. Forage utilization on summer cattle ranges in eastern Oregon. *U. S. Dept. Agr. Cir.* 796.

Range Term Glossary Committee. 1964. *A glossary of terms used in range management.* Denver: American Society of Range Management.

Reed, M. J., and R. A. Peterson. 1961. Vegetation, soil, and cattle responses to grazing on northern Great Plains range. *U.S. Dept. Agr. Tech. Bull.* 1252.

Reid, E. H., and G. D. Pickford. 1946. Judging mountain meadow range condition in eastern Oregon and eastern Washington. *U.S. Dept. Agr. Cir.* 748.

Riewe, M. E. 1961. Use of the relationship of stocking rate of gain of cattle in an experimental design for grazing trials. *Agron. J.* 53: 309–313.

——, J. C. Smith, J. H. Jones, and E. C. Holt. 1963. Grazing production curves. I. Comparison of steer gains on Gulf ryegrass and tall fescue. *Agron. J.* 55: 367–369.

Rogers, L. F., and W. S. Peacock, III. 1968. Adjusting cattle numbers to fluctuating forage production with statistical decision theory. *J. Range Mgmt.* 21: 255–258.

Sampson, A. W. 1919. Plant succession in relation to range management. *U.S. Dept. Agr. Bull.* 791.

Sharkey, M. J. 1970. The carrying capacity of natural and improved land in different climatic zones. *Mammalia* 34: 564–572.

Shaw, N. H. 1970. The choice of stocking rate treatments as influenced by the expression of stocking rate. *Proceedings of the 11th International Grassland Congress,* pp. 909–913.

Smith, D. R. 1967. Effects of cattle grazing on a ponderosa pine-bunchgrass range in Colorado. *U.S. Dept. Agr. Tech. Bull.* 1371.

Smoliak, S. 1956. Influence of climatic conditions on forage production of shortgrass rangeland. *J. Range Mgmt.* 9:89–91.

Sneva, F. A., and D. N. Hyder. 1962. Estimating herbage procution on semiarid ranges in the Intermountain Region. *J. Range Mgmt.* 15: 88–93.

Stoddart, L. A. 1946. Some physical and chemical responses of *Agropyron spicatum* to herbage removal at various seasons. *Utah Agr. Expt. Sta. Bull.* 324.

Valentine, K. A. 1970. Influence of grazing intensity on improvement of deteriorated black grama range. *N. Mex. Agr. Expt. Sta. Bull.* 553.

Weaver, J. E., and F. W. Albertson. 1944. Nature and degree of recovery of grassland from the great drought of 1933 to 1940. *Ecol. Monog.* 14: 393–479.

Woolfolk, E. J. 1949. Stocking northern Great Plains sheep range for sustained high production. *U.S. Dept. Agr. Cir.* 804.

Workman, J. P., and D. W. MacPherson. 1973. Calculating yearlong carrying capacity— an algebraic approach. *J. Range Mgmt.* 26: 274–277.

Young, V. A., and G. F. Payne. 1948. Utilization of "key" browse species in relation to proper grazing practices in cutover western white pine lands in northern Idaho. *J. For.* 46: 35–40.

Chapter 9

The Mix
of Animal Species

The practice of grazing two or more species of domestic animals together or separately on the same range in a single growing season has long been known as *common use* or *dual use*. Common-use ranges should have mixed vegetation and should support at least two kinds of domestic animals that will fully use a wide spectrum of plants. Before the free-range era and even following it, when little management was practiced, common use was discouraged because often it resulted in double use. It carried the connotation that grazing by more than one species was undesirable. Essentially ignored until recently were the grazing influences of large, herbivorous wild animals.

Attitudes toward common-use management have changed gradually. A few experiments using cattle and sheep, sheep and goats, or all three together proved more profitable on ranges with mixed vegetation than did the grazing of any one animal species alone (Cook, 1954; Merrill and Miller, 1961). Perhaps even more influential in changing people's attitudes towards mixed-species grazing has been the growing vast interest in preservation of wild animals, game meat products, and

135

recreational services from wildlife. Because of these changes in attitudes, management of a mixture of animal species, some of them wild, presents new and challenging problems.

In national parks, national forests, and other recreational areas, man—the hunter, the builder, and the recreationist—has become a part of the producing system as well as a harvester of its produce. If one man reaps the beautiful view but in so doing blocks the view of another, he becomes a part, in this example, a negative part, of the producing system. Therefore the original range concept of *common use* is extended from its early reference to livestock to include wild animals and man. In this context, all rangeland is and will continue to be commonly used. A mixture is assumed to be inevitable and desirable. Selecting, maintaining, and manipulating the mix of species using rangeland presents major management problems that are explored in this chapter.

DOMESTIC OR WILD ANIMALS?

While proponents of either game or domestic animals usually agree that mixtures of species are more productive than monospecific populations, they disagree in many respects as to whether game and domestic species should be mixed. Claim and counterclaim seem to be based more on opinion—or at least on incomplete information—than on fact. In general, debate runs about as follows.

Skyrocketing tourism, based largely on the hunting, viewing, and photographing of wild animals, and predictions of high production of game meat, skins, horn, and hair, increasingly support contentions that large areas of rangeland should be devoted to raising a mixture of wild animals. Worldwide, the biomass of game animals, including a variety of species filling a wide array of ecological niches, has been estimated as high as 18,000 kilograms per square kilometer. Implied is high efficiency in the conversion of a large spectrum of forage plants into animal products without damage to soil and vegetation. Reproductive and growth rates of many game species are high, killing-out percentages are good, and little wasteful fat is mixed with the lean meat. Some wild species do not need frequent access to water, so trailing and trampling are less than with domestic animals. Game can use areas in Africa where tsetse flies prevent livestock grazing. Wild species are resistant to many other diseases that plague livestock (Talbot, 1966).

Conversely, it can be argued that several species and breeds of domestic animals contribute variety to the appearance of the countryside, consume most of the available forage species, and contribute the only or the principal support to many pastoral peoples. Where pastoralism is of the subsistence type, as in parts of Africa and the Near East, incomes from wild animals usually accrue to the nation as a whole and to industries other than pastoralism. Furthermore, in these areas, production from viable herds of game often or usually is compared with that from poorly managed livestock. Biomass of properly and intensively managed livestock can be as high as or much higher than that of game. So long as livestock provide the daily food and secure the pastoralist's place in the social structure, he has little incentive to change his system. Many pastoral peoples do not interfere with the wild populations that have shared their lands for centuries.

Subsistence pastoralism evolved using mixed herds. Market pastoralism is rapidly learning how to use mixtures of animal populations. The mix of species that the land manager selects for any given situation results from the interplay of many constraints such as tradition or custom, laws, market demands, handling facilities, food habits of different animals, and biological relationships among species. Other people with a sincere interest in animals, as well as those with direct land-management responsibility, approach these constraints in different ways. They have various objectives, attitudes, and opinions. The following analysis of views toward animals is given to help clarify man's differing actions toward them.

ATTITUDES TOWARD ANIMALS

Man's attitudes toward animals determine the way he manages and uses them. For purposes of discussion, three attitudes are described here. The first attitude is one of protection of animals. Man protects animals in many different ways: by preservation in game reserves, parks, and zoos; by laws against cruel treatment and killing of animals; by regulations (even in international trade) against the use of skins, meat, hair, and horn; and by his religious beliefs and taboos. This protectionist view regards wild animals as pets. And no pet should be eaten. Only a few cannibalistic peoples eat their pets. Pets are to be enjoyed and protected as living creatures, as part of the family of man, and are to be killed mercifully only after all efforts to save them have failed.

Included in this attitude is the idea that if a wild-animal population goes through a buildup and crash cycle during which it has major detrimental effects on its habitat and on other species, so be it. Catastrophe due to drought or disease is natural and expected. Any efforts of management must aim at improving the habitat and minimizing such problems as disease transfer to man and domestic animals, while not disturbing the animals themselves. Support for this view is likely to be highly emotional and to include the advocacy of not taking animals for research purposes and the refusal to eat game meat, to use game skins, or to admire mounted trophies. Oddly, this crusading spirit for preservation is likely to be only in the interest of the crusader's favorite species.

The ultimate goals of people who have this attitude are to prevent extinction of endangered species, to keep other species from becoming endangered, and to maintain balanced biological systems. Carried to extreme, this attitude suggests attainment and maintenance of the conditions of animals and environment as they were, say, 20,000 years ago. An immediate purpose of preservation activities is maintenance of animal populations for sightseeing and photography. Fortunately, most people have this attitude to some degree; otherwise many more species would be extinct and the world's wealth of wild animals not so rich as it is today.

A second attitude toward animals has led man to domesticate them for food, clothing, transport, and work (Fig. 9-1). He was highly successful with cattle, sheep, donkeys, horses, yaks, reindeer, poultry, etc., bringing forth many subspecies or varieties best suited for different purposes in different environments. Animal breeding, a large and effective discipline, aims to improve domestic animals through application of genetic principles. A rancher who selects and keeps the cows in his herd for better adaptation to his particular rangeland practices this science.

For several thousand years, few serious attempts were made to domesticate new wild species. Within the last 50 years, eland have been domesticated in Russia and Africa and bison raised as ranch animals in the United States. In the last two decades, there has been a surge of interest in ranching many kinds of game animals, principally in parts of Africa and the United States. This interest is based on the proposition that man can preserve valuable and profitable species.

Domestication aims at complete control of breeding, health, growth rates, herd composition, and production. When applied to game animals, it requires elimination of population cycles caused by fluctuations of food supplies, disease, and wild predators. Domestication substitutes a highly developed predator-prey relationship in which man is the sole predator for natural population controls. Society applies high health standards in slaughtering, processing, and transporting of game meat. Domestication of new species places them in direct competition

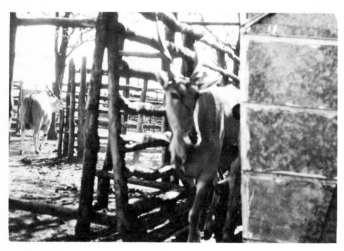

Figure 9-1   This eland is domesticated to such a degree that it is handled in a chute of the type used by cattle.

with species already domesticated. Ultimately the marketplace determines the winner or combination of winners. The term *game ranching* expresses this approach to game.

A long-term result of wild-animal domestication may be private ownership of game and perhaps no wildlife at all, but conversely, efficient meat production. Since the wise manager uses his animals as tools in the management of his range vegetation, regulation of the whole vegetation-animal system becomes easier as the domestication process becomes more complete.

Man's third attitude is one of maintaining animals in a wild state but cropping them to keep populations in check and to reduce cyclic extremes in numbers. This viewpoint extends the traditional hunter approach and commonly is known as *game cropping*. Sale of all types of animal products makes profitable the keeping of game on extensive areas, usually in competition with livestock. Man, as a predator, controls populations only after disease, natural predators, and stress do not exert sufficient pressure. Populations continue, with diverse herd compositions and at densities that prevent overgrazing of food supplies. Wild animals exercise full competition with each other, have freedom of movement, and follow natural behavioral patterns. The ultimate management objectives are to protect the species and their habitats by taking over formerly natural controls and at the same time, but secondarily, to produce as many products and services as possible. The profit motive is of minor importance.

Probably no person limits his views to any one of these attitudes, but most people tend more to one attitude than to another. For example, hunting clubs and safari businesses tend more to the third attitude. Ranchers and agriculturalists who raise domestic animals need to control the wild animals, so they favor domestication of wild species. National park administrators and tourists looking for game usually take a protectionist attitude and look on the animals as pets. Most people agree about saving certain species; for example, in recent years, few have argued against efforts to save the mountain zebra in South Africa and the California condor, although laws and management procedures as yet may not match the requirements for long-term preservation of these species.

Unfortunately, considerable discord exists among persons with different attitudes and objectives toward wild and domestic animals; thus the rate of accomplishment in the whole field of range-animal management is slow. Since no two wild species present the same needs for survival, the same values to society, and the same opportunities for management, attitudes toward wild and domestic animals will continue to be varied, but they need not conflict.

FORAGE AND ANIMAL COMBINATIONS

In a general way the proportions of grass, broad-leaved herbaceous plants, and browse determine the desirable kinds of animals on a given range. Cattle and horses, among the domestic animals, prefer grass to a greater extent than do sheep and goats. Goats are known for their browsing habits, and, to a lesser extent, so are sheep, but both eat much grass and do well without browse. Neither cattle nor horses thrive on strictly browse feed. Most foraging and browsing animals exhibit a wide range of preferred dietary plants and shift from one or a few species to others as forages change in their availability and growth stages. The larger grasses should be used by cattle; fine grasses make excellent sheep feed; browse is used mainly by certain game, sheep, and goats; and sheep do well on many weedy, broad-leaved plants. Exceptions to these generalizations occur in specific locations. For example, food habits of deer in northwestern California suggest that they require grass ranges in the winter–early-spring period but not at other times of the year. Deer in other areas have different food preferences.

The fact that several kinds of animals occupy the same region, pasture, or even vegetational type does not indicate that they occupy the same niche and are in direct competition with each other. More likely, they occupy separate but overlapping parts of the total area. Lamprey (1963), after lengthy study of numerous grazing and browsing animals in north central Tanzania, suggested that the separation is accomplished in six different ways:

1   Species concentrate in different parts of the vegetational mosaic.
2   Species select different types of food.
3   Species separate topographically on a seasonal basis.
4   Species select the same area but at different seasons.
5   Species select different feeding levels in the vegetation.
6   Species separate on a vegetational basis according to season of food stress.

The first two of these principles are illustrated in Figure 9-2, which shows that occupied habitat is not the same as food selection. The third principle, topographic separation, is accomplished in the dry season, when impala and Grant's gazelle use upland areas because they can live without free drinking water while other species move to lower areas near water. Elephants illustrate the fourth principle by their ability to range more than 40 kilometers from water in the dry season, placing them on forages that are used by other species only in the wet season. Black rhino, dikdik, and giraffe illustrate the fifth principle because they browse, but they feed at different levels in the woody vegetation. The sixth type of separation is illustrated by zebra and wildebeest, which live closer together and near water in the dry season but separate to different parts of the grassland in the wet season. These separations illustrate types of horizontal and vertical stratification among animals.

Three combinations of animals that use the total land resource efficiently and profitably are as follows. Use by mule deer, elk, and cattle on a section of the Missouri River Breaks in central Montana showed minimal interspecific competition, although the three species occupied the same general area (Mackie, 1970). In

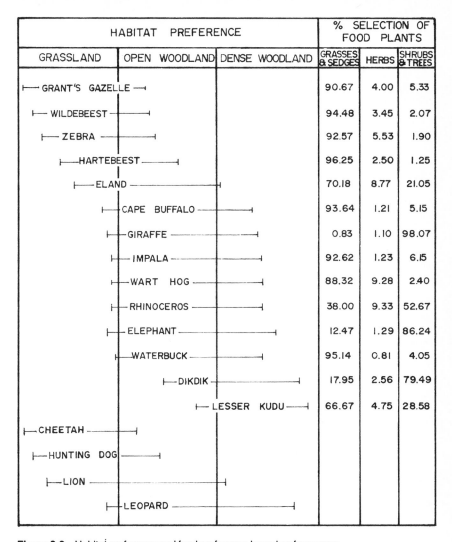

| HABITAT PREFERENCE | | | % SELECTION OF FOOD PLANTS | | |
GRASSLAND	OPEN WOODLAND	DENSE WOODLAND	GRASSES & SEDGES	HERBS	SHRUBS & TREES
⊢— GRANT'S GAZELLE —⊣			90.67	4.00	5.33
⊢— WILDEBEEST —⊣——⊣			94.48	3.45	2.07
⊢— ZEBRA ——⊣——⊣			92.57	5.53	1.90
⊢—HARTEBEEST———⊣			96.25	2.50	1.25
⊢—ELAND ———————⊣			70.18	8.77	21.05
	⊢CAPE BUFFALO——⊣———⊣		93.64	1.21	5.15
	⊢GIRAFFE ———————⊣——⊣		0.83	1.10	98.07
	⊢— IMPALA ——————⊣———⊣		92.62	1.23	6.15
	⊢—WART HOG ———⊣———⊣		88.32	9.28	2.40
	⊢— RHINOCEROS ————⊣——⊣		38.00	9.33	52.67
	⊢- ELEPHANT———————⊣——⊣		12.47	1.29	86.24
	⊢WATERBUCK—⊣———⊣		95.14	0.81	4.05
		⊢—DIKDIK⊣————————⊣	17.95	2.56	79.49
		⊢— LESSER KUDU——⊣	66.67	4.75	28.58
⊢—CHEETAH ———⊣					
⊢—HUNTING DOG ———⊣					
⊢—LION ——⊣————⊣					
	⊢LEOPARD ————⊣————————⊣				

Figure 9-2 Habitat preference and food preference based on frequency observations along transects in two areas of Tanzania *(adapted from Lamprey, 1963)*. Recordings were made almost daily for four years.

the summer, deer concentrated in ponderosa pine–juniper, elk selected *Sarcobatus-Agropyron smithii* in the bottomlands, and cattle grazed the sagebrush-grass type. During winter and spring, all three species occupied the sagebrush-grass type. Deer preferred steep southerly slopes all year; elk moved from southerly exposures in the winter to northerly slopes in the summer; and cattle spent at least 80 percent of their time in all seasons on slopes of less than 10 percent. Deer and elk overlapped in their preference for forbs in the summer. Deer and cattle separated completely, since they concentrated in different parts of the vegetational mosaic, they grazed on slopes of different steepness, and they preferred different foods. Elk and cattle were more competitive, since both ate grass, but they still selected different winter habitats.

Banff and Jasper National Parks in the Canadian Rocky Mountains had abundant elk in 1880, and the elk were very few in 1915, when bighorn sheep, deer, and moose were common. In the 1950s, abundance, from highest to lowest, was elk, bighorn sheep, moose, and deer. These population changes related to changing food supplies due to fires and to the elk overgrazing their habitats (Flock, 1964).

Work with cattle, sheep, and goats on the Sonora Experiment Station and adjacent ranches in Texas indicated that raising the species in combination yields more profit than does raising any of them singly (Merrill and Miller, 1961). White-tailed deer constitute a fourth species of value on many ranches in the area.

The Dye Creek Reserve in northern California is a cattle ranch with some 4,000 Hereford cows as the basic producing herd. During the 1960s, the ranch added new services, including hunting of California black-tailed deer, wild pig, valley quail, ringneck pheasant, and several waterfowl species; and picnicking, hiking, and general outdoor enjoyment for individuals, families, and clubs. While capital investment for cattle raising helped develop the other products, the new ventures provide income that makes the whole operation more profitable than it was before. Management turned problem areas in the cattle operation into other uses.

Maintenance of Forage and Animal Combinations

Other factors being equal, an animal species with specific food habits finds its best habitat to be the one furnishing these foods to the greatest degree. As the number of grazing species increases, the spectrum of consumed forages broadens and increasingly overlaps. Therefore, each combination of animal species needs a certain combination of forages and other range conditions which involves three sets of factors: (1) the manager's choice of animals and operating procedures; (2) those vegetational, soil, and other physical factors that constitute the rangeland habitat; and (3) feedback influences that the consumer animals exert on their habitat.

A change in the numbers of one animal species influences the population numbers of other species because it changes vegetation. These relationships may be used for managerial purposes. However, widely varying cause and effect responses must be recognized. Herein lies the major problem in the ranching of mixed animal populations. For too long, the general question in range management, when a second animal was used, has been, ''What can it do for the first?''

The view developed here emphasizes that each species of animal should be managed for what it can produce and how it can influence total production. Succinctly, goats should be raised for goat products, not just to control brush.

Several examples that illustrate the close relationship between changing habitat and changing animal populations are described below. They illustrate situations where, for the most part, the changes were remembered or recorded in hindsight. The ultimate objective in management is to predict changes in vegetation and animals and to plan for their best use.

That vegetation and animal populations change as a result of management is illustrated by experiences in Kruger National Park in South Africa. From 1902 to 1947, an area near Numbi Gate was burned annually and became open grassland with numerous wildebeest and zebra as dominant grazers. Fire was eliminated from 1947 to 1954, during which time bush increased, as did impala and greater kudu, but wildebeest, sable and roan antelope, and zebra decreased (Pienaar, 1969). This example illustrates an effect of fire on vegetation and the close relationship between kinds of animals and kinds of feed available. Animal populations were not controlled but were left to adjust naturally with the habitat changes. Undoubtedly impala and kudu tended to slow the change or to improve the habitat for wildebeest and zebra by eating the bush. The latter two species, preferring grass, probably had the reverse effect.

For at least two decades, winter deer range condition in northeastern California has been declining. Elimination of cattle from the area of winter deer range aimed to improve the browse (mainly *Purshia tridentata)* supply for deer. However, browse regeneration was minimal, and grasses increased considerably. When heavy early-spring cattle use of grass in experimental areas was followed by no summer grazing, stands of grass were reduced and bitterbrush increased. Apparently this range needs grazing by cattle to remain in acceptable condition for deer (U.S. Forest Service, 1970). Careful management properly serves both cattle and deer.

Following exceptionally widespread wildfires in 1910, elk and deer populations in northern Idaho and western Montana increased rapidly. Elk reached an estimated 11,000 head in the Selway River drainage alone by 1935. As coniferous trees replaced the shrubs and as shrub fields produced less browse in their older growth stages, elk feed became less and elk populations decreased. If the elk herds are to be maintained or increased, timber management must continually create new elk habitat, including shrubs producing abundant browse (Mueggler, 1967). A further decrease in mule deer in western Montana is expected as the tree canopy continues to increase (Klebenow, 1965).

Increasingly, management of forested lands for timber production in the southwestern United States aims to include practices that promote understory vegetation usable by deer and livestock (Reynolds, 1969). A succession of forest openings that have browse and grass but are no larger than 12 to 18 hectares can be maintained by patch clear-cutting. Openings of that size can be seeded to browse and grass and used efficiently by deer and livestock. Thinning, which enhances timber yields, also favors deer food. Leaving slash promotes a better habitat for deer than does cleaning up completely. Cattle and sheep favor grass, gentle slopes, and areas where the slash is cleared. A compromise may be needed between management for *Pinus ponderosa* timber, *Quercus gambelii* for browse (less than 20-centimeter-diameter stems), and *Quercus* for mast (40-centimeter-diameter stems) (Reynolds et al., 1970).

Changes in animal populations and habitats may be naturally cyclic. In 1900, during the building of the railroad through the area that now includes Tsavo National Park in Kenya, lions endangered the workmen but few elephants were seen. Grassland more nearly dominated the landscape than it did later. Bush increased in density for several decades. Elephant population increased even faster than the supply of browse and went beyond it, recently causing destruction of trees and shrubs. Grasses increased as the *Commiphora-Acacia* cover thinned, first near water and later at considerable distance from water, in response to the browsing and playfulness of the elephants. Fires speeded the change toward more grassland (Napier Bax and Sheldrick, 1963). Although grasses favor the plains game species, these vegetational changes discouraged rhinoceros, which suffered heavily during the 1961 drought (Goddard, 1970). Elephants, being taller than rhinoceroses, could reach sufficient browse to remain alive when the grass was gone. Nutritional quality of grass feed is lower than that of browse feed during the dry season. With less and less browse available, suggesting that the quality of diet was lowered and less feed was available, the next drought caused the death of many elephants and, afterwards, a rapid increase in grazing species of the open grassland (Laws and Parker, 1968). Perhaps as plains animals increase and overgraze the grassland, woody plants will be encouraged. And so the cycle, partly observed and partly predicted, might carry on, except that man, with his increasing influence, is unlikely to permit the full circle. For example, with continued heavy grazing and reduced fire, the *Commiphora* woodland will regenerate rapidly (Agnew, 1968). With light grazing and frequent burning, the grasses will dominate. Thus, the manager can combine the use of animals and fire to produce the species he wants.

Suggestions of elephant cycles exist in other sanctuaries. Elephants were absent from the Serengeti Plains for at least 40 years previous to 1955 (Lamprey et al., 1967). Their next earlier recorded occurrence there was in 1882 (Fosbrooke, 1968). Their increase was largely through immigration and coincided, to a considerable degree, with elephant increases in Tsavo Park. By 1966, Serengeti's elephants were destroying trees at the rate of at least 6 percent per year. The Murchison Falls area of Uganda is another location where elephants have modified their habitat in the past 20 years (Laws, 1968). Other damaged areas include Ruaha Park in Tanzania (Savidge, 1968), Kruger Park in South Africa (Pienaar, van

Wyk, and Fairall, 1966; van Wyk and Fairall, 1969), and Kibale Forest Reserve in Uganda (Wing and Buss, 1970).

In the future, man will exert his influence on these cycles by controlling animal numbers, by hampering migrations and lesser movements, by controlling fire, and by grazing domestic animals on the vegetation. However, the choice of techniques to control the cycles presents a question secondary to the choice of objectives. Are changes caused by elephants and other animals to be considered destructive or desirable according to today's and future values? Is the aim to stop the cycle and to maintain a certain combination of animals and plants? Choice among the alternatives determines if steps should be taken to control the elephant populations or if nothing should be done so one can marvel as the system changes. If the manager selects elephant control at a certain level as his objective, he should do so on the basis that a stipulated mixture of animals and combination of vegetational types also will be maintained.

Little information on the relative influence of many wild species on their habitats is available. Therefore, opportunities need to be expanded for gathering knowledge in parks, nature reserves, and extensive pastures where large numbers of wild animals can be managed in grazing experiments. For example, at Percy Fyfe Nature Reserve in the Transvaal, South Africa, 500 blesbok, 41 tsessebe, and 18 roan antelope grazed in separate pastures. A fourth pasture contained greater kudu, zebra, impala, eland, waterbuck, sable antelope, black wildebeest, and a number of smaller species. These pastures gave the opportunity for determining the separate influences of several animal species on their feed supply, the effects of grazing systems in which one species follows another on a seasonal basis, and the techniques for handling or semidomesticating each kind of animal.

The feed on a given range may support a single grazing species or a combination of species. One species may be intentionally used to develop a habitat for another. In order to be useful, a mixture of species needs an information base that will permit the manger to recognize and predict changes in vegetation and soil.

Introduction of Exotic Range Animals

Man intentionally has transplanted grazing animals to new lands wherever he has gone (Fig. 9-3). Fourteen species of large herbivores were liberated in New Zealand, beginning with releases of goats and pigs by Captain Cook in the eighteenth century (Wodzicki, 1950). Horses became a wild animal of central North America following Coronado's expedition in the sixteenth century. By accident or carelessness of the keeper, any enclosed animal may escape. Thus importing a new foraging species, even if it is enclosed in a small pen, adds a potentially wild species to the rangelands of that region.

All domestic grazing animals in the United States have become feral on rangelands. Wild horses are the best known of such animals. At their peak they

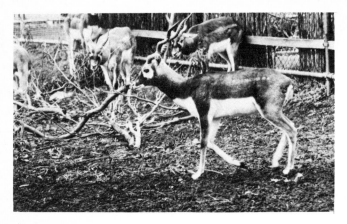

Figure 9-3 Blackbuck antelope have been introduced successfully from Asia to Texas rangelands.

numbered many thousands. Wild burros are problem animals in parts of Arizona, California, Nevada, and New Mexico and exist in small groups in several other states (McKnight, 1958). They may number as many as 13,000 (Presnall, 1958). Feral cattle and sheep are not so persistent. Feral goats have caused extensive damage to range vegetation on several islands along the California coast. All of these species provide sport hunting and profit, but the feral pig is the most likely to become a managed game species. Managers have crossed it with wild boar from Europe to enhance its sporting values.

Although federal law prevents import and release of animals, import to and maintenance on private lands has been permitted, subject to state laws. Local laws on feral animals vary from complete protection, as the burro is protected in California, to stipulation in Texas that a game species must be an indigenous species. In the latter state, no exotic grazing species, birds excepted, are subject to game laws and regulatory responsibility by a state agency. In 1968, Texas was reported to have 26 species of large exotic herbivores which totaled over 37,000 animals (Ramsey, ca 1969). Six of these species that numbered more than 1,000 each were as follows:

Mouflon sheep	10,000
European wild boar	10,000
Axis deer	6,450
Blackbuck antelope	4,125
Nilgai antelope	4,000
Aoudad	1,300

These numbers can be only approximate because some animals escape unreported. The interbreeding of mouflon sheep with domestic sheep further complicates censusing. Most of the buildup in numbers has occurred since 1950.

California has had a center of animal releases at the Hearst Ranch in San Luis Obispo County, where several deer and sheep species and other animals have been held in large range pastures (Presnall, 1958). However, none has developed into a large herd. Wild pigs have become established as the second (after deer) most important big game species in California (Craighead and Dasmann, 1966).

Only a few herbivorous species have become successful and beneficial immigrants to any country. Most either have been unsuccessful or have expanded to nuisance levels, as have the red deer in New Zealand. The successful species would appear to be the opportunist animals that can take advantage of widely varying habitat conditions. Specialized species transplant with difficulty and are unlikely to become pests (Ramsey, ca 1969). Disease, poor physical condition of animals at release time, lack of adaptation to new habitats, too few numbers, and shock from handling cause failures (Bump, 1968).

High hunting fees from guests who want something different encourage importation of game species. Some advocates of importation claim that more meat, better hunting, and higher profits can be obtained with additional species that fill vacant niches. Other advocates claim that newcomers improve upon the complexity of nature and help to prevent extinctions of rate species. However, faunas should not be mixed because genetic changes soon take place in imported animals. Undesirable consequences of introducing animals cannot be predicted at reasonable risk levels. Regardless of controversy over introducing new species, exotic animals are increasing rapidly in numbers and more species are likely to be added, endangering physical resources and native animals.

Alternative regulations for exotics include declaring them private rather than public property, exterminating them altogether, giving them protection, placing them in sanctuaries, and including them as game animals. None of these can be a final answer to importation and management of all species or even one species in all places. A species imported, raised, and managed on a ranch should be private property, as blackbuck are in Texas or as ringneck pheasant are on game farms. In different situations, one or more of these regulations may be required, but they seldom can be stated in advance of importation.

Without brands or other ownership markings, escaped individuals on public land traditionally become public property and subject to regulation by public agencies, as have wild horses. Private regulation of game animals can be successful on private lands, but public rangelands will continue to require public regulation of exotics as publicly owned animals. Those species (horse, burro, goat) that have little value for hunting should not be declared to be game.

Several points concerning exotic and feral animals seem clear. Many foreign species have made permanent homes in new areas, and more are likely to be added to the list. Exotic game birds and exotic forage plants have been highly beneficial on rangelands. New game animals also can be beneficial, but problems will develop. Their control and even elimination will be needed where habitats are required for other purposes.

Each introduction brings a need to determine the ecology and management of the species in its new situations. Mixtures of exotic species and domestic species on rangeland have been profitable in Texas, largely because of careful management by all interests. Further development of exotic range animals, especially on public lands, requires careful consideration of policy matters, statutory regulations, and biological relationships.

Exchange Ratios Among Animal Species

If management requires a switch from one kind of animal to another or a change in proportions of animal types, the concept of equivalent grazing pressure among species is useful. Thus, "How many sheep equal one cow?" The cow is taken as the standard and called an *animal unit*.

Various methods of obtaining exchange ratios among species have been used, but none has been completely satisfactory. If the feed eaten is reasonably the same for both species being compared, the ratio of metabolic weights, gives the exchange. Although variation exists among individuals and species, the ¾ power of weight in kilograms defines the metabolic size of an animal (Kleiber, 1961). It expresses the fact that smaller animals produce more heat and consume more food per unit of body size than do larger animals. For example, a 500-kilogram cow and a 50-kilogram sheep have metabolic sizes of 105.74 and 18.8, respectively (Maynard and Loosli, 1969). The ratio of live weights is 1:10, but the ratio of metabolic weights is approximately 1 cow to 5.6 sheep, which is a better expression of the relationship of their feed needs. A cow-sheep ratio of 1:5 has been used on rangeland more than any other has and appears to be a reasonable expression of the relative impact of the two upon the range. Table 9-1 gives animal unit equivalents for a number of species and for animals of different sizes within a species, e.g., 1.5 animals weighing 272 kilograms equal 1 animal unit.

Food habits, ages of animals, and differences among species alter exchange ratios. For example, little competition and, therefore, little basis for exchange exists between moose and cattle in southwestern Montana, where the former has a diet of 98 percent browse and the latter mainly graze (Dorn, 1970). Giraffe and cattle in the same African pasture exert little competition with each other because one feeds on browse and the other on grass and forbs. The proper number of each in a pasture depends upon the amount of grass and browse available, not upon the notion that it takes 3 cows to weigh as much as 1 giraffe or that their ratio of metabolic sizes is approximately 1:2. In fact, the manager may desire to use excess giraffe to overbrowse the woody plants; so he might start with 1 giraffe to 2 cows. As the brush disappears so must the giraffe, until the final result is grassland with cattle alone. Each species properly grazes or overgrazes its own food supply and not that of the other species, except for species that have overlapping food habits.

Table 9-1 Approximate number of individuals per animal unit based on ratios of metabolic weights (wt. kg$^{0.75}$) for mature animals

	Approx. wt.			
	lb	kg	kg$^{0.75}$	Ratio, 98/x	No. per animal unit
Cape buffalo	1,200	545	112	0.87	0.9
Bison, cow, eland, horse	1,000	455	98	1.00	1.0
Elk, zebra	600	272	67	1.46	1.5
Waterbuck, wildebeest	400	182	50	1.96	2.0
Hartebeest, topi	300	136	40	2.45	2.5
Mule deer	150	68	24	4.08	4.0
Sheep, impala	120	55	20	4.90	5.0
Pronghorn antelope, goat	100	45	17	5.76	6.0
Thomson's gazelle	50	23	10	9.80	10.0
Dikdik	12	5	3	32.00	33.0
Black-tailed jackrabbit	5	2.8	2	49.00	50.0

Any use of exchange ratios among range animals should be limited to those with similar diets and to the initial exchange. Table 9-1 is only a guide, since wide dietary differences exist among the animals included. Manipulations in proportion of species should depend upon changes in range condition which are caused by each species.

HARVESTING OF WILD ANIMALS

Harvestable Numbers

Determination of a percentage off-take or harvest that will maintain a maximum productive herd without destructive changes in soil and vegetational resources constitutes a major problem in game ranching. Theoretically the herd has a density at which all its environmental needs are met to the fullest and increase in annual biomass is the greatest. Off-take is maximized in balance with the increase in annual biomass.

Unfortunately only a few guidelines, based on experiments and experience, exist for harvesting wild-animal populations. After many years of study and control, an annual off-take of 40 percent of the autumn herd has been recommended for the saiga antelope in Russia. This species has a high twinning rate and a relatively low rate of loss in the young (Bannikov et al., 1961).

For 19 years, the average annual number of white-tailed deer removed from the George Reserve in Michigan was 39 percent of the fall herd (Chase and Jenkins, 1962). Average annual decrease of a white-tailed-deer herd in northern

Michigan amounted to 32 percent of the fall herd. This decrease was composed of 12 percent through natural losses and 20 percent through hunting (Arnold and Verme, 1963). Mule deer on the National Bison Range in western Montana sustained an annual removal of a third of the herd; fawn and predator losses were light (Nellis, 1968). After examination of available biological information of various kinds, Dasmann and Mossman (1961) recommended 16 to 30 percent annual off-takes of the several ruminant species of Rhodesian herds. These estimates later had to be revised downward because of errors in censusing and unknown losses to predators and drought. Annual yield was estimated at 10 percent of the population in a game cropping scheme at Loliondo, Tanzania (Watson, Graham, and Parker, 1969). It should be noted that heavier predation and poaching occurred in the African situations than in the examples from Russia and Michigan.

Game eradication in Africa for the purpose of removing the food of the tsetse fly *(Glossina* spp.) and thereby eradicating the fly and the disease, trypanosomiasis, has special reference to the problem of determining harvestable numbers of game animals. Game removal first became a national program in South Africa in 1929. The suggestion that game elimination would reduce tsetse-infected areas originated from the fact that fly areas diminished after the rinderpest epidemic of 1896, which decimated both game and livestock populations. Other countries that have employed game shooting for tsetse control are Nigeria, Uganda, Kenya, Tanzania, Zambia, Botswana, and Rhodesia. Estimates based on recorded kills in the Umfolozi area of South Africa suggest biomass of game animals at about 280 kilograms per hectare before the first eradication program in 1929, 244 kilograms per hectare in 1942 before the second kill program, and 488 kilograms per hectare from a 1967 census. Over 29,000 animals were shot in the 1929 campaign and 70,000 between 1942 and 1950 (Mentis, 1970). Species such as eland, wildebeest, and zebra were easily eliminated or reduced to near zero, and others, such as cape buffalo, greater kudu, and waterbuck, were greatly decimated, but some survived. Smaller antelopes and nocturnal animals such as bushbuck, duiker, and bushpig were curtailed but perhaps for only a brief time. In no case was eradication of the fly achieved, although reduction, as in Uganda, has permitted livestock to use the land.

Problems of reducing or maintaining each animal population at a certain level are illustrated in all tsetse control-hunting operations. In eastern Zambia, two years of hunting duiker were insufficient to change age composition in the herd. Feeding habits were changed, and the animals became more difficult to find (Wilson and Roth, 1967). In Rhodesia, after killing 10,838 duiker over 310,000 hectares in a 29-month period, hunters were shooting as many as at the beginning (Lovemore, 1963). After 23 years of organized game shooting to control tsetse in a 775-square kilometer area of Botswana, only one of a dozen hunted species was reduced in numbers (Child et al., 1970).

These failures to eliminate species support the proposition that wild-animal populations could produce considerable meat if their harvest was sustained. Although many approximations went into the estimate, the 1942–1950 program in South Africa produced about 1.2 kilograms of meat per hectare per year in an overkill situation. Advance of tsetse probably could be reduced in other areas so that prophylactic drugs could maintain cattle there. Presently in Rhodesia, removal of selected hosts of the tsetse flies, spread of insecticides on preferred tsetse habitats, and limited brush clearing constitute the tsetse control program (West, 1972). Production of meat from game could be a valuable product in tsetse control.

Problems basic to harvesting of animals in parks and reserves are illustrated by data from Kruger Park and the combined Hluhluwe and Umfolozi Reserves in South Africa (Table 9-2). Recommended off-takes for maintainance of herds of five species in Kruger Park are based on observed annual population increases. The difficulty in determining numbers of animals causes wide variation in recorded populations between species and between years. For example, impala are difficult to count in their bush habitat. However, their annual increase directly reflects the removal rate because numbers are near grazing capacity.

The annual increase of zebra in Kruger Park has changed from 4.8 to 9 percent in a few years. Immigrations enlarge the elephant population in this park. Each species presents a separate problem in managing numbers.

Table 9-2   Game numbers in Kruger National Park and two reserves, South Africa[*]

	Kruger National Park			Hluhluwe and Umfolozi Reserves	
	Estimated annual increase, %	Estimated population[†]		Estimated population[†]	Recommended removal
		1968	1970		
Impala	5.0	97,400	180,000	4,500	1,500
Elephant	11.3	7,701	8,852		
Blue wildebeest	4.8	14,143	16,000	3,446	800
Zebra	9.0	14,710	17,000	1,687	350
Cape buffalo	2.5–4.0	15,867	21,500	1,060	0
Warthog		4,000	4,330	6,000	2,200
Nyala		750	750	4,500	350
Square-lipped rhino				1,208	200

[*]Data selected from Pienaar (1969), a published brochure about Kruger Park, and conference with administrative personnel for both areas.
[†]Population estimates are based on aerial counts.

At the Hluhluwe and Umfolozi Reserves, the aim was to keep each species from damaging its habitat. Off-takes were high for the species near overpopulation and low or nonexistent for the others.

Whether the determination of off-take numbers is approached on a basis of herd increase or maintenance of a specified herd size, the actual harvest will vary from year to year. It must be sensitive to habitat changes and to annual variation in reproductive rates.

Harvesting or removal of animals from parks and reserves necessitates careful attention to public opinion. The public permits reduction of animal populations only after long and careful enunciation of reasons. Less public opinion against reduction often is associated with more concern for increased water and feed to support more animals and to prevent the ravages of droughts.

The successful examples of animal population controls are the continuous reduction programs in Kruger Park in South Africa, among elk in or near Yellowstone Park in Wyoming, and among hippopotamus in Ugandan parks. In the last example, 1.4 million kilograms of undressed carcasses were taken during a 10-year period.

Generally, killing and capturing should be done by park personnel or under their close supervision (Leopold et al., 1963). Tourists have not been allowed to witness the taking and processing of animals in most parks. An exception was the reduction of hippopotamus numbers in Queen Elizabeth Park in Uganda, which continued for approximately 10 years in full view of many tourists.

Capturing of Various Species

Domestic animals normally are dehorned, castrated, branded, checked for health, and sorted in a set of corrals. Cattle and sheep, being of different sizes and behavior, require handling facilities of different designs; for example, permanent structures for shearing sheep have minimum usefulness for other purposes. Designs for livestock handling facilities, although highly varied, are readily available and will not be described here. Facilities for wild-animal capture and handling in quantity are relatively new and will be discussed.

The number of animals to be handled in part determines the harvesting technique. The rifle and capture-gun are used to take small numbers of all species and all of the large, dangerous animals such as elephant, rhinoceros, hippopotamus, and cape buffalo.

Live-trapping procedures, usually including baited traps of many designs, serve in the study of smaller wild species. For example, deer and pronghorn antelope have been trapped, measured, marked, and retrapped in numerous studies.

Except for a few species, mass catching of wild animals has not been perfected. Corrals to handle springbok and blesbok are shown in Figure 9-4.

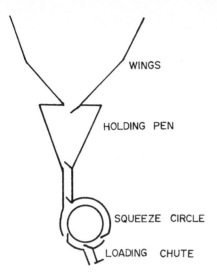

WINGS

HOLDING PEN

SQUEEZE CIRCLE

LOADING CHUTE

Figure 9-4 Design of a portable corral for catching springbok, blesbok, zebra, and wildebeest, animals that are not high jumpers *(adapted from Riney and Kettlitz, 1964)*. The wings are dark plastic and at least 1.5 meters high. The chute into the squeeze circle and the squeeze itself are wood or wire panels as needed to hold the animals, but they are open so that the herd leaders (blesbok) can seen through the material or solid so that horns will not tangle in them (springbok). The inside circle gives capacity to the chute and at the same time keeps the animals milling rather than bunching them into a corner. The circle has gates or baffles at two or three points so that only a few animals can be caught at once and all can be handled easily. Blesbok will not jump a 1.5 meter fence. They are caught by the horns by a person reaching over the fence, then led through the gates into shipping crates. A straight chute is used for wildebeest. All pens should have rounded corners and posts on the outside so animals will not be injured in handling. A helicopter has been effective in driving animals into the first compartment.

Wildebeest and zebra have been captured by being driven into corrals of similar design. These animals are larger than blesbok, so corral construction needs to be more substantial than for the smaller species. Corrals to hold bison should be as heavily constructed as the best of cattle facilities. The usual methods of mass capture of several African species are shown in Table 9-3.

Hunter Harvest of Game on Ranches

By 1965, sale of shooting preserve licenses to private landowners in Texas had increased to more than 13,000. Teer and Forrest (1968) estimated that these ranchers sold hunting rights on 8,900,000 hectares of rangeland for at least $13 million. Sales were for seasonal privileges, day hunting, animals in the bag, and secondary leasing through a broker or outfitter. Income varied from a few cents to

Table 9-3   Methods of mass capturing of several
African game species

	Driving into one or two nets[*]	Driving into corrals or pens	Drugs[†]
Impala[‡]	X		
Sable	X		
Zebra	X	X	
Kudu	X		
Waterbuck	X		
Reedbuck	X		
Wildebeest	X	X	
Warthog	X		
Nyala	X	X	
Tsessebe	X		
Blesbok		X	
Eland		X	
Springbok		X	
Ostrich		X	
White rhinoceros			X
Black rhinoceros			X
Elephant[§]			X
Hippopotamus			X
Giraffe			X
Roan			X
Cape buffalo			X

[*]Some animals, especially nyala, will jump a net, so a second net is placed behind the first. The animal will be caught before it can gain the momentum to make a second leap.

[†]All wild animals may be taken with the aid of tranquilizer drugs. Those species marked in the *Drugs* column usually are taken only with drugs and by shooting because of their large size and difficulty in handling.

[‡]Impala can be blinded with a spotlight at night during the dark of the moon and caught by hand or shot at close range with a small-caliber gun.

[§]Collecting of elephants in Kruger Park is done with an overdose of drugs (usually succinylcholine chloride), administered by a hunter operating in a helicopter.

$5.40 per hectare. Advantages of leased hunting included reduced poaching, hunters' compliance with safety standards, and evenly distributed hunting pressure. Managed hunter harvest tended to reduce kill below the level of that from full public hunting. Except for the private owner of big game—principally exotic species of the United States—the landowner complies with dates and bag limits in state and federal hunting regulations. He, in effect, sells to others the right to trespass on his land. States vary in these regulations, but none permits adequate management and harvest of native game as an integral part of a ranch operation.

Field Slaughter of Game Animals

Field slaughter for market presents problems of cleanliness and health. High standards set for the meat from domestic animals are costly when applied to game meat. Commonly, wild animals are shot in the head or neck, bled on the spot, and hauled to a farm abattoir for skinning, eviscerating, cooling, and short-term storage. The carcass may be dirty on arrival at the abattoir, taxing facilities and labor to produce acceptable products. Many ranchers live too far from meat inspectors for regular service, although high standards of cleanliness and thorough inspection result in public safety and confidence in the meat products.

Farm slaughtering facilities require hot water, refrigeration, concrete floor space, and adequate enclosure against insects. Power for continuous operation is difficult to maintain, especially in areas without reticulated electricity. Equipment failures in remote areas cause spoilage of meat and add extra cleanup costs. Adequate floor space in the cooler depends upon the amount of storage needed between trips to market. The cooler and the refrigerated truck or trailer may be the same equipment, such as that commonly used in handling kangaroo meat in Australia.

Many unexpected events can occur between field slaughter and delivery of meat to market. Animal migrations cause fluctuations in the kill, muddy roads hamper transport from field to abattoir and from abattoir to market, and equipment failures have already been mentioned. Each irregularity in delivery favors the competitor who can deliver clean meat on a regular basis.

Few ranchers in Africa have been able to surmount these meat-handling problems, and several ranchers are moving away from the game meat business, saying they need higher prices for the meat in order to cover continous operational costs. Probably game meat that passes equivalent health standards for meat from domestic animals will be as costly to deliver as is domestic meat. If live game animals could be delivered to the abattoir, and held and fed until slaughtered, many problems with game harvesting would be solved. The driving, capturing, holding, and feeding of zebra, wildebeest, and gazelle as done in the Hluhluwe Game Reserve, South Africa, leads to solutions of these problems.

Holding and Hauling Facilities

All commercial animal industries require facilities for the holding and transportation of live animals. Otherwise new herds cannot be established, crossbreeding or other herd improvements cannot be obtained, and the conveyance of animals to slaughter cannot be maintained on an even flow. Considerable demand exists for animals to restock game ranches in South Africa, for bison on ranches in the United States and for animals to restock parks and reserves. Because live capture and delivery to new sites can seldom mesh as to time and type of needed animals, a holding, feeding, and quieting period is necessary. Each species requires special facilities. For giraffes, the hauling crate is built like a horse trailer with high sides and a tall, windbreaker front to accommodate their long necks. The feed box is placed high in the holding pen. For gazelle, antelope, and zebra, the designs shown in Figures 9-5 and 9-6 have emerged after much trial and error at Hluhluwe Nature Reserve in the Natal region of South Africa.

For domestic animals, trucks and pens holding a few to 100 or more animals have been sufficient. Usually these holding facilities are without roofs because the animals are not high jumpers. For wild animals, transport facilities require individual crates for the larger antelope, zebra, etc., and crates holding two to five individuals for the smaller species, especially those, such as Thomson's gazelle and springbok, which have highly developed herding instincts.

Regulations Concerning Game Meat

Game meat is a staple in the diets of many African peoples, a taboo for others, and a delicacy in much of the world. Venison, although meaning different kinds of

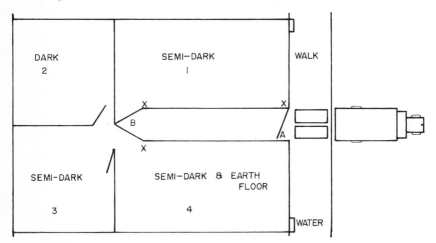

Figure 9-5 Floor plan of roofed holding pens for animals awaiting shipment. Darkness or semidarkness helps to quiet the animals. The gate at A is longer than the width of the passageway so animals crowding it will never push it open and escape is less likely during feeding and cleaning of pens. Hinges are marked X. Gates at B swing to block the passage and to allow pens 1 and 4 to hold animals while other animals are loaded out of pens 2 and 3. Normally animals are loaded into crates at the end of the passageway. The floor and walk level is close to the height of a truck bed for ease of loading and unloading crates of animals. This type of facility is used for gazelles, where two to five are loaded per crate.

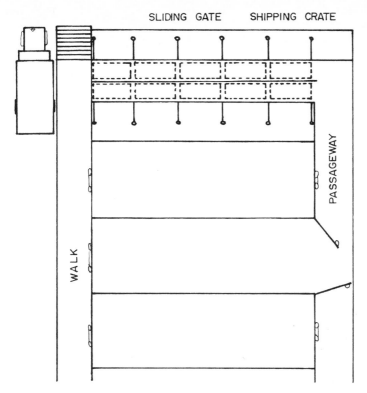

SLIDING GATE   SHIPPING CRATE

Figure 9-6 Covered holding pens and loading-unloading equipment for zebra. Crates are made to fit into the chutes so that they form a continuous single-file pen. Two such pens with five crates each are shown. Control of animals in the separate crates is accomplished with sliding doors as well as with the end gates on the crates, which lift upward. When the crates are filled, they are moved on rollers across the walkway to the truck. Side loading is preferred to end loading with crates of this size. Normally one zebra is loaded per crate. Three holding pens are shown, but the total facility may include many.

meat in different parts of the world, is unmarketable by law or so highly controlled that it has considerable novelty value in the United States and Europe. Biltong and other dried or processed game meats pass through highly controlled markets in South Africa. International regulations reduce trade in beautiful animal skins, horn, hair, feathers, and products made from them. These regulations and the tremendous concern for wild animals which supports them prohibit the complete and wanton slaughter of animals. The laws foster easier control of poaching and do much to prevent extinction of endangered species.

Rightfully, there is tremendous reluctance to open general markets in game meat which could lead to the demise of any wild-animal resource. The problems of separating products to protect one animal and harvest another are unsolved. Their solutions involve the highly controversial attitudes toward protection, ranching for profit, safari hunting, and the use of wild animals for other recreational purposes. The physical problems of harvesting this wild and remote resource seem easier to solve.

ANIMAL DAMAGE TO TREES

Grazing animals damage plants grown for purposes other than grazing. Browsing of forest seedlings, newly planted trees, and larger growing stock may reduce growth and delay timber harvesting. In a study of damage to conifers in Oregon and Washington, nearly all animals inhabiting the forests were found to be potentially harmful to the trees (Crouch, 1969). Foliage browsing, stem and root barking, and trampling were the major types of damage. Rodents and birds ate seed, either extracted from cones or gathered after natural or artificial seeding. Deer, livestock, and black bear did most of their damage during the growing season, but other animals destroyed plants in the dormant season. In order of greatest to least damage on planted forest were deer, porcupine, pocket gopher, rabbit and hare, elk, livestock as a group, mountain beaver, beaver, and a few other rodents. Significantly, in Oregon and Washington, livestock did relatively little browsing on tree species. Planted *Pseudotsuga menziesii* sustained major browsing by rodents, mountain beaver, snowshoe hare, deer, elk, and bear, while *Pinus ponderosa* was subject to gnawing by jackrabbit, pocket gopher, deer, elk, livestock, and porcupine. Planted stock received more browsing than did natural regeneration.

In Oregon and Washington, major animal damage occurred on clear-cut areas, but in California, partial cuttings were most harmed. The problems of animal damage are complex, varying from little effect that rights itself quickly to influences that accrue over long periods (Dimock and Black, 1969). In eastern Oregon, grazing on a ponderosa pine–grass plantation by elk, deer, elk and deer, and cattle neither harmed nor benefited growth and survival of the trees (Edgerton, 1971). Properly managed domestic animals do little harm to conifer reproduction.

MANAGEMENT PROBLEMS WITH MIXED SPECIES

Seasonal Restrictions Related to Kind of Animal

If a breeding herd of one species, say sheep, obtains efficient use of range during the winter season, the rancher must provide sheep feed during spring, summer, and fall also. He may be obliged to graze sheep during the summer months on coarse grass or other ranges that are better suited to cattle. If he changes to cattle, his summer range may be more efficiently used than is the winter range, but he gains little. Usually, developing appropriate yearround feeds is preferable to combining species of animals in situations of widely different seasonal restrictions or efficient range use.

Grazing influences in one season carry over to grazing by other animals at a different time. This fact was illustrated by a situation in the Blue Mountains of Oregon. Cattle used the range from June 15 to October 15; mule deer, for 8 or 9 months in spring, summer, and fall; and elk, in spring (May–June) and early winter (November–January). Cattle influenced elk more than deer (Fig. 9-7) because there is a greater overlap of selected foods between cattle and elk than between cattle and deer. Moderate cattle grazing affected deer use minimally but discouraged elk use. Sustained maximum use by the three kinds of animals required light cattle and elk stocking. It mattered little that the animals were using the range at different times (Skovlin, Edgerton, and Harris, 1968).

In mountainous regions where deer migrate, their winter range at low altitudes coincides with spring and fall livestock ranges. Either species can overgraze the range, but usually damage results from one or the other. Since parts of the winter deer range may be owned privately, and the deer are public property, many controversies arise over the causes of and solutions to overuse. As food habits, behavioral characteristics of animals, and responses of vegetation to different influences become better known, these seasonal uses by different animals can be made to complement each other.

Diseases and Parasites

Deer and sheep in northwestern California are known to have at least 45 species of internal and external parasites of which 21 occur in both host animals (Longhurst et al., 1954). This large number of parasitic species suggests that either deer or sheep may harbor parasites that do little damage to themselves but great damage to the other species. However, less than half a dozen species cause major damage to either host. Physiological differences seem to restrict or even prevent actual transfer of several gastrointestinal nematodes from one host species to the other (Baker et al., 1957).

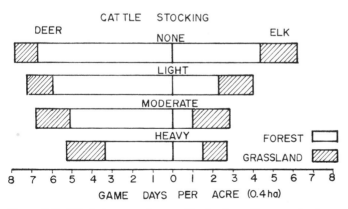

Figure 9-7 Effect of summer forage utilization by cattle on use by deer and elk grazing during different seasons *(Skovlin et al., 1968).*

Brucellosis, or contagious abortion, may be one of the more troublesome diseases that appear when wild and domestic species graze together. This disease occurs in wildebeest, zebra, giraffe, hartebeest, and eland in Africa; and in bison and elk in North America. Neither the seriousness of the disease to each wild species nor its transferability to other species, including domestic animals, is well known. For example, the bison herd in Yellowstone Park has brucellosis (Tunnicliff and Marsh, 1935), but the herd almost never contacts domestic animals because fall and spring migration patterns keep the bison away from livestock. Other bacterial diseases common to wild and domestic animals include hemorrhagic septicemia, tuberculosis, and tularemia.

Anaplasmosis, a widespread protozoan parasite of red blood cells, occurs in cattle and deer in warm climates of the United States (Stiles, 1942). Under natural conditions, external parasites, mainly ticks, transfer it from infected or carrier animals to healthy ones. Deer, at least the Columbian black-tailed, constitute a reservoir of this disease. Values of deer for hunting and viewing preclude reductions to achieve anaplasmosis control, especially since the danger of transferring the disease to cattle cannot be assessed with accuracy.

Four viral diseases of game and domestic animals in East Africa are very relevent to the proposals for ranching mixtures of species (Plowright, 1968). Rinderpest, more or less continuously present in the tropics and subtropics, potentially is the greatest killer of cloven-hoofed animals. Domestic animals can be immunized against rinderpest, but in wild animals the disease remains uncontrolled. Quarantines against the widespread and widely feared foot-and-mouth disease prevent imports of uncooked meats and other animal products from entering many countries. Signs of these two viral diseases appear in a wide spectrum of domestic and wild species.

Two other viral diseases, African swine fever in the giant forest hog, bush pig, and wart hog and malignant catarrhal fever in the wildebeest, cause no visible symptoms in those animals. However, domestic pigs and cattle are highly susceptible, having mortality rates as high as 95 percent. Transfer of the viruses from wild to domestic animals can be prevented through isolation of the domestic from the wild species.

Trypanosomiasis control in Africa illustrates the complicated nature of disease problems on extensive rangeland. Techniques of control have included removal of the game reservoir; removal of man until the infecting trypanosomes disappeared; removal of tsetse flies through trapping, insecticides, and habitat manipulations; and treatment of infected animals. Slaughter of some 60,000 game animals in the Ankole District of Uganda made cattle raising possible there. However, the disease persisted because of natural game increase, and continued slaughter was required. Some tsetse fly species were not completely dependent on game, and others changed their feeding habits as host populations changed

(Glover, 1967). Expensive fly habitat controls that alter vegetation need continuous maintenance. With the advent of immunizing drugs, the use of all other controls gradually has diminished.

Changing from sheep to cattle may eliminate problems of foot rot, certain ticks, and blow flies. Since Indian cattle are more resistant to tropical parasites and diseases than are temperate breeds, much effort in the tropics aims at establishing hardier breeds with combinations of various *Bos indicus* blood lines. Sheep and goats are less likely than cattle to contract trypanosomiasis. While the presence of disease in any animal or species is potentially dangerous and must be of concern to game and livestock managers alike, evidence suggests that the threat of transfer of most diseases between domestic and wild animals is not great. It has become less prevalent since the advent of vaccines such as those for trypanosomiasis, brucellosis, and rinderpest, and effective tick control. Management of mixed species requires continuous attention to disease problems.

Poaching

Managed production of any animal always is subject to thievery, whether the situation is one of snaring of a wild animal in violation of game laws, cattle rustling, or taking of a pet in a metropolitan area. Both wild and domestic animals remain tempting and frequent targets for poachers, who take animals for their own food, for profit, for spite, and for sport. Poaching seriously restricts the management of wild species for two reasons. Because the number of poached animals is unknown, poaching prevents determination of population sizes, increase rates, and harvestable off-takes. Also, poaching loss decreases profit by increasing costs and decreasing returns. Preservation of diminishing species, game ranching, and cropping of wild animals require prevention of poaching.

Predation

Predation on grazing animals is a part of the natural system, whether the predator is a man or an animal of the range. For man to profit most from his husbandry, he must eliminate or reduce his competition, the other predators. Predatory species on rangeland are subject to elimination through diminishing habitat, less prey, and direct human efforts. Species differ in their ability to meet these increasing pressures. The coyote, for example, does well in close proximity to population centers, but the wolf and the grizzly bear have been eliminated from most of North America. Lion and cheetah in Africa appear more vulnerable than are leopard, hyena, and jackal.

General attitudes toward predators resemble those toward game: these animals are to be preserved in parks and reserves, to be eliminated in game ranching, and to be taken, at least as trophies, along with their prey in game-cropping situations.

Intensive livestock-game programs cannot tolerate much loss to predators. However, livestock raisers have been prone to condemn all predators when only a few individuals prey on their livestock. Most predators feed on competing foragers such as rabbits, rodents, and other native animals. A predator-control program should concentrate on the troublesome individuals rather than on a species as a whole (Leopold et al., 1964). Coyote control in cattle country is seldom needed, and, if trouble develops, it is likely to be with one or a few individuals. Sheep, are much more susceptible than are cattle to predation by coyotes. Government and conservationist support for selected control in problem situations could maintain both predatory species and profitable husbandry.

The domestic dog is one of the most troublesome predators on livestock. Many people in the world make little effort to control their dogs, with the result that some become hunters. One grazing experiment in Israel which used sheep in small flocks also had dogs in one or more of the adjacent ungrazed pastures. These animals, known as *anti-dog dogs,* were trained to bark as a warning to the herdsman when other dogs approached (Fig. 9-8).

Although expensive, fencing against hyenas and predators of the dog family provides effective long-term control. Predator fences must be buried in the ground

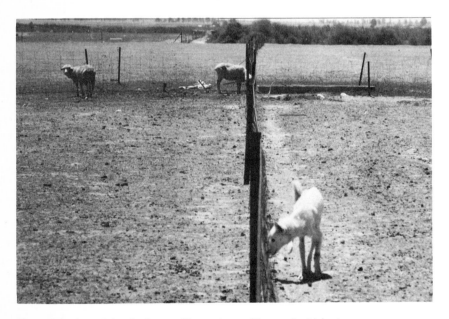

Figure 9-8 An anti-dog dog in one of the pastures of the grazing trials at Migda, Israel. This animal barks when strange dogs approach.

and carefully maintained, but need not be stronger than fences to keep out deer and rabbits. Fences against cats must be higher than those for dogs and must have a device to prevent climbing. Australia has a number of barrier fences to protect sheep from dingo predation and to prevent emus from grazing range forage and planted crops. The longest of these "dog" fences is some 8,500 kilometers. It is located in the states of South Australia, New South Wales, and Queensland. This fence forms a major boundary between areas used for cattle and sheep (McKnight, 1970).

A fencing program to exclude predators often inadvertently includes a number of them, especially nocturnal species such as coyotes, jackals, and hyenas, within the enclosure. Quick elimination of enclosed predators prevents large losses. Enclosed prey species become highly vulnerable because fences restrict their movements. For example, 2 of 15 tsessebe calves were lost to jackals the first year in fenced pastures at Percy Fyfe in South Africa. Jackals and hyenas killed several fully grown Thomson's gazelle in the beginning of fenced experiments in Kenya. Survival of blesbok young near Pretoria, South Africa, increased from 37 to 85 percent when black-backed jackals were removed from their pastures (du Plessis, 1970).

Observations of predator behavior and analysis of recorded kills by predators in Kruger Park, South Africa, suggest that populations of predators are controlled by intraspecific densities that affect reproductive rates and survival of young (Pienaar, 1969). Other controlling factors include cannibalism, floods, fires, army ants, diseases, injuries inflicted by the prey, and parasites, much the same factors that control numbers of prey animals.

The need for a program to cull herbivorous animals in Kruger and other parks indicates that predators alone cannot maintain a balance between the prey species and their habitat. Much predation has little depressing influence on the prey populations, since losses from different causes tend to compensate each other and to increase reproductive rates. In parks and game reserves, the herbivores are more likely to reach overpopulation levels than are the carnivores. Except for elimination of troublesome individuals, carnivore control should be avoided.

Noxious Plants

If rangeland is properly maintained in excellent condition, losses from poisonous plants can be effectively reduced. Most animals avoid noxious species and seldom graze them if palatable species abound. However, this is not always true. Potential trouble for cattle always exists where poisonous varieties of *Delphinium* occur, but sheep can safely graze there. In contrast, sheep are more susceptible than are cattle to *Zygadenus* and to *Lupinus*.

Mechanically injurious plants cause shifts in animal species grazing certain ranges. *Erodium* seed in California foul the wool and burrow through the skin of sheep. *Heteropogon contortus* and species of *Stipa* are especially bad in this respect. Large increases in *Heteropogon* following thinning of *Eucalyptus* forests in east central Queensland, Australia, forced many ranchers to change from sheep to cattle. Noxious plants of any type which have properties more damaging to one kind of animal than to another determine, or at least influence, the mix of species.

Topography

Sheep and goats normally do better than cattle on steep slopes and stony areas. Cattle will graze among rocks, as has been shown in northern Israel. However, given free choice, cattle spend most of their time on the flattest land available to them, rapidly crossing the steep land between preferred level areas. With unherded grazing, patterns of range use depend upon the willingness of animals to graze the land evenly and not upon their ability to do so.

Steepness and roughness of slope appear to have little direct effect on mule deer distribution, but steep slopes may be little used because they produce unsuitable forage (Julander, 1966). Many wild animals show preference for specific topographic situations, as the moose for marshy or wet areas and the klipspringer for rocky locations. Regardless of what causes these location preferences, they offer opportunities for efficient mixing of animal species to achieve favorable use on land with varied topography.

MAN AS A DIRECT USER OF RANGELAND

Man's increasing direct use of rangeland for recreational services such as hunting, fishing, camping, snow sports, motorcycle events, and shooting clubs give rangelands new values. The manager can make these activities profitable through land development and the collection of fees or sale of use privileges. Hunting rights and campground rentals are notable examples of leased services. One ranch in California charges trail riders to help move a cattle herd between the ranch and summer range. Fees provide for profit and expenses such as insurance, horses, riding equipment, food, and camp cooking facilities. The rider receives a week's outing that has much western historical flavor to it. The recreational pursuits finally picked for development survive the same selective and competitive processes as do other land developments and uses.

Management for recreational use in principle resembles management of rangeland for grazing animals. Problems and destruction of resources by man result from the presence of too many people on the land, from their poor distribution, from their presence in the wrong season of the year, and from wrong kinds of recreational use of the site (Fig. 9-9). These are the main problems with domestic and game animals on ranges. Although techniques of controlling recreationists and grazing animals differ, management of both gives attention to numbers, distribution, season of use, and kind of use.

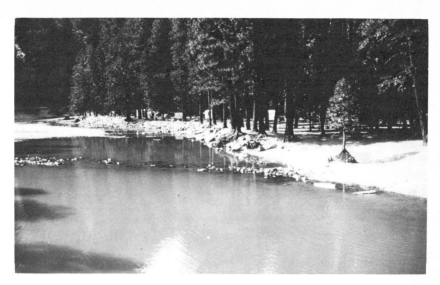

Figure 9-9   The presence of too many people along the Merced River in Yosemite National Park destroyed the stream-bank vegetation, permitting severe erosion.

ECONOMIC FACTORS

Cost often prevents a manager from changing animal species and adding new types of operations to his long-established productive system. The costs of change include the risk of loss in selling one species and purchasing another and in the capital changes in equipment and facilities. The latter do not add to capital values if they replace undepreciated facilities.

Among the economic considerations of producing a mixture of animal species are several different kinds of decisions. One presumes that the manager has a limited amount of money to spend on development. He needs to spend that money on the animal or practice that will be most effective. He must choose the best combination of practices and apply them at optimum intensity.

PERSONAL FACTORS

Managers give personal preference as a major reason for their particular mix of animals. Cattlemen and sheepmen normally remain in the same business as long as they stay on the same ranch. They may have been trained at a university, by family tradition, or by their own experience to manage one species. Whatever their backgrounds, they often do not have confidence with a second kind of animal or even a second type of animal within the same species.

Groups of people or communities commonly select the same species. While this choice seldom results from a vote, neighbors do influence each other's decisions. They find that problems of transportation, marketing, and health diminish when faced on a community basis. The manager of a minority animal can be at a competitive disadvantage within his locality. Simply, a man may like one kind of animal better than another and be satisfied with it alone, so foregoes profits that could be produced by changing or mixing animals.

LITERATURE CITED

Agnew, A. D. Q. 1968. Observations on the changing vegetation of Tsavo National Park (East). *E. Afr. Wildl. J.* 6:75–80.

Arnold, D. A., and L. J. Verme. 1963. Ten year's observation of an enclosed deer herd in northern Michigan. *Trans. N. Am. Wildl. and Nat. Res. Conf.* 28:422–430.

Baker, N. F., W. M. Longhurst, and J. R. Douglas. 1957. Experimental transmission of gastrointestinal nematodes between domestic sheep and Columbian black-tailed deer. *Trans. N. Am. Wildl. Res. Conf.* 22:160–168.

Bannikov, A. G., L. V. Zhirnov, L. S. Lebedeva, and A. A. Fandeev. 1961. *Biology of the Saiga.* Translated from Russian. U.S. Department of the Interior and National Science Foundation.

Blair, W. F., A. P. Blair, P. Brodkorb, F. R. Cagle, and G. A. Moore. 1968. *Vertebrates of the United States.* New York: McGraw-Hill.

Bump, G. 1968. Exotics and the role of the State-Federal Foreign Game Investigation Program. In *Symposium: Introduction of exotic animals,* Texas A. & M. Univ., pp. 5–8.

Chase, W. W., and D. H. Jenkins. 1962. Productivity of the George Reserve deer herd. *Proceedings of the 1st National White-tailed Deer Disease Symposium,* Univ. of Georgia, Athens, pp. 78–88.

Child, G., P. Smith, and W. von Richter. 1970. Tsetse control hunting as a measure of large mammal population trends in the Okavango Delta, Botswana. *Mammalia* 35:34–75.

Cook, C. W. 1954. Common use of summer range by sheep and cattle. *J. Range Mgmt.* 7:10–13.

Craighead, F. C., Jr., and R. F. Dasmann. 1966. *Exotic game on public lands.* U.S. Dept. Int., Bur. Land Mgmt.

Crouch, G. L. 1969. Animal damage to conifers on national forests in the Pacific Northwest region. *U.S. Dept. Agr. Forest Service Resource Bull.* PNW-28.

Dasmann, R. F., and A. S. Mossman. 1961. Commercial utilization of game animals on a Rhodesian ranch. *Annual meeting, The Wildlife Society, California Section, Davis, Calif.*

Dimock, E. J., II, and H. C. Black. 1969. Scope and economic aspects of animal damage in California, Oregon, and Washington. *Symposium Proceedings on Wildlife and Reforestation in the Pacific Northwest,* Ore. State Univ., pp. 10–14.

Dorn, R. D. 1970. Moose and cattle food habits in southwest Montana. *J. Wildl. Mgmt.* 34:559–564.

du Plessis, S. S. 1970. Predation by black-backed jackals on newborn blesbok lambs. *Trans. N. Am. Wildl. and Nat. Res. Conf.* 35:85–92.

Edgerton, P. J. 1971. The effect of cattle and big game grazing on a ponderosa pine plantation. *U.S. Dept. Agr. Forest Service Research Note* PNW-172.

Flock, D. R. 1964. Range relationships of some ungulates native to Banff and Jasper National Parks, Alberta. In *Grazing in terrestrial and marine environments,* ed. D. J. Crisp, pp. 119–128. Oxford: Blackwell.

Fosbrooke, H. A. 1968. Elephants in the Serengeti National Park: An early record. *E. Afr. Wildl. J.* 6:150–152.

Glover, P. E. 1967. The importance of ecological studies in the control of tsetse flies. *World Health Org. Bull.* 37:581–614.

Goddard, J. 1970. Age criteria and vital statistics of a black rhinoceros population. *E. Afr. Wildl. J.* 8:105–121.

Julander, O. 1966. How mule deer use mountain rangeland in Utah. *Utah Acad. Sci., Arts, and Letters* 43(2)/22–28.

Klebenow, D. A. 1965. A montane forest winter deer habitat in western Montana. *J. Wildl. Mgmt.* 29:27–33.

Kleiber, M. 1961. *The fire of life: An introduction to animal energetics.* New York: Wiley.

Labuschagne, R. J., and N. J. van der Merwe. 1968. *Mammals of the Kruger and other national parks.* Pretoria, South Africa: National Parks Board.

Lamprey, H. F. 1963. Ecological separation of the large mammal species in the Tarangire Game Reserve, Tanganyika. *E. Afr. Wildl. J.* 1:63–92.

———, P. E. Glover, M. I. M. Turner, and R. H. V. Bell. 1967. Invasion of the Serengeti National Park by elephants. *E. Afr. Wildl. J.* 5:151–166.

Laws, R. M. 1968. Interactions between elephant and hippopotamus populations and their environment. *E. Afr. Agr. For. J.* 33 (special issue): 140–147.

———, and I. S. C. Parker. 1968. Recent studies of elephant populations in East Africa. *Symp. Zool. Soc. Lon.* 21:319–359.

Leopold, A. S., S. A. Cain, C. M. Cottam, I. N. Gabrielson, and T. L. Kimball. 1963. Study of wildlife problems in national parks. *Trans. N. Am. Wildl. and Nat. Res. Conf.* 28:28–45.

———, ———, ———, ———, and ———. 1964. Predator and rodent control in the United States. *Trans. N. Am. Wildl. and Nat. Res. Conf.* 29:27–49.

Longhurst, W. M., J. R. Douglas, and N. F. Baker. 1954. Parasites of sheep and deer. *Calif. Agr.* 8(7):5–6.

Lovemore, D. F. 1963. The effects of anti-tsetse shooting operations on the game populations as observed in the Sebungwe District, Southern Rhodesia. In Conservation of nature and natural resources in modern African states. *I.U.C.N. Pub. New Series* 1:232–234.

Mackie, R. J. 1970. Range ecology and relations of mule deer, elk and cattle in the Missouri River Breaks, Montana. *Wildl. Monog.* 20:1–79.

Maynard, L. A., and J. K. Loosli. 1969. *Animal nutrition,* 6th ed. New York: McGraw-Hill.

McKnight, T. L. 1958. The feral burro in the United States: Distribution and problems. *J. Wildl. Mgmt.* 22:163–179.

———. 1970. Biotic influence on Australian pastoral land use. *Yearbook: Assoc. of Pac. Coast Geog.* 32:7–22.

Mentis, M. T. 1970. Estimates of natural biomasses of large herbivores in the Umfolozi Game Reserve area. *Mammalia* 34:363–393.

Merrill, L. B., and J. E. Miller. 1961. Economic analysis of year-long grazing rate studies on Substation No. 14, near Sonora. *Texas Agr. Expt. Sta.* MP-484.

Mueggler, W. F. 1967. Trees, shrubs and elk. *Idaho Wildl. Rev.* Jan.-Feb.: 12–13.

Napier Bax, P., and D. L. W. Sheldrick. 1963. Some preliminary observations on the food of elephant in the Tsavo Royal National Park (East) of Kenya. *E. Afr. Wildl. J.* 1:40–53.

Nellis, C. H. 1968. Productivity of mule deer on the National Bison Range, Montana. *J. Wildl. Mgmt.* 32:344–349.

Pienaar, U. de V. 1969. Predator-prey relationship amongst the larger mammals of the Kruger National Park. *Koedoe* 12:103–176.

———, P. van Wyk, and N. Fairall. 1966. An aerial census of elephant and buffalo in the Kruger National Park, and the implications thereof on intended management schemes. *Koedoe* 9:40–107.

Plowright, W. 1968. Inter-relationships between virus infections of game and domestic animals. *E. Afr. Agr. For. J.* 33 (special issue): 260–263.

Presnall, C. C. 1958. The present status of exotic mammals in the United States. *J. Wildl. Mgmt.* 22:45–50.

Ramsey, C. W. ca 1969. Texotics. *Texas Parks and Wildl. Dept. Bull.* 49.

Reynolds, H. G. 1969. Improvement of deer habitat on southwestern forest lands. *J. For.* 67:803–805.

———, W. P. Clary, and P. F. Ffolliott. 1970. Gambel oak for southwestern wildlife. *J. For.* 68:545–547.

Riney, T., and W. L. Kettlitz. 1964. Management of large mammals in the Transvaal. *Mammalia* 28:189–248.

Savidge, J. M. 1968. Elephants in the Ruaha National Park, Tanzania—Management problem. *E. Afr. Agr. For. J.* 33 (special issue): 191–196.

Skovlin, J. M., P. J. Edgerton, and R. W. Harris. 1968. The influence of cattle management on deer and elk. *Trans. N. Am. Wildl. and Nat. Res. Conf.* 33:169–181.

Stiles, G. W. 1942. Anaplasmosis: A disease of cattle. In *U. S. Dept. Agr. Yearbook,* pp. 579–587.

Talbot, L. M. 1966. Wild animals as a source of food. *Bur. Sport Fisheries and Wildl. Special Sci. Rep.—Wildlife* No. 98.

Teer, J. G., and N. K. Forrest. 1968. Bionomic and ethical implications of commercial game harvest programs. *Trans. N. Am. Wildl. and Nat. Res. Conf.* 33:192–204.

Tunnicliff, E. A., and H. Marsh. 1935. Bang's disease in bison and elk in the Yellowstone National Park and on the National Bison Range. *Am. Vet. Med. Assoc. J.* 86:745–752.

U.S. Forest Service. 1970. *Research progress, 1969.* Berkeley, Calif.: Pacific Southwest Forest and Range Expt. Sta.

van Wyk, P., and N. Fairall. 1969. The influence of the African elephant on the vegetation of the Kruger National Park. *Koedoe* 12:57–89.

Watson, R. M., A. D. Graham, and I. S. C. Parker. 1969. A census of the large mammals of Loliondo controlled area, northern Tanzania. *E. Afr. Wildl. J.* 7:43–59.

West, O. 1972. The ecological impact of the introduction of domestic cattle into wild life and tsetse areas of Rhodesia. In *The careless technology,* eds. M. T. Farvar and J. P. Milton, pp. 712–725. Garden City, N.Y.: The Natural History Press.

Williams, J. G. 1967. *A field guide to the national parks of East Africa.* London: Collins.

Wilson, V. J., and H. H. Roth. 1967. The effects of tsetse control operations on common duiker in eastern Zambia. *E. Afr. Wildl. J.* 5:53–63.

Wing, L. D., and I. O. Buss. 1970. Elephants and forests. *Wildl. Monog.* 19:1–92.

Wodzicki, K. A. 1950. Introduced mammals of New Zealand. *N. Z. Dept. Sci. and Ind. Res. Bull.* 98.

Chapter 10

Animal Distribution

The ideal distribution of animals extends their area of proper utilization over as large a range area as possible. This ideal requires reducing the sizes of places where animals congregate and the numbers that congregate; the animals must be spread to seldom-grazed areas. Judicious fencing, watering, salting, riding, or herding; one-night bed-grounds for sheep; vegetational manipulations; and other practices aid in improving distribution. Failure to account for uneven distribution of grazing pressure results in considerable range damage (Phinney, 1950). Correct livestock numbers on a range do not ensure correct utilization of forage.

In the development of new country for grazing purposes and in the initial steps of establishing a range program, stock-watering facilities usually receive first attention. During the free-range era in the western United States, control of water signified control of the land. Available water determined grazing capacity.

Fencing was the next range facility to become common; at first, the purpose of fences was to prohibit abusive trespass and later, it was to attain even forage utilization. Other grazing-management practices, such as specialized grazing systems, prescribed burning, fertilization, and seeding, require control of livestock movements to be effective. Division of large range units into small ones and increased water usually increase grazing capacity and have value in themselves without seasonal grazing plans, brush control, etc.

Faulty livestock distribution caused much rangeland abuse during the latter half of the last century and early part of the 1900s. Early recommendations and requirements for improved range management on national forests included many suggestions for improved livestock distribution (Jardine and Anderson, 1919; Chapline and Talbot, 1926; Talbot, 1926). These recommendations need to be continuously updated and applied to all rangelands (Williams, 1954; Skovlin, 1965).

FACTORS INFLUENCING ANIMAL DISTRIBUTION

Geographical locations of climates, vegetational types, soils, and slopes influence animals distribution and management. Informed management requires knowledge of the location of resources and of the uses made of them. Grazing animals distribute themselves unevenly over the land. Their physical impacts, selection of foods, and intensity of eating often result in irregular patterns of use.

Vegetational Types

All animal species prefer certain vegetational types to others. For example, domestic animals normally stay away from dense timber, except for shade. Although forage quantities within a timber stand may be small, proper use of it may not be attained. Arnold (1950) found that regrowth of trees in a mosaic with grassland after logging and fire reduced the area available for grazing. Patches of thick trees restricted livestock movement, making uniform grazing difficult to attain. Mule deer in northern Montana consistently used the bunchgrass type more than any other in spring, willow-meadow vegetation in the summer, and alfalfa in winter. White-tailed deer in the same area used woody deciduous vegetation and alfalfa more than did mule deer (Martinka, 1968). In another study in Utah, cattle, deer, and elk on summer range all used aspen and mixed shrub types. However, cattle continuously grazed the grass-forb types, elk used them in midsummer, and deer used them hardly at all (Julander and Jeffery, 1964). Clearly, the distribution of animals correlates with vegetational type. Reference is made to Chapter 9 for additional dicussion of this subject.

Topography

The steepness and length of slope influence the use of forage by domestic animals. In 1944, Glendening reported forage utilization of 80 percent on *Muhlenbergia montana* at the bottom of 20 percent slopes and zero use 1.6 kilometers away. Those slopes greater than 40 percent had little value for cattle grazing. Mueggler (1965) found that as an average on 38 bunchgrass areas in southern Idaho, 75 percent utilization was attained 32 meters above the foot of 60 percent slopes, while the same utilization occurred 740 meters above the foot of 10 percent slopes (Fig. 10-1).

Steepness of slope significantly influences distribution of cattle, but this factor does not operate alone. Water usually occurs at the bottom of slopes, causing animals to congregate there. Plants near the streams stay green and palatable for a longer time than do those on slopes, especially those facing the sun. Mueggler (1965) recognized these complicating factors. Cook (1966) found significant correlations between herbage utilization and percentage of slope, distance to water, percentage of palatable plants, thickness of brush, position of salt, and others. No single factor accurately measured the influence of slope, and all 21 factors studied by Cook (1966) accounted for only 55 percent of the variability in results.

Different species of animals prefer different positions on the topography. In Utah the greatest summer deer use occurred on slopes between 30 and 40 percent and on major ridgetops; elk selected slopes less than 30 percent and cattle mostly used slopes of less than 10 percent (Julander and Jeffery, 1964).

Animal Behavior

Animal behavior influences distributional patterns. Sheep graze into the wind, causing concentration and overuse in the southeastern corners of pastures near Broken Hill, Australia, where wind prevails from the southeast. When disturbed, as when being corralled, blesbok of South Africa run uphill, so the mustering point

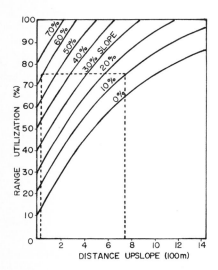

Figure 10-1 Influence of slope steepness and distance upslope on use of range by cattle *(Mueggler, 1965)*.

of their pastures should be at the highest place. Rambouillet traveled farther than did Targhee sheep when unherded on mountainous summer range (Bowns, 1971). Santa Gertrudis cattle walk farther than Herefords, resulting in even use of a large area (Herbel et al., 1967). Many studies, illustrated by Doran (1943), have shown that animals travel farther on poor than on good range. To improve range condition by any means alters animal behavior, just as the reverse is true. Solutions to distributional problems must consider the habits of the animals being managed.

After several generations, hill sheep in Scotland were found to gather in subflocks or family groups that were restricted to certain parts of the pasture. This segregation resulted in some groups being heavier than others and furnishing most of the replacement ewe lambs (Hunter, 1964). The home ranges seemed to be related to soil and vegetational types, but crowding intensified peck orders that forced some animals to establish new groups. The location of improvements altered established patterns of animal behavior. Failure by the manager to consider animal habits reduces the effectiveness of range improvements and results in overuse near points of animal concentration.

CONSEQUENCES OF FAULTY ANIMAL DISTRIBUTION

Animal concentrations near water, near shade, near salt, and on relatively level areas within steep topography destroy vegetation. A permanent water source, such as a spring or well, serves as a focal point for grazing animals. They trail to and from water and repeatedly graze along the way. Lange (1969) showed that the concentration of their grazing varied as the square of the distance from water. Sheep trails between 1,600 and 3,200 kilometers long radiated from water in the center of 260-hectare area. Populations of *Atriplex* increased in density as distance increased from water (Barker and Lange, 1970).

Measurements of forage utilization in several vegetational types illustrate the effects of animal concentrations. In eastern Montana, percentage utilization of *Agropyron smithii* on cattle winter range was 100 percent at water, 54 percent 180 meters away, and 28 percent 1,460 meters away. In the same study at the same distances from water, cattle used *Bouteloua gracilis* 100, 38, and 19 percent, respectively (Holscher and Woolfolk, 1953). Cattle used 100 percent of the bunchgrasses at water, 78 percent 180 meters away and 32 percent 900 meters away in a southern Idaho study (Mueggler, 1965). Semidesert grassland in southern New Mexico showed an average of 50 percent use within 0.8 kilometer of water but only 12 percent use between 3.2 and 4 kilometers distant (Valentine, 1947). Use of *Festuca arizonica* and *Muhlenbergia montana* in Arizona decreased to zero at 5.6 to 8 kilometers from water and 0.4 to 0.8 kilometer from established trails (Glendening, 1944). With heavy camel grazing in Saudi Arabia, no perennial vegetation occurred within 15 to 20 kilometers of water and occasionally the distance was over 50 kilometers (Heady, 1963). Agnew (1966) suggested that the proportion of land in animal trails indicates the degree of grazing.

Development of water without control of livestock results in range destruction. This range improvement and others that tend to concentrate animals require careful livestock management and can be advantageous only in conjection with control of animal numbers, seasonal grazing, and other aspects of a total range program.

PRACTICES TO LESSEN ANIMAL CONCENTRATIONS

Range management includes many practices to spread animals in accord with the herbage resources. Several practices such as development of water, construction of fences, and building of roads, trails, and windbreaks, are considered range improvements. Others, including herding, spreading of salt, and vegetational practices, directly influence animal distribution. In the following sections, each of these practices will be discussed as to its location and effectiveness. Specifications for construction are not included because they are readily available in several field manuals used by federal government agencies. However, a few of the newer developments in construction will be described in detail.

Development of Water

Water for livestock and game has been developed with dams, man-made ponds or tanks, wells, opening of springs, pipelines, troughs, metal tanks, and guzzlers with sealed runoff aprons. The water has to be found, stored, and delivered in adequate amounts at the right times and places (Fig. 10-2). The problems of discovery, storage, and delivery of range water have been present for centuries; only the means of dealing with them have changed.

Wherever practicable, new water facilities should be located where grazing has been lightest and where grazing capacities are high. Barnes (1914) recommended that cattle not be forced to go more than 3.2 kilometers to water in relatively flat country and 1.6 kilometers in rough topography. Hamilton and Jepson (1940) stated the need for water on each 800 to 1,200 hectares. Talbot (1926) suggested slightly longer distances between watering points, but Goebel (1956) claimed that 0.8 to 1.2 kilometers is ideal. No place on the Starkey Experimental Range in eastern Oregon exceeds that distance from water. Between 1949 and 1953, the number of watering places on the Range was increased from 9 to 52. In planning for that development, it took several years to coordinate water with cattle behavior. Water was used to attract cattle to little used forage resources, to divide large herds into smaller ones, and to reduce trailing. No more than 50 animal units per watering facility is a commonly used rule of thumb. Matching requirements with site feasibility for reservoir development takes close study of animal movements, soil, topography, and geology.

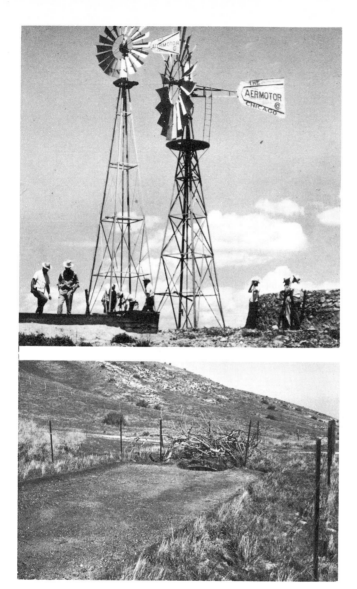

Figure 10-2 Upper photo: The large windmill pumps water from a deep well and the smaller one lifts it to a storage tank from which gravity flow supplies several watering points. Lower photo: A guzzler for quail is shown with its protective fence and brush covering the water.

Herded sheep can make even use of rangeland with water at greater distances than the maximum distance for cattle (Jardine and Anderson, 1919). Where sheep are pastured without herding, as in Australia and parts of the United States, they need water as close as cattle do if efficient range use is to be attained. Lange (1969) claimed that number of animals on a watering point has more importance in proper management than does number of points per pasture.

Discovery of water depends on interpretation of the geology. Dug wells have served the Bedouins of Arabia for many centuries and were an early form of water development on rangeland. These wells are limited to relatively shallow water tables. Drilled wells and windmills facilitated livestock expansion into many semiarid and arid parts of the world. Welchert and Freeman (1973) reported the use of horizontal wells to tap seepages and small flows of water on the San Carlos Apache Indian Reservation. A liter flow per minute was enough for a single water point, and 20 to 25 liters per minute supported storage and pipeline development for several troughs. The wells were cased and capped for water control because most flowed by gravity. Advantages of horizontal wells include storage of water in the soil with a minimum of loss, sanitary water, usually low-cost development since the wells are shallow, and high success rate. Larger, naturally flowing springs have similar advantages when they are boxed and fenced and the water is piped to troughs (Hendricks, 1938).

Storage of water in open dirt tanks has developed into a pond hydrology with specifications for construction under varying situations of runoff, soil, geology, vegetation, land use, size, sedimentation, water quality, evaporation, and seepage (Monson, 1939; Peterson and Heath, 1963). These small stock-water structures duplicate in miniature many of the values, such as gully control, recreation, and garden irrigation, and problems such as control of streamflow, water rights regulations, and downstream values, of larger reservoirs.

Much water is lost by evaporation from open dirt tanks. In dry, hot climates, that may amount to 3 meters or more in a year. Deep reservoirs with little surface area in relation to depth reduce but do not eliminate evaporation losses. In the southwestern United States, these deep reservoirs are called *charcos*. A desilting basin above them traps the silt. Covering the water surface with a monomolecular film of alcohol reduces evaporation, but wind, which breaks the film and piles the material to the lee side of the ponds, makes it of questionable value (Waldrip, 1960). Any facility must provide sufficient water for animals after losses. Louw (1970) summarized information on minimum water requirements (in liters per 100 kilograms of body weight) among several animal species when they were subjected to temperatures of 40 °C during the day and 22 °C at night:

Hereford	6.42
Waterbuck	6.00
Eland	5.49
Wildebeest	4.81
Cape Buffalo	4.58
Grant's gazelle	3.86

Zebu cattle	3.22
Oryx	3.00
Thomson's gazelle	2.74

These data do not, in themselves, indicate need for drinking water because feeding habits and use of water in the feed differ among the species. Commonly a mature cow requires about 45 liters and sheep, between 2.2 and 4.5 liters per day, varying with location and season of the year.

Sand trapped above a dam holds water in the voids among the sand grains. In coarse sand, water space amounts to 25 to 30 percent of the volume (Sykes, 1937). Evaporation proceeds at a slow rate after the top 2 or 3 decimeters of sand have become dry. No plants of any kind should be allowed to grow on the sand because transpiration uses much water. Water in the sand tank may be obtained from a well on the upstream side or from a pipe in the bed of the dam. Desert-sand tanks have been developed and used for a century or more in the southwestern United States, Mexico, and parts of Africa. Bedouins in Arabia have dug wells into sand river beds for centuries. The African elephant is noted for his ability to dig for water in sandy river beds.

Paved or otherwise sealed drainage areas that lead to covered storage cisterns accumulate considerable water from small drainages (Humphrey and Shaw, 1957). These watering devices first became known in California as guzzlers for quail (Glading, 1943); over 2,000 were in use by 1953 (Edminster, 1954). Precipitation of 10 centimeters on a 1,000-square meter area provides 10,000 liters of water, enough for over 200 cow days. A common formula is to make the apron such a size that half the average rainfall fills the storage tank. Water for game and livestock can be provided in this way, but the installations are expensive. Efficient use of water requires a trough and float valve to control the flow, covered storage, and maintenance of the seal on the drainage apron. Frost, particularly, may be a problem.

Plastic pipe has made possible range pipeline systems for watering livestock. Commonly the system begins with a well and pump to lift the water into a storage tank located on a high point where gravity flow may be utilized. For safety purposes, the storage capacity should be at least a 7-day supply for motor-driven systems or a 14-day supply for wind systems (Patterson, 1967).

Line routing and placement of drinking facilities depend upon number of animals and topography. Troughs placed at 800-meter intervals along the line tend to spread cattle into small bunches. Troughs may be opened or closed to attain rotational grazing and to relieve heavy use near water. Martin and Ward (1970) claimed that water points must be separated by the maximum daily cattle travel distance for water to serve as a device to keep them away from certain areas.

Ingram (1930) described the hauling of water for livestock in eastern Oregon, beginning in 1918. The practice has gained in popularity in recent years. A 1.5-ton truck with two 2,275-liter tanks and space for nested troughs permits use of rangeland for distances of 20 to 30 kilometers from permanent water (Costello and Driscoll, 1957). Livestock on winter range in the Great Basin regions, of necessity, receive water in this manner when snow is not available (Hutchings, 1958). With an adequate range road system, hauling of water should be looked upon as a partial replacement for the range rider. Animals soon learn to come to water when the truck arrives. This system provides an opportunity for close inspection and accurate count of animals as well as for the placement of water in a new place each day.

Fencing

Efficient use of fences requires an initial concept of the boundaries and different use of the landscape on either side of the boundary. Well-defined property boundaries make good neighbors. Division fences are discussed here, since their value is not as widely appreciated as is that of boundary fences.

Obviously, cropland and hayland must be separated from grazing resources. Different classes of livestock require separate pastures for animal management. Fences confine animals to certain areas and exclude them from others. However, the number of pastures and locations of fences often depend upon availability of water and upon other facilities. Regulation of access to areas by animals and people requires fencing.

Fences should be located on ridges, approximately on the contour that animals tend to follow but avoiding steep slopes, and should be placed where they serve their purposes with the least upkeep. Fences will aid management if they can be placed between different range-condition classes so that high- and low-value vegetational types are separated (Skovlin, 1965). Before any fence is constructed, the need for that fence, in terms of conserving soil and added use of forage to repay the cost of the fence, should be determined. Roughly, 1.6 kilometers of new fence should add the equivalent of 1 AU in grazing capacity.

Fences that cross drainages cause concentration of animals on one side. If they must be located near water on rough cattle range, they should cross drainages at elevations below the water because cattle usually graze outward and upward (Miles, 1951). Narrow corners tend to create ungrazed areas on cattle range, but on sheep range they may be overgrazed if they point toward the prevailing wind.

Fence construction varies as much as the builders do. Electric fences have many advantages on rangeland. They can be used as temporary barriers to eroded places, new seedings, creek bottoms, stands of poisonous plants, extremely palatable forage, and new water facilities. A single wire about 1 meter above the ground holds mature cattle and permits calves to cross underneath to better feed. Electric fences cost relatively little, since posts are widely spaced and the one wire strings easily. Juniper or local woods (Meagher, 1940) may be used for fence posts in range areas and the wire placed on them for the grazing season only. This practice avoids damage by snow and reduces problems with game. An electric fence that has whitewashed posts and glitter strips on the wire and is cleared of brush has discouraged elephants in Tanzania (Vesey-Fitzgerald, 1968).

Fencing where wild animals need to be permitted full movement or prevented from entering presents special problems. Deer control requires straight, vertical fences about 2.5 to 3 meters in height. Slanting, overhanging, and outrigger types of construction, which prevent deer from approaching the fence base, discourage them from jumping (Blaisdell and Hubbard, 1956; Longhurst et al., 1962). Pronghorn antelope will not jump a fence much over 80 centimeters in height unless they are pursued or stressed. They tend to go under rather than over most fences (Spillet et al., 1967). Zobell (1968) suggested low fences, the highest possible lower wire, and narrow passes for them to go through. Mapston et al. (1970) recommended a grill (1.8 square meters) over a 35-centimeter-deep pit as a cattle guard that antelope will cross. High-tensile-strength smooth wire stretched very tight and threaded through holes in posts 50 meters apart provides a fence that gives way when hit by large game and then returns to position. The anchor posts may be as much as 800 meters apart with stays about 2 meters apart between the wires. Wires are tightened with ratchets on the anchor posts. This type of fence has been effective in holding livestock and letting wild animals pass unharmed in Kenya.

After many designs failed, a moat-type barrier was effective in preventing trespass by elephants, cape buffalo, and jumping animals from the Aberdare National Park, Kenya, onto adjacent farmland. The spoil from a 3-meter-deep trench with a 2-meter fence on top was placed on the farm side. A sloping trench bank on the park side permits animals to escape (Woodley, 1965). Covering moats reduced rainfall damage, promoted growth of mosses and creeping plants, and bluffed the game. Costs of such a barrier are high.

Fencing for seasonal grazing plans on relatively level country with high grazing capacity presents special problems because the pastures may need to be divided a second time as the plans develop. Watercourses can be blocked into small pastures on each side and larger units located toward the hills. Triangular shapes that extend from a central watering point divide more efficiently than do square pastures.

Roads and Trails

Construction of livestock trails and roads over rough, rocky areas, through dense timber, and across other barriers increases efficiency in use of rangeland. Grazing ceases away from trails in dense timber and shrub stands (Glendening, 1944). Livestock distribution in large areas of marsh and overflow land, as near the Gulf of Mexico, improves with the construction of earthen dikes for walkways (Williams, 1959) and windbreaks (Shiflet, 1963). When water covers the land, cattle graze near firm ground. The dike should be at least 2 meters at settled height and 2 meters across the top and should have slopes of 1.5:1. The barrow pit furnishes a permanent aquatic habitat for waterfowl and stock water through the dry season. Rather than always being on one side of the dike, the barrow pit should be staggered on both sides of about 100-meter intervals. Windbreaks have the same construction as do the dikes but have wings toward the lee side.

Range roads have many values for the landowner, recreationists, and wildlife. Pioneer plants and insects along the track furnish food, and the culverts become warrens for wild species. Roads, as open strips through the vegetation, are lines of sight for predators and people, fuel breaks, and escape routes (Pienaar, 1968).

Another method of distributing animals is trailing. Hockmuth and Franklin (1942) described extensive trailing of sheep and cattle between winter and summer ranges in the intermountain region. Trailing reduces weight gains in livestock, increases death loss, and causes considerable damage to vegetation and soil on the trails (Ares, 1941a). Stock routes still exist throughout the world, but their use has decreased as trucking has increased (Fig. 10-3).

Herding

Herding of cattle keeps them spread onto all parts of the range, where they use the forage evenly and according to the grazing capacity. Skovlin (1965) suggested that one rider could take care of approximately 500 head or 125 square kilometers. The rider needs to know range condition, effects of grazing, and animal habits. Cattle can be trained to use certain areas and will repeat that use year after year (Skovlin, 1957). Duties of the range rider include repairing fences, maintaining adequate water and salt, caring for sick animals, preventing death losses, keeping bulls distributed, and assuring proper forage utilization.

Herding sheep in bands of nearly 1,000 ewes plus lambs in the summer and roughly double that number in winter remains a common practice in the western United States. Even use of a range by sheep depends almost wholly upon the herder and the methods that he used. Such practices as open herding, one-night bed-grounds, and proper use of mixed timber and grass types are at the option of the herder (Fig. 10-4). The sheep should be allowed to graze in open formation, with only their direction determined. This type of grazing means little use of dogs and quiet handling so that the band will spread over the area to be grazed. Herding in this manner increases weight gains over those attained with close herding.

Bedding bands of sheep on national forest in a new place each night increased weight gains, decreased damage to bed-grounds, wasted little forage, and resulted in even forage use (Fleming, 1922). During the free-range era, bands of sheep stayed in one location every night for three or four weeks. Open herding, slow moving of the bands, and one-night bed-grounds became regulations in the use of

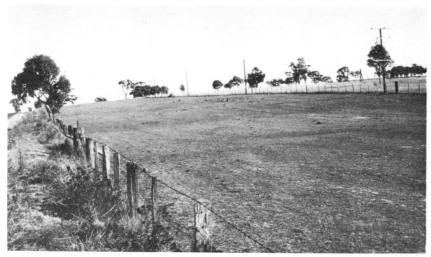

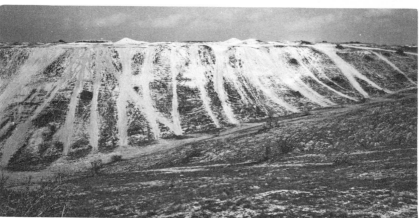

Figure 10-3 The upper photo shows a stock route between a highway and private land in Australia badly abused by trailing sheep. The lower photo shows damage by motorcycles.

national forests by sheep and were shown to be a means of range improvement (Heady et al., 1947; Pechanec and Stewart, 1949). Herding of sheep offers closer control of forage use than does herding of cattle.

On ranges where tree and meadow types of vegetation exist in a mosaic, each type of vegetation should be used in proportion to the forage produced. Usually the open areas are grazed early and late in the day and the forested areas, in late morning and again in early afternoon after the midday resting period. Thus the

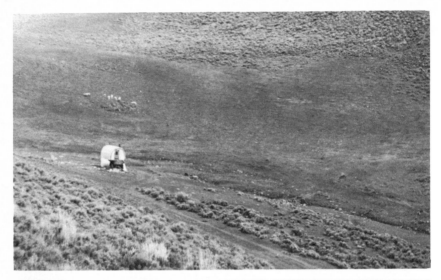

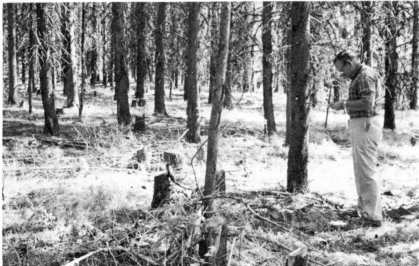

Figure 10-4 Upper photo: A severely overgrazed sheep bed-ground. Lower photo: A pine type that tends to be overgrazed in spots and undergrazed in other places.

sheep are kept in open country during the times of greatest danger from predator loss and in shade during the hottest part of the day.

In Australia, where sheep are pastured within fences and not herded, distributional problems become similar to those of cattle. Bowns (1971) found that unherded sheep damage their resting places on approaching them rather than on leaving them. Large pastures with few watering points leave many parts of the pastures essentially unused. Additional fencing and water would relieve the badly damaged areas where animals congregate for water and resting. In much of Africa, small groups of domestic animals are herded into the bush each morning and returned to a central corral at night. Village sheep and goats in Arabia follow the same pattern. Using widely spread corrals for a day or so at a time in rotation reduces trailing of animals and permits range improvement.

Light aircraft and helicopters are aids to counting, capturing, and gathering wild and domestic animals. Wildebeest, eland, and many other African animals have been herded into temporary corrals by helicopters. Aerial photos and aircraft provide means for counting deer, elk, waterfowl, etc. Numerous Australian sheepmen use light fixed-wing aircraft to find sheep in large pastures and to herd them toward the ground crew. Brushy and rough country deters quick finding and easy gathering of animals, except with the aid of aircraft.

Salting

Salting is the planned distribution of the amount of salt required by livestock for the grazing period. Cattle movement can be altered effectively by proper salting. Locations for salting should be selected so that animals are drawn away from overgrazed or heavily trampled areas. Well-placed salt grounds are reached easily by animals. Likely, these salt grounds will be on flat places, near shade, on accessible ridges, on level spots on slopes, in lightly used openings in forests, in patches of vegetation with low palatability, and in accessible corners of ranges where animals seldom graze. Common mistakes in salting include placing too much salt in one place, locating salt grounds over 1.6 kilometers apart, salting in the same location year after year, placing salt closer than 400 meters from water, and not showing animals salt at new locations (Jardine and Anderson, 1919; Chapline and Talbot, 1926). In forested areas, salt should be placed so as to attract cattle away from the meadows and onto the dry slopes. As slope and distance from water increase, more salting locations should be used (Skovlin, 1965).

Where abundant dissolved salts exist in soil, water, and vegetation, free salt may have little attractive value for animals. Ordinarily one salt ground should be established for each 30 to 40 head of cattle in flat country and for each 25 head on rough range. Enough salt should be placed in each bunker to last until proper use is attained or until ten days before animals are moved. Salt-hungry cattle readily will accept new locations at moving time.

Amounts of salt taken by animals vary between seasons and years. Woolfolk (1944) reported more consumption of salt-bonemeal mixture in the fall than in early or midsummer on short-grass ranges in eastern Montana. If precipitation were higher than normal during a particular season, salt consumption tended to increase (Houston, 1963).

Herded sheep in bands on open rangeland should be salted at or near their bed-grounds in the evening, away from overused sites near water. If this is done, the band will settle for the night and stay on the bed-ground, with less tendency to leave than when salting occurs in the morning.

Salt (20 percent) and cottonseed meal (80 percent) distributed on rangeland in self-feeders serve to maintain livestock condition as well as to improve the utilization of the forage (Fig. 10-5). Movable self-feeders, bunkers and troughs, permit flexibility in attaining an effective proper-use plan for the entire pasture. Ares (1953), after several years of study of forage use attained with different distributional patterns of a 4:1 meal-salt mixture, reported that the area of proper use increased from 32 to 59 percent of the pasture when no feeding site was closer than 800 meters from water. Feeding near water resulted in more supplement and less grass consumption than feeding away from water. Martin and Ward (1973) used a 3:1 meal-salt mixture on the Santa Rita Range Experiment Station and attained similar results. Animals consumed 900 grams per day of the mixture near water and about 200 grams per day 1.6 to 4 kilometers away from water.

Salting and watering behavior of cattle varies from having no apparent need for water after licking salt (Bentley, 1941) to going directly to water after consuming large amounts of salt in meal-salt mixtures. The necessity for placing salt near water has not been demonstrated, and salt away from water will not decrease the calf crop because animal distribution is widespread (Ares, 1941b).

Elk in northern Idaho consumed salt distributed for cattle, especially after two to three weeks on succulent spring feed. However, elk did not change their movements from winter range to summer range in response to salting that aimed to retard their trek to high elevations (Dalke et al., 1965).

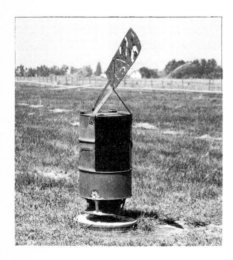

Figure 10-5 Homemade facilities often serve best. This movable salt bunker, made from a discarded oil drum and a wheel, rotates with the wind, thereby reducing blowing of rain onto the salt.

Vegetational Practices

Seeding highly palatable species away from water and less palatable ones near water has been suggested as a means of improving animal distribution (Hurd and Pearse, 1944). Suitable species and sites limit the usefulness of this scheme. However, seeding of plants with low palatability near areas of livestock concentration has value in soil conservation and range rehabilitation.

Fertilization and prescribed burning away from water may serve the same purpose as seeding. Livestock are known to be attracted to both treatments. Smith and Lang (1958) fertilized a strip 100 meters wide and 1.6 kilometers long going outward from a watering point. Forage utilization adjacent to the strip increased from 15 percent before fertilization to 55 percent afterward. Hooper et al. (1969) claimed that increased utilization and better livestock distribution are as valuable as the added forage from fertilization and that profitability comes from the combined results.

Fires in the California chaparral, in dense sagebrush, in slash after logging, and in cacti facilitate use of the land by livestock and game animals and increase forage supplies. Fires in dry grasslands and marshlands make available new green growth, which soon attracts both livestock and game to graze.

Combination of Practices

Fencing can be hardly worthwhile without assurance of adequate water. Conversely, water developments can improve the evenness of forage use without fencing. Half a dozen or more practices give numerous alternative combinations. The amount of money that can be expended for range improvements to increase livestock distribution depends upon increased production from the land. Increased grazing capacity stems from newly available range, even use, and a longer grazing season, rather than from added facilities. These practices should increase the weight of animal products, reduce labor and machinery, and decrease the nonrange feed requirements (Roberts and Wennergren, 1965). Economic evaluation of cattle distribution on mountain rangelands suggested for one location that water development, trail construction, salting, and herding were more profitable than was fencing (Workman and Hooper, 1968).

LITERATURE CITED

Agnew, A. D. Q. 1966. The use of game trails as a possible measure of habitat utilization by larger animals. *E. Afr. Wildl. J.* 4:38–46.

Ares, F. N. 1941a. Trucking versus trailing cattle from ranch to railroad. *Southwestern For. and Range Expt. Sta. Research Note* 94.

———. 1941b. Does salting away from water decrease calf crops? *Southwestern For. and Range Expt. Sta. Research Note* 95.

————. 1953. Better cattle distribution through the use of meal-salt mix. *J. Range Mgmt.* 6:341–346.

Arnold, J. F. 1950. Changes in ponderosa pine bunchgrass ranges in northern Arizona resulting from pine regeneration and grazing. *J. For.* 48:118–126.

Barker, S., and R. T. Lange. 1970. Population ecology of *Atriplex* under sheep stocking. In *The biology of* Atriplex, ed. R. Jones. Australia: CSIRO.

Barnes, W. C. 1914. Stock-watering places on western grazing lands. *U.S. Dept. Agr. Farmers' Bull.* 592.

Bentley, J. R. 1941. Automatic recording of salting and watering habits of cattle. *J. For.* 39:832–836.

Blaisdell, J. A., and R. L. Hubbard. 1956. An outrigger type deer fence. *Calif. For. and Range Expt. Sta. For. Research Note* 108.

Bowns, J. E. 1971. Sheep behavior under unherded condition on mountain summer ranges. *J. Range Mgmt.* 24:105–109.

Chapline, W. R., and M. W. Talbot. 1926. The use of salt in range management. *U.S. Dept. Agr. Cir.* 379.

Cook, C. W. 1966. Factors affecting utilization of mountain slopes by cattle. *J. Range Mgmt.* 19:200–204.

Costello, D. F., and R. S. Driscoll. 1957. Hauling water for range cattle. *U.S. Dept. Agr. Leaflet* 419.

Dalke, P. D., R. D. Beeman, F. C. Kindel, R. J. Robel, and T. R. Williams. 1965. Use of salt by elk in Idaho. *J. Wildl. Mgmt.* 29:319–332.

Doran, C. W. 1943. Activities and grazing habits of sheep on summer ranges. *J. For.* 41:253–258.

Edminster, F. C. 1954. *American game birds of field and forest.* New York: Scribner's.

Fleming, C. E. 1922. One-night camps vs. established bed-grounds on Nevada sheep ranges. *Nev. Agr. Expt. Sta. Bull.* 103.

Glading, B. 1943. A self-filling quail watering device. *Calif. Fish and Game* 29:157–164.

Glendening, G. E. 1944. Some factors affecting cattle use of northern Arizona pine-bunchgrass ranges. *Southwestern For. and Range Expt. Sta.* Report 6.

Goebel, C. J. 1956. Water development on the Starkey Experimental Forest and Range. *J. Range Mgmt.* 9:232–234.

Hamilton, C. L., and H. G. Jepson. 1940. Stockwater developments: Wells, springs, and ponds. *U.S. Dept. Agr. Farmers' Bull.* 1859.

Heady, H. F. 1963. Report to the government of Saudi Arabia on grazing resources and problems. *FAO Expanded Prog. of Tech. Assistance* No. 1614.

————, R. T. Clark, and T. Lommasson. 1947. Range management and sheep production in the Bridger Mountains, Montana. *Montana Agr. Expt. Sta. Bull.* 444.

Hendricks, B. A. 1938. The conservation of water of small seeps, springs, and earth tanks in the Southwest. *Southwestern For. and Range Expt. Sta. Research Note* 3 (revised).

Herbel, C. H., F. N. Ares, and A. B. Nelson. 1967. Grazing distribution patterns of Hereford and Santa Gertrudis cattle on a southern New Mexico range. *J. Range Mgmt.* 20:296–298.

Hockmuth, H. R., and E. R. Franklin. 1942. Sheep migration in the Intermountain Region. *U.S. Dept. Agr. Cir.* 624.

Holscher, C. E., and E. J. Woolfolk. 1953. Forage utilization by cattle on northern Great Plains ranges. *U.S. Dept. Agr. Cir.* 918.

Hooper, J. F., J. P. Workman, J. B. Grumbles, and C. W. Cook. 1969. Improved livestock distribution with fertilizer—A preliminary economic evaluation. *J. Range Mgmt.* 22:108–110.

Houston, W. R. 1963. Salt consumption by breeding cows on native range in the northern Great Plains. *J. Range Mgmt.* 16:12–16.

Humphrey, R. R., and R. J. Shaw. 1957. Paved drainage basins as a source of water for livestock or game. *J. Range Mgmt.* 10:59–62.

Hunter, R. F. 1964. Home range behaviour in hill sheep. In *Grazing in terrestrial and marine environments,* ed. D. J. Crisp, pp. 155–171. Oxford: Blackwell.

Hurd, R. M., and C. K. Pearse. 1944. Relative palatability of eight grasses used in range reseeding. *J. Am. Soc. Agron.* 36:162–165.

Hutchings, S. S. 1958. Hauling water to sheep on western ranges. *U.S. Dept. Agr. Leaflet.* 423.

Ingram, D. C. 1930. Ranges are made usable by hauling water for livestock. *U.S. Dept. Agr. Yearbook.* pp. 446–449.

Jardine, J. T., and M. Anderson. 1919. Range management on the national forests. *U.S. Dept. Agr. Bull.* 790.

Julander, O., and D. E. Jeffery. 1964. Deer, elk, and cattle range relations on summer range in Utah. *Trans N. Am. Wildl. and Nat. Res. Conf.* 29:404–414.

Lange, R. T. 1969. The piosphere: Sheep track and dung patterns. *J. Range Mgmt.* 22:396–400.

Longhurst, W. M., M. B. Jones, R. R. Parks, L. W. Neubauer, and M. W. Cummings. 1962. Fences for controlling deer damage. *Calif. Agr. Expt. Sta. Cir.* 514.

Louw, G. N. 1970. Physiological adaption as a criterion in planning production from wild ungulates. *Proc. So. Afr. Soc. Ani. Prod.* 9:53–56.

Mapston, R. D., R. S. Zobell, K. B. Winter, and W. D. Dooley. 1970. A pass for antelope in sheep-tight fences. *J. Range Mgmt.* 23:457–459.

Martin, S. C., and D. E. Ward. 1970. Rotating access to water to improve semidesert cattle range near water. *J. Range Mgmt.* 23:22–26.

———, and ———. 1973. Salt and meal-salt help distribute cattle use on semidesert range. *J. Range Mgmt.* 26:94–97.

Martinka, C. J. 1968. Habitat relationships of white-tailed and mule deer in northern Montana. *J. Wildl. Mgmt.* 32:558–565.

Meagher, G. S. 1940. Service life of untreated juniper fence posts in Arizona. *Southwestern For. and Range Expt. Sta. Research Notes* 89.

Miles, A. D. 1951. Electric fence for distribution of cattle on a range grazed by sheep and cattle. *J. Range Mgmt.* 4:228–232.

Monson, D. W. 1939. Small reservoirs for stock water and irrigation. *Mont. Agr. Expt. Sta. Cir.* 154.

Mueggler, W. F. 1965. Cattle distribution on steep slopes. *J. Range Mgmt.* 18:255–257.

Patterson, T. C. 1967. Design considerations for small pipelines for distribution of livestock water on rangelands. *J. Range Mgmt.* 20:104–107.

Pechanec, J. F., and G. Stewart. 1949. Grazing spring-fall sheep ranges of southern Idaho. *U.S. Dept. Agr. Cir.* 808.

Peterson, H. V., and V. T. Heath. 1963. Stock water facilities for the Pacific Southwest. *J. Soil and Water Cons.* 18(3):103–108.

Phinney, T. D. 1950. How grazing capacity of mountain range lands is affected by range condition and usability. *J. For.* 48:106–107.

Pienaar, U. de V. 1968. The ecological significance of roads in a national park. *Koedoe* 11:169–174.

Roberts, N. K., and E. V. Wennergren. 1965. Economic evaluation of stockwater developments. *J. Range Mgmt.* 18:118–123.

Shiflet, T. N. 1963. Earthen windbreaks, a new management device for salt marsh rangelands. *J. Range Mgmt.* 16:332–334.

Skovlin, J. M. 1957. Range riding—The key to range management. *J. Range Mgmt.* 10:269–271.

———. 1965. Improving cattle distribution on western mountain rangelands. *U.S. Dept. Agr. Farmers' Bull.* 2212.

Smith, D. R., and R. L. Lang. 1958. The effect of nitrogenous fertilizers on cattle distribution on mountain range. *J. Range Mgmt.* 11:248–249.

Spillet, J. J., J. B. Low, and D. Sill. 1967. Livestock fences—how they influence pronghorn antelope movements. *Utah Agr. Expt. Sta. Bull.* 470.

Sykes, G. G. 1937. Desert water tanks. *Southwestern For. and Range Expt. Sta. Research Note* 18.

Talbot, M. W. 1926. Range watering places in the Southwest. *U.S. Dept. Agr. Dept. Bull.* 1358.

Valentine, K. A. 1947. Distance from water as a factor in grazing capacity of rangeland. *J. For.* 45:749–754.

Vesey-Fitzgerald, D. F. 1968. An experiment in adopting an electric fence to elephant behavior. *E. Afr. Agr. For. J.* 33 (special issue): 185–190.

Waldrip, W. J. 1960. Evaluation of chemical films for retarding evaporation under field conditions. *Texas Agr. Expt. Sta. Prog. Rept.* 2158.

Welchert, W. T., and B. N. Freeman. 1973. Horizontal wells. *J. Range Mgmt.* 26:253–256.

Williams, R. E. 1954. Modern methods of getting uniform use of ranges. *J. Range Mgmt.* 7:77–81.

———. 1959. Cattle walkways: An aid to coastal marsh range conservation. *U.S. Dept. Agr. Leaflet* 459.

Woodley, R. W. 1965. Game defence barriers. *E. Afr. Wildl. J.* 3:89–94.

Woolfolk, E. J. 1944. Salt-bonemeal mixture used by breeding cows on shortgrass ranges during four summer and three winter seasons. *N. Rocky Mtn. For. and Range Expt. Sta. Research Note* 32.

Workman, J. P., and J. F. Hooper. 1968. Preliminary economic evaluation of cattle distribution practices on mountain rangelands. *J. Range Mgmt.* 21:301–304.

Zobell, R. S. 1968. Field studies of antelope movements on fenced ranges. *Trans. N. Am. Wildl. and Nat. Res. Conf.* 33:211–216.

Chapter 11

Management of Seasonal Grazing

Seasonal management implies that, whether a range is being used by livestock, by game, or even by recreationists, a portion of the range will be free of animals for a sufficient time during a particular season so that the vegetation will benefit from not being grazed, trampled, or otherwise disturbed. The reasons for moving grazing animals from one place to another are to minimize sacrifice sites, improve ranges in poor condition, maintain high-quality ranges, and achieve high animal production. To carry out the moves according to schedules of efficient rangeland use requires workable physical layouts of such facilities as fences and roads.

Jared Smith (1895) first suggested seasonal grazing plans on rangeland when he advocated rotation grazing as one means of improving range conditions in the southern Great Plains. Sampson (1913, 1914), after considerable ecological research in the Wallowa Mountains of Oregon, recommended deferred-rotation grazing as a general practice. Shortly thereafter, Jardine (1915) and Jardine and Anderson (1919) presented that schedule in diagram form and suggested it for use on national forests. Since that early beginning, recommendations for variously designed plans have been a part of most practical range management programs.

Moreover, problems in design of plans and unknown seasonal grazing effects have been the subjects of considerable research. Until the recent shift of attention toward seasonal manipulations that maximize returns from excellent condition ranges, the emphasis in both management and research was on range improvement or rehabilitation.

A rationale for seasonal grazing is that many grasslands in the world evolved under intermittent grazing pressure from migrating herbivores, for example, bison in North America and wildebeest in East Africa. These animals used a given range during a short period, perhaps overused it, then moved to a new range in a pattern that more or less repeated itself yearly. Migrations became fixed in the behavior of many species and, consequently, exerted seasonal grazing pressures to which vegetation became adapted through natural selection. Not all animals migrated in a regular pattern. Some species moved at random, and others remained in a location to graze yearlong. Seasonal grazing plans developed as land managers attempted to fit their domestic animal species into naturally evolved plant and animal systems. The belief was that range productivity could be increased and damage decreased if grazing patterns were as near as possible to those under which the vegetation evolved.

OPTIMAL GRAZING SEASON

Modifiers of the word *range,* such as *spring, spring-fall, summer, winter,* and *yearlong,* define areas that are grazed primarily during those seasons. For example, *summer range* may be in mountains at high elevations or in climates where grazing is restricted to summer. The sagebrush-grass type is frequently called *spring-fall range,* because animals use it before they are moved to summer range in the mountains and during their return to lower elevations in the fall. Some sagebrush-grass ranges are used during summer and winter. In warm climates, *wet* and *dry seasons* describe periods of range use.

Although grazing of any range vegetation seldom is completely restricted to a certain season, these range -use terms imply that an optimal grazing season exists for many range types. The idea stems from the fact that there are differential plant responses to defoliation at different seasons. However, every grazing plan that takes advantage of an optimal grazing season in one place normally includes less than ideal seasonal grazing in another.

Variation in Growing Period

An earlier chapter described plant responses to defoliation at different points in the growth cycle. Some plant species and, hence, some range types are damaged more by grazing at certain times of the year than by grazing at other times. Conversely, other species show little differential response in herbage growth to moderate-intensity defoliations in different seasons. Therefore, seasonal grazing may foster range improvement in one range type while changing another hardly at all.

Grasses respond to defoliation by changing production of seed and organic material. Generally, herbage removal within the rapid-growth periods reduces total growth more than do either earlier or later removals. During the first few decades of range management, it was believed that relatively more damage resulted from too early grazing than later studies showed to be the case. Single, early defoliations do little damage to plant vigor, but destruction becomes severe if they are repeated.

The opportunity to improve range by correlating grazing use with vegetational phenology varies from one vegetational type to another (Fig. 11-1). Yearlong grazing is practiced throughout the tropics and subtropics. Low temperatures cause plant dormancy at high elevations. Most tropical highlands have cool-season forage species with yearlong growth and potentially excellent grazing. If periods of dormancy occur in the tropical highlands, they are caused by lack of rainfall. At lower tropical elevations, two rainy seasons and two dry seasons each year result in two growing periods. Different grasses may produce the major growth in the two seasons. The subtropics are characterized by single dry and wet seasons each year. Tropical and subtropical grasslands at low elevations are dominated by warm-season species, mainly the *Andropogoneae*.

In temperate regions with dry summers, the rapid-growth period occurs in spring after temperatures become warm. In semidesert grasslands, late-summer rainfall results in rapid late-summer growth. A mixture of species maturing in the cool and warm seasons grows in the true prairie of central North America, where a combination of spring soil moisture and summer rainfall fosters a long growth period.

In annual grasslands of the Mediterranean climatic type, growth begins at the start of winter rains and ends when summer arrives. Since there is a new generation of annual plants from seed each year, no possibility exists for plants to develop vigor that carries from one year to the next. Maintaining a desirable botanical composition in the annual grasslands depends almost entirely upon intensity of utilization and very little upon season of grazing.

Since seasonal differences in plant development vary from location to location, seasonal grazing schedules must be correlated with the growth characteristics of the particular species and vegetation at hand. No grazing plan is likely to have worldwide application. The expected vegetational composition as well as animal production from a specialized grazing plan must be carefully determined for each region or even for each ranch. For example, one grazing plan may be used to increase cool-season grasses over warm-season species in the true prairie, while a second plan does the opposite and a third favors both plant growth pattern but in different pastures.

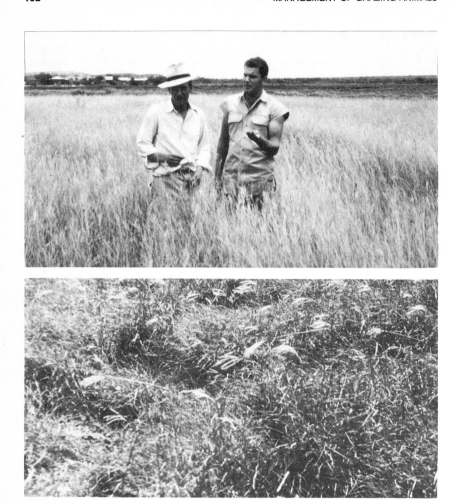

Figure 11-1 These two photos of an ungrazed *Andropogon is-chaemum* stand show several-fold differences in herbage growth between consecutive years.

Range Readiness

Range readiness defines *that point in the plant growth cycle at which grazing may begin without permanent damage to vegetation and soil.* It implies that earlier grazing will cause range deterioration and that little feed will be available for livestock at an earlier time. During the early history of rangeland grazing in the United States, severe range destruction resulted from intense and often continuous early grazing when green growth first appeared and from trampling when the soil was wet. To counter that situation, guidelines to range readiness were developed for much of the forested rangeland in the Western states (Table 11-1). These standards indicate that grazing without damage to the range may begin (1) when certain showy spring flowers are fading; (2) when growth by key perennial grasses has reached a stipulated height or number of leaves; and (3) when a standard proportion of full growth has been made by the leaves and twigs of browse species. Normally, these phenological stages indicate soil moisture sufficiently low to prevent animals from making deep tracks.

Only a few other countries have made use of the range-readiness concept. Native pastures in Switzerland are ready to graze when *Taraxacum officinale* begins to flower and hay is ready to cut when *Chrysanthemum leucanthemum* flowers (Caputa, 1968). Where domestic animals graze year long, the question of range readiness in the sense of a beginning time for grazing never arises. Range readiness has received little attention in the subtropical- and tropical-range regions.

Range-readiness guides are useful where the beginning of range grazing is completely controlled, as on forest ranges of the western United States, where severe weather prevents winter grazing. Federal lands grazed according to a permit have a turn-in date stipulated in each lease. This date represents an average of year-to-year variations in range-readiness dates. The practice is for lessor and lessee each year to decide upon the actual opening date of grazing according to vegetational development.

Ranch managers often are impatient with range-readiness dates on federal land, claiming that the ranges should be grazed earlier. Clipping studies have

Table 11-1 Selected examples of range readiness for national forests in California (*Wood et al., 1960*)

Achillea lanulosa	Leaves 5–10 cm; flowers in bud
Agropyron spicatum	Leaves 10–20 cm
Amelanchier alnifolia	Current twigs 5–10 cm; leaves 50% developed; buds opening
Balsamorhiza sagittata	Leaves 3/4 developed; buds opening
Cercocarpus betuloides	Twigs 5–10 cm; leaves 50% developed; flowers in bud
Erodium cicutarium	Plants 5–10 cm tall; flowers in bud
Festuca idahoensis	Leaves 7.5–10 cm; flowers in boot
Koeleria cristata	Leaves 12 cm; panicles mostly emerged
Poa secunda	Leaves 5–7.5 cm; heads all emerged
Prunus emarginata	In partial leaf and flowering
Purshia tridentata	Full leaf; twigs 7.5–15 cm; flowers opening to full
Ranunculus occidentalis	Plants 30–40 cm; flowers faded
Symphoricarpos albus	Leaf buds opening; flowers in bud

tended to support these contentions that early grazing is not damaging if perennial grasses are given relief from grazing during culm elongation and maturation. Beginning use at the earliest time that will not damage the range relieves dependence on costly conserved feeds, grain crops, and planted pastures. Minor damage from early grazing that cannot be avoided usually can be corrected with seasonal grazing plans, adjustments in stocking rates, or other management practices, not the least of which is seeding of early-growing species to be used only for early grazing. The time for increased flexibility in the beginning date of grazing through the use of seasonal grazing plans appears to have arrived.

Plant species vary greatly in their ability to withstand early grazing. *Agropyron desertorum* is much less sensitive to early use than is *Agropyron spicatum*. Spring grazing of the former should be set by animal welfare or the time when livestock can get a full feed each day. Sharp (1970) suggested that time as a standing crop of 225 kilograms dry matter per hectare and a daily increment of approximately 11 kilograms. Before that time, animals will have difficulty obtaining a full feed from young grass.

Movement of animals from one pasture to another, time of fertilizer applications, haying operations, and other events in the annual livestock management operation are dependent upon determination of plant growth stage. Whether it is called *range readiness* or some other name, measurement, as well as ocular estimation, of growth attained is desirable. Jagtenberg (1970), working with seeded pastures, used the height to which the new growth supported a ½-meter-diameter disk as a measure of growth. This measure of height closely correlated with temperature summations and took the guesswork out of time for fertilization. A range manager could use such an objective measure to advantage in determining when to begin grazing and when to move livestock in a grazing system. However, such a measure may be difficult to use in vegetation of low density.

Yearly Changes

Although each range type may have an optimum time for grazing, many factors necessitate use at other times. Ranchers must provide feed for 365 days of the year, and seldom can an optimum green-feed supply move in concert with that need. In range operations, green feed is oversupplied during the rapid-growth period, and some of it must be saved for future times when growth is slow or nonexistent. As the botanical composition changes, for whatever reason, the time of optimum grazing also changes.

Range vegetation presents a wide variety of growing periods from place to place and of optimal times when the range can be used. Also, at any place, production and development vary from year to year. Within a year, the manager is faced with making the best of cyclic situations in demand for feed and production of forage quantity and quality; therefore some ranges are used under less than optimum conditions. Ranchers must employ practices that reduce animal losses in drought years and forage losses in wet years.

Forage-Supply Cycle

Daily increments of herbage on rangeland are small at the beginning of plant growth. They increase rapidly during a short period of flush growth and cease at plant maturity, when the standing crop is highest. Upon maturity, there begins a period of decrease in herbage supply, whether or not the range is grazed by domestic and game animals. This decrease is the result of shattering of seeds; leaching by rain and snow; breakage of leaves and stems by wind; grazing and breakage by insects, rodents, and birds; and decomposition. In many vegetational types, the whole herbage crop can disappear in a year because of these factors. In others, a mulch will accumulate, but in all grassland and forb types the turnover of organic matter is rapid. The rate of disappearance increases with moisture supply. This cycle goes on whether or not man allows his animals to harvest some of the feed. Consequently, he must harvest the feed or lose it. He is very much at the mercy of this natural cycle since he can neither irrigate most range vegetation to lengthen the growth period nor mow it to conserve feed.

Forage-Quality Cycle

A second cycle of major concern to management is that of nutrient quality in the feed. New growth is high in percentages of crude proteins, carbohydrates, vitamins, and water on a dry-matter basis, so it must be low in fiber, lignin, and those items that generally suggest low nutritional quality. As the growing season progresses, these two groups of substances gradually reverse their positions, and poor-quality feed results after plant maturity. Nonstructural carbohydrates may be highest at midgrowth. Fine grasses and short species often retain greater nutritional quality when cured than do tall, coarse grasses. In all range types, the quality of feed for larger herbivores decreases as the available quantity of forage decreases after plant maturity.

During the early part of the growing period, especially in mornings with heavy dew and after rain, the water content of young forage may be so high that an animal cannot consume enough dry matter to be properly nourished. At these times, the highly favorable content of crude protein, as determined on a dry-matter basis, may not measure feeding values accurately. Usually the weight of desirable nutrients per hectare reaches its peak near the time of plant maturity, but percentages in the feed are low at that time. Conversely, the amount of nutrients per hectare is low during the early growth period, when dry-weight percentages of nutrients are high. Both amounts and percentages are low after leaves have matured and shattered or have been leached by rain.

Forage-Demand Cycle

A third cycle of concern to range managers is the amount of needed forage. An operation that runs cows and calves or maintains a breeding herd of any species must provide feed yearlong. The amount needed for each mature animal changes only slightly from day to day as requirements vary for pregnancy, fattening, lactation, growth, and general good health. Normally, as young animals grow, the demand for high-quality feed increases, thus there are peak needs at or near sale time. When animals are sold, the total demand for feed in the operation takes a corresponding drop. Other types of producing systems, steer production, for example, need larger quantities of feed for shorter periods and may not require feed for certain parts of the year when no animals are present.

Combining the Cycles

Grazing management aims to combine the cycles of forage supply, quality, and demand to obtain the highest profit from the operation consistent with maintaining excellent condition range. Although the cycles describe continuously changing situations, their union is divided into four periods for ease in discussing the matching of grazing schedules with forage resources.

In Period 1, vegetation produces inadequate green forage to meet all the demands of grazing animals. This is the beginning of growth and a time of slow herbage increment. Animals avidly seek the new green material, but its low availability forces grazing on old growth. Much care should be taken to prevent overuse and trampling during this period because new growth can be reduced rapidly and the capacity of the plants to recuperate may be endangered. The concept of range readiness resulted from concern with too early grazing that also was too intense.

Specialized grazing plans that concentrate livestock in a few areas and rotate them among pastures tend to foster overuse or at least heavy grazing pressure during Period 1 (Fig. 11-2). The manager must redress the balance between green-forage supply and animal needs on a day-to-day basis to avoid damaging the range more in this period than can be repaired in later ungrazed periods. Bunching of animals, hence less available green feed per animal during this period of scanty supply, may be a major reason why widely spaced animals often show more weight gains in the early growing season than do those in rotations. The former have more feed available and more chance to select quality feed without so much competition from other animals.

Period 1 is a time when the manager often pushes his interlocking cycles to their limit. He needs the less expensive range forage as a relief from winter feeding of hays and concentrates. Young animals and lactating mothers need high-quality green feeds for rapid production. Bunching of animals accentuates the possibility for stress on both the livestock and the range. So that possible damage can be

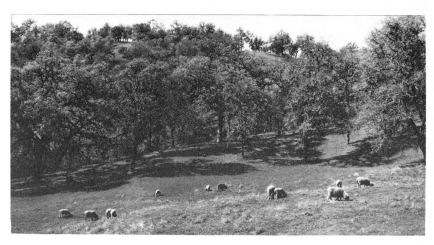

Figure 11-2   Sheep grazing on young plants in the California annual grassland during late winter.

relieved, the grazing time in the rotations should be shortened or the animals distributed in several pastures. In yearlong-grazing situations, the beginning of Period 1 is a time to start rotations and to move animals rapidly. Often, 20 or more millimeters of rainfall signals that time.

Period 2 is the span of time when demand for and growth increment of forage are about equal. This period is short, perhaps no longer than a day or a week, on most rangeland. In contrast, on improved pastures, where the manager has more control over daily herbage production by using planted species, fertilization, and irrigation, there is a long period when increment and demand are similar. If forage production on irrigated pastures gets too rapid, the manager harvests and conserves some forage as hay. Period 2 is difficult to define, but it appears to be the beginning of rapid growth. It is a key time for changing the schedules of specialized seasonal grazing plans.

Period 3 is that part of the growth cycle when daily increment of new herbage exceeds demand. It is the flush growth period. In general, rangelands with low rainfall have short rapid-growth periods. Rapid growth may occur over a long period of time on irrigated pastures and in tropical areas that have long rainy seasons. Period 3 is the span of time when ungrazed forage is accumulated for later use, either as cured standing feed on the ground or as hay.

In practice, range can get little overuse during this period unless too many animals are concentrated in a pasture and left there too long. If herbage is accumulating, grazing pressure is light and the possibilities of range damage slight, in contrast with Period 1. Clipping treatments that remove herbage to a low stubble height too late in Period 3 for regrowth have shown that vegetation can be damaged by defoliation at this time. Such a situation can be duplicated with grazing only if large numbers of animals are kept in a small area, which often means other areas are ungrazed. Few studies of repeated seasonal grazing during Period 3 or any other time are available to give field answers to this question of relative damage by grazing during different parts of the growth cycle. Without extremes of animal concentration and forage utilization, it would seem that the plan of grazing would make little difference to either plant vigor or animal production during Period 3.

Period 4 is a time without forage increment and with considerable natural herbage losses, including gradual loss of nutrients. Demand for forage by domestic animals normally is reduced at this time by sale, but needs of wild animals remain high or even increase. Before the end of Period 4, hunting, losses to predators, disease, and lack of feed normally will have reduced the wild animal populations to their annual low. Grazing consequences on mature vegetation generally are considered minimal, but trampling, reduction of stubble heights, changes in litter amounts, and laying of standing dead material may profoundly influence the next crop through altering the environment near the soil surface. Much work is needed on this point. Effects from the absence of grazing, overgrazing, and rotation of grazing during Period 4 are unclear.

The highest animal production probably would come from grazing only during Period 3. With this plan forage would be used when it was palatable and when it had the highest yield per hectare of dry matter with adequate nutrient content. Summer ranges in mountainous areas frequently are harvested in Period 3, and livestock on any ranch may graze all the feed from a pasture or two at this ideal time. However, ranches that maintain breeding herds normally graze the range during all four periods. Any problems of maintaining a yearlong balance between feed supply and needs must be met. An important aspect of good management is that numbers of animals and the time they are allowed in each pasture are such that overgrazing is minimized at all times. If overgrazing cannot be avoided, the overused areas should be allowed periods of recovery without grazing.

The need to keep specialized seasonal grazing plans coordinated with the three cycles is obvious. Dates of grazing and stocking rates should be planned so that expected needs and emergencies requiring last-minute change can be met. The manager should not hesitate to combine different grazing plans to take advantage of all kinds of available feed. Grazing schedules improve effectiveness of these changes.

TERMINOLOGY FOR GRAZING PLANS

Terms commonly employed in conversation and literature dealing with grazing management have been loosely defined and irregularly used. Misunderstandings have arisen. For example, the words *ungrazed, deferred,* and *rested* are synonyms in many situations but have different and precise meanings in other contexts. The resulting confusion limits communication among range workers and retards development of range practices. Precise definition is especially important for those terms that apply to specialized seasonal grazing plans. The objective of this section is to define terms for grazing management so that the number of synonyms is reduced and ambiguities are minimized. Therefore, each term is limited to a single concept and designed for broad rather than for local or regional application. For these reasons, the definitions differ from those of Sampson, 1951; Range Term Glossary Committee, 1964; Booysen, 1967; Heady, 1970; and Shiflet and Heady, 1971.

Grazing plan is used in preference to *grazing system.* A schedule for moving grazing animals from one pasture to another is more appropriately a plan than a system, notwithstanding long-term usage. The concepts of *grazing management system* and *rangeland management plan,* as employed here, encompass the day-to-day seasonal grazing plan and much more. A grazing management system might include grazing of improved pastures and crop aftermath, feeding of hay and concentrates, health precautions, rangeland improvements, and many more practices. A rangeland management plan centers on keeping a resource inventory, planning for range improvements, and scheduling. Planning and establishment of range improvements may be needed before a schedule for grazing pastures in sequence can be accomplished, but improvements are separate from the seasonal grazing plan and have value in themselves. This chapter concentrates on the characteristics and values of seasonal grazing unconfounded with other range practices.

Grazing Season and Grazing Period

The *grazing season* is *that portion of the year when grazing is feasible on a specific area.* Throughout the tropics and subtropics, the grazing season is the whole year; but in cold climates or at high elevations, grazing may be possible for only a portion of each year. The length of the grazing season is controlled by environmental influences on the animals and normally is longer than the plant growing season. Yearlong range has a 12-month grazing season. On public lands, the established time for which grazing permits are issued approaches the grazing season.

The *grazing period for a specific area* is *that portion of the grazing season within which grazing actually occurs.* It is the time span of actual grazing. Yearlong range may or may not have yearlong grazing. The beginning and ending dates of one or more grazing periods on each land unit are stipulated by grazing plans, so they seldom are the same from year to year. The term *grazing period* makes no distinction between grazing by different groups or kinds of animals at different times. Modifiers, such as *for cows and calves,* should be used to make the meaning specific for time, land unit, and animals.

Deferred, Rested, and Ungrazed

Deferred specifies that *a pasture is not grazed until seed maturity is assured or a comparable growth stage has been reached* and that *it is grazed after seed maturity.* Deferment permits gain in plant vigor, increased seed production, storage of food materials in roots and stems, and generally improved health of the range. A second consecutive year of deferment permits additional gain in vigor and, presumably, establishment of seedlings from the first seed crop. Improvement of perennial grass range by reproduction from seed happens irregularly and is poorly documented.

Rested, as a term in range grazing plans, stipulates that *a pasture is not grazed at all in a given year; not even the mature forage is harvested.*

Periods of no grazing which are not specifically scheduled as deferred or rested treatment are left without a name. A plan that employed one herd in four pastures, each with a two-month grazing period, would have at least one deferred pasture and perhaps three other treatments that did not meet the specifications of *deferred.* For lack of a better term, these latter are called *ungrazed* treatments.

The three terms, *deferred, rested,* and *ungrazed,* separate different periods of no grazing on the proposition that vegetation responds differently to grazing and the absence of grazing at different stages in the growth cycle. The term *ungrazed* permits specific definition of the other two terms. The loose application of these three terms as synonyms in descriptions of ungrazed periods of any length should be avoided. *Controlled, delayed,* and *strategic* also have been used as labels for all the nongrazing treatments.

Continuous, Repeated Seasonal, and Rotational Grazing

Continuous grazing is *unrestricted livestock grazing through the whole of the grazing season,* i.e., grazing in which the grazing season and the grazing period are the same. Grazing occurs during the whole period that plants are growing as well as during part or all of the dormancy period. Continuous grazing is yearlong grazing in warm climates. *Set Stocking* is the term employed outside North America.

Grazing after the growing season depends upon forage accumulated during Period 3, the time of rapid growth. Therefore, pressure on the vegetation from continuous grazing must be light in Period 3, although it can be heavy when growth begins, as for example, in winter use in Mediterranean-type annual grasslands. Continuous grazing has been criticized because grazing occurs throughout the growing season, and it is argued that even light grazing during the growing season encourages overuse of the preferred species. Many areas, however, have received continuous grazing for long periods without permanent damage to the resource. The proposition that continuous grazing means complete defoliation is fallacious. Continuous grazing can result in any degree of forage utilization.

Repeated seasonal grazing defines *a situation in which a pasture is grazed at the same time each year.* Migratory game animals usually follow a repeated seasonal grazing plan. This plan is rotation of grazing on an annual basis. Ranchers who save pastures for grazing during a certain season each year are using this plan.

When animals are moved from one pasture to another on a scheduled basis, this plan is called *rotational grazing.* If the grazing period is short and the pastures few, each pasture will be alternately grazed and ungrazed several times during a grazing season. Longer rotations result from longer grazing periods, more pastures, or both. Short rotations are used widely for the harvesting of forage on improved pastures but seldom are employed on extensive rangeland. A variant of rotation grazing in southern Africa is short-duration grazing. It uses a grazing period of two weeks maximum in rotation with an ungrazed period of approximately six weeks minimum.

Combinations of Terms

Commonly used combinations of these terms are *deferred-rotation, rest-rotation, rotational deferment, rotational resting, rotational grazing and resting, rotated-deferred, deferred and rotated, rotated and deferred,* and *rotation of deferred grazing.* Most of these combinations of terms have been applied to specific grazing plans that their authors have emphasized as being somewhat different from traditional deferred-rotation grazing. Nearly all grazing plans on rangeland in North America have been called *continuous, deferred-rotation,* or *rest-rotation grazing,* almost without regard to their actual design. Obviously, one name for all plans is not desirable, nor is a separate name for each of the hundreds of plans that now exist. Every author and speaker needs carefully to describe his plan, including number of herds, number of animals in each herd, number of pastures, size of pastures, and especially dates or plant phenological stages when animals are to be moved. It is nearly impossible from the published description of most specialized seasonal grazing plans to correlate movement of the livestock with growth characteristics of key plants and changes in range condition.

As a step toward better terminology and usage, the definitions given in preceding sections are strictly employed in the discussion that follows. Further, in the following examples, each term is applied to the grazing treatment of a pasture. A grazing plan often combines several treatments: for example, a five-pasture, two-herd plan may have a rested pasture, a deferred pasture, a continuously grazed pasture, two pastures in a short grazed-ungrazed spring rotation, and yearly rotation of all pastures. Such a plan as this might be called either *rest-rotation* or *deferred-rotation.* Neither name is adequate because other grazing treatments are included in the plan and contribute to its effectiveness. Responses by livestock and vegetation are most likely the results of the plan as a whole.

EXAMPLES OF GRAZING PLANS

In the following examples, a plan is described under the term that applies to the grazing treatment of greatest emphasis. Except for continuous grazing, every grazing plan has grazed and ungrazed pastures at most times. Some plans include continuous grazing as one of the rotated treatments.

Continuous Grazing

Perhaps the simplest of all plans is continuous grazing. It might be called a single-pasture plan. In two experimental tests, one with sheep in the coastal ranges of northern California (Heady, 1961) and the other with cattle in the southern Sierra Nevada foothills (Duncan and Heady, 1969), continuous grazing, yearlong in these examples, gave greater and more consistent livestock returns without detrimental changes in the range than have any other tested plans of rotation and deferment. These results are consistent with general practice where the grazing is entirely on the California annual-type grassland.

Continuous grazing has been and still is used widely, although condemned as causing range deterioration because of grazing pressure on preferred sites and species. In tests in which degree of range use has been controlled and proper distribution attained, continuous grazing has shown excellent results. Short grasses, annual grasses, sod grasses, and grasslands with few species of extreme palatability have responded well to continuous grazing. Unless vegetation and livestock are under stress due to overgrazing, continuous grazing produces as well as any other plan in most situations.

Repeated Seasonal Grazing

Seasonal variations in forage resource and animal husbandry may require repeated seasonal use. Vegetational types with coarse, unpalatable herbage and seeded stands of one or two species often are grazed on a repeated seasonal basis, as proposed by Campbell (1961) for grazing on a grass-alfalfa mixture in the prairie of south central Canada. Valentine (1967) suggested the term *seasonal suitability grazing* for a plan that embodies opportunistic principles in grazing range types such as *Distichlis stricta*. Each year, *Distichlis* is grazed in Periods 1 and 2 because those are the only times it is palatable. Abundant annuals and short-lived perennials that grow after scattered rains in arid areas furnish forage best used at the time of growth (Herbel and Nelson, 1969). Because of differences in palatability and response, *Hilaria mutica* repeatedly is grazed in summer and *Bouteloua eripoda* in fall (Paulsen and Ares, 1962). Another example of repeated seasonal grazing is repeated spring use on *Agropyron desertorum,* which has low palatability and nutrient content in mature forage. Still another example is the marsh vegetation along the Louisiana coast, which is winter-grazed after fall burning each year. Animals are moved to forest land for high-quality summer grazing (Shiflet, 1966).

Migratory game often graze the same area at the same time each year. Winter deer ranges in the western United States repeatedly are grazed in the same season. Caribou, with their linear routes in Alaska (Skoog, 1968), and wildebeest, with their circular routes in East Africa (Talbot and Talbot, 1963), follow more or less the same yearly pattern in their migrations, but with some unexplained variations. For example, caribou in Alaska migrate with long treks twice a year to their summer range and return to winter range. The herds are more dispersed on the seasonal ranges than on the treks. These seasonal movements may be in great herds or in almost unnoticed small groups, and they may follow the same route for ten years, more or less, but another route for the next period. Their range goes ungrazed for a part of each year but all gets grazed at the same time every year. Much has been said about rotational grazing by herds of bison in the United States and the tendency of the bison to follow circular migratory routes (Matthews, 1954). One suspects that they, too, might have followed certain regular routes, perhaps in response to available water and feed, and might have grazed in about the same place at the same time year after year.

Ranchers throughout the world save certain pastures for grazing during the same season year after year. They do this because they need to have animals close to headquarters during winter weather, near roads in the spring when the young are born, accessible to water in dry seasons, and feeding on high-quality forage when animals are being readied for market. Some of these seasonal grazing plans are at variance with the proposition that a range should be ungrazed at key times so that plant regeneration and high production can occur.

Wild animals in natural settings do not follow rest- or deferred-rotational treatments in most instances. Their plan is repeated seasonal grazing. This plan has resulted in excellent range that still supports abundant wild and domestic animals. Overgrazing by wild animals occurs where high animal density persists for too long.

Unrotated deferred grazing on a pasture year after year is a type of repeated seasonal grazing. Common practice in the northern Great Plains is to have animals on the same summer and winter ranges year after year (Clarke and Tisdale, 1936; Hurtt, 1951). Another excellent example of this type of grazing occurs on the steep slopes and benches in Hell's Canyon of Snake River in eastern Oregon (Fig. 11-3). The canyon furnishes protection from winter storms because it is at lower elevation than are surrounding ranges and has less snow cover. The result is that grazing is deferred until late fall or winter every year. There may be some grazing in early spring, but none is allowed during Periods 2 and 3.

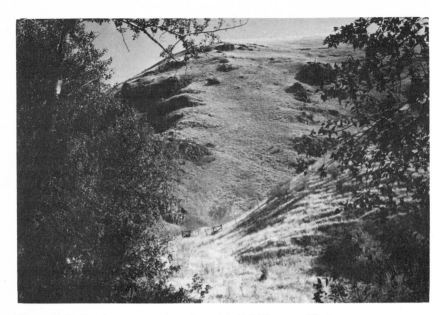

Figure 11-3 Bunchgrasses on steep slopes into Hells' Canyon of Snake River between Idaho and Oregon are grazed on a repeated seasonal basis during winter.

On mountainous range in western Montana, a once-over grazing that followed seasonal vegetational development resulted in more range improvement than did an early, light grazing followed by a second grazing in late summer from low to high elevations (Heady, et al., 1947).

Generally, repeated seasonal use has not been a treatment included in experiments with grazing plans. It is a widely used practice that needs measurement. Varying responses to seasonal use could indicate when grazing is damaging to the vegetation and when it is not. Repeated seasonal use could be the control against which the results from separate parts of other plans are measured. These kinds of comparisons are needed to furnish the building blocks in designing grazing plans in general. The ideal plan provides the greatest improvement or production in the favored pasture as well as the least deterioration or the maintenance of production in other pastures. To promote range improvement, a well-operated seasonal plan considers the grazed as well as the ungrazed pastures. The effects of both grazing and the absence of grazing at every season are needed as foundation knowledge in designing grazing plans.

Rotational Grazing

Rotational grazing plans are used in specific rangeland situations, especially in the early growing season, when forage supplies and growth rates are low. Types of rotational grazing plans include daily strip grazing in pastures, short rotations of a few days, complementary rotations with different species, and repeated seasonal grazing. Every rotation plan encompasses sequential stages of plant growth on a variety of sites. Normally on rangeland, short rotations of one or two complete cycles span growth period 1 and are used to prevent overgrazing during that period. One example of a short-rotation plan is a two-pasture switchback arrangement on *Agropyron desertorum* in which each pasture is grazed in early and late spring in alternate years. If three or four pastures are available, the plan employed with this species may be a strict rotation of short grazing periods in each pasture (Fig. 11-4) or a deferred-rotation plan.

Other types of rotations on rangeland are being used in Africa. One such plan was known first in South Africa as *nonselective grazing* or the *Acocks-Howell plan,* in which intensive grazing for two weeks or less was followed by ungrazed periods of six weeks to five months (Acocks, 1966). Later, especially in Rhodesia, a similar plan was labeled *short-duration grazing* (Goodloe, 1969). It has been called the *multicamp plan* in southern Africa, where *camp* means *pasture.* If several herds are used, the pastures are grouped for each herd under the name *groupcamp plan* (Roux and Skinner, 1970).

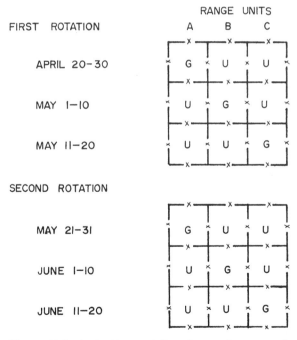

Figure 11-4 A short-term rotation plan on *Agropyron desertorum,* showing each unit grazed twice during the 60-day spring period *(Frischknecht and Harris, 1968).* Abbreviations are G = grazed, U = ungrazed.

Short-duration grazing puts heavy grazing pressure on a pasture for a short time to reduce the unpalatable species, to reduce competition against the better species, and to prevent grazing on the first regrowth. Long ungrazed periods give regrowth ample time for considerable recovery before the pasture is grazed again. In the dry season, the aims are to reduce standing dead material, loosen the soil surface by trampling, and prevent the development of large ungrazed bunches of grass filled with dead stems. Seed production and seedling establishment are emphasized objectives. Proponents suggest that, as a rangeland reclamation procedure, short-duration grazing should begin after good rains and a year of rest (Howell, 1967).

The implications of nonselectivity of forage with high livestock density make this grazing plan controversial. People on both sides of the controversy agree that light grazing use is selective and heavy use is nonselective. One side claims that high livestock density, as with large herds in small areas, reduces selectivity and that use of the unpalatable species can be attained without overuse of the palatable plants (Howell, 1967; Anderson, 1967a). The other side maintains that selectivity decreases more with increased forage use than it does with increased stocking density and that continued heavy use leads to disaster. This side cites failures during drought in semiarid vegetation where highly unpalatable shrubs have invaded grassland as a result of overuse (Roux, 1968). Where the plan has been successful, herbage residues have remained on the soil surface, and the presence of these residues suggests moderate forage utilization.

Another aspect of the controversy is whether or not grazing the unpalatable species gives a competitive advantage to the palatable plants. One side states that climax species will return if given relief from heavy use, independent of the competition. The other claims that nonselective grazing hastens changes toward climax by reducing competition. Periods without grazing in the short-duration plan logically should favor the palatable and unpalatable species alike, but it is argued that selective grazing gives the ungrazed species an advantage of starting from a more vigorous condition. However, much experience has shown that reduction of overgrazing promotes range improvement by allowing change in the species composition. In addition, selective grazing usually gives animals forage materials of high quality. They reject the poorest herbage, protecting seedlings and soil and promoting the climax species. The preponderance of evidence is in favor of the view that heavy use reduces the desirable species by defoliation more than it helps them by lessening competition.

However, these results have come from experiences with vegetational types that have narrow ranges or species palatabilities. Types with wide palatability spectra, such as the false karoo of South Africa and tall-grassland types generally, may respond differently. Selective grazing is a major problem in the sour and mixed velds of southern Africa because it tends to decrease the palatables such as *Themeda, Tetrachne,* and *Digitaria* while promoting less desirable species

(Acocks, 1966). The resolution of this controversy lies in the relative responses to defoliation by different species. If the unpalatable species are less susceptible to deterioration by defoliation than are the palatable species, heavy utilization will cause range deterioration. If the palatable species are less susceptible than are the undesirable, the range will improve with heavy use. The speed and degree of response to defoliation are yet to be determined for many key species.

Where normal dry seasons and droughts prevent growth during a long period, a second dry-season grazing, or even a third grazing as required by two-month rotation cycles, has resulted in overgrazed conditions. This fact has been recognized, so in actual practice, forage utilization has been lightened to improve range condition rapidly during growing seasons and years with high rainfall. Droughts and dry seasons are times to concentrate on preventing losses in range condition.

The concept of a short, intensive period of grazing in rotation with a long period without grazing should not be confused with light or heavy utilization. Frequent light grazing gives high production on pastures where palatable species dominate and where unpalatable species decrease with competition from the desirable species. Infrequent heavy use during the dormant season or in early spring may be necessary to reduce coarse grasses and to create a uniform stand. With proper forage utilization, short-duration grazing and many of the traditional two- to five-pasture plans have given rapid range improvement and increased livestock production (Roberts, 1970).

Short-duration grazing operates with a wide variety of pasture numbers and sizes, with differing lengths of grazed and ungrazed periods, and with fluctuating numbers of livestock herds. It is highly flexible. By increasing the number of pastures, the manager also increases his control and husbandry of animals and spatial uniformity of forage utilization. He can give preference to fattening animals, lactating mothers, and others. A 16-pasture system illustrates some of the possibilities. At the beginning of plant growth, the herd can be divided for handling ease during calving or lambing. Each herd may be moved every day or two through four pastures and in two weeks to other sets of four pastures. After the young no longer need daily care, the herds can be combined into the full 16-pasture plan. As the growing season progresses, grazing time in each pasture should increase until, by late growing season, it is ten days to two weeks. Plant maturity will find some pastures ungrazed or not grazed since early spring. These pastures should furnish feed until the next growing season starts.

In years of high production, excess feed is trampled down so that soil improvement is promoted, and some pastures may go ungrazed. In drought times, the rotation must be more rapid and all pastures grazed to provide adequate forage. Unused pastures in droughts are wasteful of high-quality forage and indicate a need for more animals.

Enough rainfall after drought to bring new plant growth is one cue for moving animals to a new pasture and beginning a new rotation cycle. In fact, a strict time schedule of grazing days for each pasture and a constant sequence of pastures should not be followed. Criteria for ending grazing in one pasture and beginning in another are discussed in a later section of this chapter.

Deferred Rotation

Designs for deferred-rotation plans are numerous, and seldom are two alike. Hugo (1968) gives designs for 18 different rotational plans for various combinations of vegetational types and use objectives in South Africa. The simplest deferred-rotation plans employ one herd of animals. The number of pasture units equals the number of grazing periods and the number of years required to complete a rotation cycle. It normally is five or less.

One deferred-rotation plan is the plan for yearlong grazing by bison on the National Bison Range in western Montana (Fig. 11-5). The bunchgrasses, *Festuca scabrella, F. idahoensis,* and *Agropyron spicatum,* usually are in flower by the

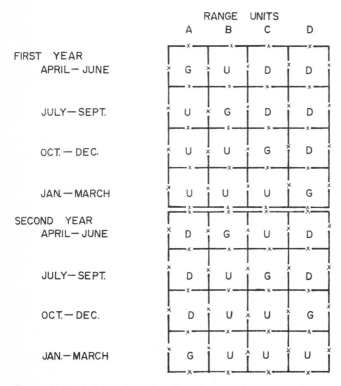

Figure 11-5 A deferred-rotation plan of grazing by bison on *Festuca scabrella* grassland at the National Bison Range in Montana. U = ungrazed, G= grazed, and D= deferred.

first of June and mature in July. Two pastures, ungrazed until fall and winter (October through March), are deferred each year. The pasture grazed early is ungrazed from July until the next January, a period of 18 months that includes the end of one growing season and all of the next. The fourth pasture, which is grazed from July through September, may or may not be deferred, depending on the earliness of the growing season. Even in late growing seasons, grazing in this pasture probably is too late to be damaging to plant vigor.

The plan tested by Herbel and Anderson (1959) on tall-grass vegetation dominated by *Andropogon scoparius* in the Kansas Flint Hills illustrates the use of ungrazed periods for cool- and warm-season plants (Fig. 11-6). The absence of grazing during May and June defers use on desirable cool-season species that are a part of this grassland. The absence of grazing from July 1 until sometime in the fall favors the warm-season grasses, although they were grazed in the spring and early summer. Consecutive years without late-growing-season grazing demonstrate that the tall species are easier to maintain or improve than are the cool-season species. Opening of all pastures to free-choice grazing in the fall provides livestock full selection of highest quality herbage in the final harvesting. Grazing spread

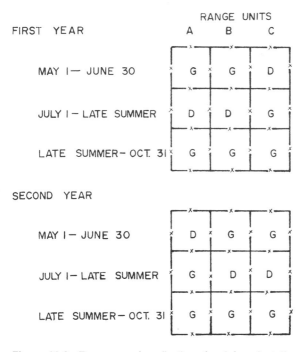

Figure 11-6 Two years of application of a deferred-rotation plan for tall-grass prairie in the Flint Hills of Kansas *(Herbel and Anderson, 1959).* U= ungrazed, G= grazed, and D= deferred.

over two pastures in May and June gives relief from concentrated early use due to high livestock density.

A plan that is called *deferred-rotation grazing* by its author (Merrill, 1954) has shown impressive results in Texas and in East Africa. It employs three herds and four pastures, each grazed continuously for a year and ungrazed for four months (Fig. 11-7). The result is a deferment plus two other ungrazed periods of four months for every pasture during a four-year period. This plan emphasizes rotation of nongrazing and deferment rather than rotation of nongrazing and grazing.

Rest-Rotation Grazing

A rest-rotation plan employed on public land in the western United States is shown in Figure 11-8. The five pasture treatments, or a five-year sequence of treatments,

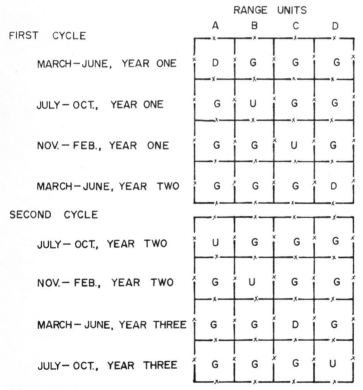

Figure 11-7 Two grazing periods per pasture in three years of the three-herd and four-pasture plan used in Texas *(Merrill, 1954; Keng and Merrill, 1960; Waldrip and Parker, 1967)*. U = ungrazed, G = grazed, and D = deferred.

and their rationale for a single pasture dominated by *Festuca idahoensis* are as follows: During the first year, close grazing makes full use of all herbage, and standing dead material, if any exists, is trampled. The second year is one of rest to restore vigor and litter supply. Deferred treatment in the third year promotes and protects the seed crop and enhances plant vigor. Grazing animals use the forage and trample seed into the soil. The second rest period in the fourth year benefits seedling establishment, further promotes vigor, and adds greatly to the litter cover. The absence of grazing until the key grass species have flowered in the fifth year ensures seedling establishment. Afterwards the whole forage crop is harvested.

This plan is extreme in that 40 percent of the available land and perhaps 40 to 50 percent of the usable forage are ungrazed every year. Increased grazing pressure on the 60 percent that has to carry the grazing load may do harm that will exceed the benefit that can be gained during the three-year sequence of rest-deferred-rest. In this plan, animals are forced to use forage on two pastures after it has lost quality. If *Agropyron desertorum* occurs in pastures grazed according to this plan, it tends to form dense clumps of straw called "wolf plants" during the years of rest. An advantage of rest is that it gives all sites and species within a pasture relief from

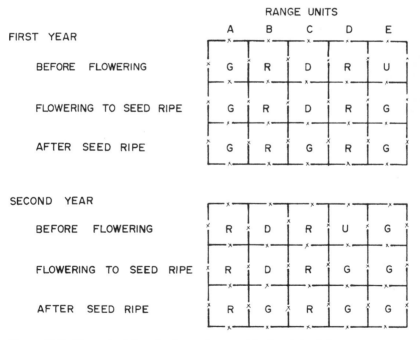

Figure 11-8 The rest-rotation plan for grazing on public domain lands in the Western United States *(Hormay, 1970).* U = ungrazed, G = grazed, D = deferred, and R = rested.

grazing, whereas with continuous grazing, some sites usually are too heavily used. Although the original test of this plan was designed with five pastures, other applications commonly have used three or four pastures.

Grazing Plans that Combine Treatments

Different native species, seeded stands, and range sites have characteristics that require combinations of grazing treatments. A plan for seeded *Agropyron desertorum* and the native bunchgrass type on public domain land in southeastern Oregon illustrates a combination of repeated seasonal grazing and rotation of deferred grazing (Fig. 11-9). Two pastures of *Agropyron* are grazed in a rotation or switchback plan during April and May. The April grazing begins as soon as feed is available and ends when sufficient soil moisture remains for regrowth of a few seed stalks. As a rule of thumb, *sufficient moisture* means about 30 centimeters of moist

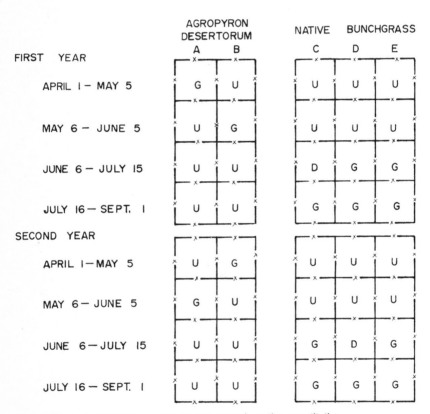

Figure 11-9 A switchback or two-pasture annual rotation constituting repeated spring grazing of *Agropyron desertorum* combined with rotation of deferred grazing on native range, principally *Agropyron spicatum,* in southeastern Oregon. U= ungrazed, G= grazed, and D= deferred.

soil, which might be at the 30- to 60-centimeter depth. This grazing treatment tends to result in heavy utilization, but it has the advantage of reducing or preventing wolf plants. Reserve feed produced on this pasture can be used in the autumn or in times of late-summer emergency.

The second *Agropyron* pasture is grazed until the utilization is 50 to 60 percent. Then, for about a month and a half, the animals are on two native bunchgrass pastures while one pasture is deferred. From July 15 until September 1, all three of the native pastures are grazed. Although dates are shown in Figure 11-9, they are only approximate since the animals are moved on the basis of soil moisture, growth stage, and degree of forage utilization.

Grazing treatments in this plan include annual rotation without deferment on *Agropyron desertorum,* continuous grazing after a delayed spring beginning, and a three-year rotation of deferment on native range dominated by *Agropyron spicatum.* This plan takes advantage of early growth and resistance to grazing of *Agropyron desertorum,* prevents all early use of *Agropyron spicatum,* and gives it a further opportunity to gain in vigor with a deferment once in every three years. In practice, the native bunchgrasses have responded rapidly, especially where *Artemisia tridentata* has been reduced.

In the northern Great Plains, seeded stands of *Agropyron desertorum* provide early-spring grazing on greed feed. All grazing is on *Elymus junceus, Agropyron intermedium,* and *Medicago* spp. rather than on the native grasses (Campbell, 1963; Lodge, 1963). For a 10-year period, seeded stands of *Agropyron desertorum* averaged 23 days and *Bromus inermis* 12 days earlier range readiness than did native range in central Montana (Williams and Post, 1945). These species usually are grazed on a repeated seasonal plan (Campbell, 1961). Smoliak (1968) suggested for southern Alberta, Canada, that 20 percent of the land should be in *Agropyron desertorum,* 50 percent in native range, and 30 percent in *Elymus junceus.* Sheep rotated themselves on a repeated seasonal basis when given free access to these grass types. These schedules have been called *complementary grazing plans* (Lodge, 1970). The plan for each pasture type may be a rotation of various durations, continuous grazing for the season, or deferred-rotation (Lodge et al., 1972).

Fertilization often increases productivity and may lengthen the period of green feed in the Mediterranean-type annual grassland. Selected sites seeded to *Phalaris tuberosa* and *Trifolium subterraneum* provide green feed before the annual grasses grow more than 2.5 centimeters or so and after they dry. The seeded mixture, fertilized annuals, and unfertilized range may be grazed in a plan that combines repeated seasonal use, rotation grazing, and deferred grazing (Miller et al., 1957) to attain the proper degree of utilization at the best time of year on the legumes, large grasses, and small grasses.

In parts of southern Africa where highly palatable and unpalatable species are mixed, seasonal grazing treatments may control the balance of botanical composition between the two groups. Spring grazing tends to reduce and deferment to increase the species that are unpalatable late in the growing season, as shown in pastures B and C, Figure 11-10. Rotation of grazing in pasture A reduces the top growth of all species and gives the shorter palatable species an advantage because they tend to grow rapidly and mature earlier (late summer) than the unpalatables

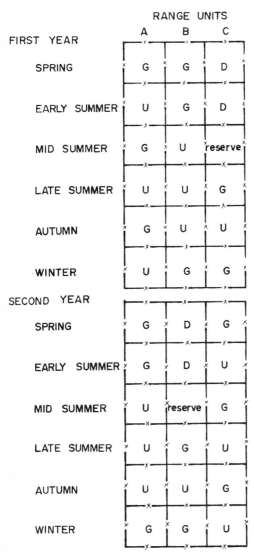

Figure 11-10 Rotational grazing in different patterns for maintenance and use of a mixture of palatable and unpalatable species in southern Africa *(Hugo, 1968)*. U= ungrazed, G= grazed, and D= deferred.

(autumn). The absence of grazing in early summer provides for seedling establishment, especially of the palatable species. The absence of grazing during late summer and autumn promotes seed production and vigor. These treatments, for different purposes combine a rotated pasture, one grazed early and ungrazed late, and one deferred.

Grazing of salt marshes and forest vegetation in the southern part of the United States combines rotations of burning and animals. Winter grazing on the marshes follows burning every second year. Spring and summer forest grazing is controlled by burning at three-year intervals. Newly cutover lands are burned in May, but forested areas are burned in March so that damage to timber stands is prevented. After six years under test, forage utilization averaged 78, 31, and 18 percent, respectively, on the current, one-year, and two-year burns in the forest, amounting to a rotation of animals as they follow the burning. This combination of burning and rotational grazing improves the quality of forage where quality rapidly declines as coarseness of herbage increases (Duvall and Whitaker, 1964; Duval, 1969).

Yearlong forage supplies for cattle in the longleaf–slash pine region of the southeastern United States consist of native range and improved pastures used in combination. The grazing schedule begins with grazing on native ranges in spring and summer. The first growth on improved pastures is cut once or twice for hay. Ranges and pastures are grazed alternately in late summer and fall. Feeding of hay commonly supplements poor-quality range and pasture in winter (Halls et al., 1964).

RESPONSES TO SEASONAL GRAZING PLANS

Seasonal grazing plans reclaim deteriorated ranges, increase yield of livestock products, facilitate animal husbandry, and improve profits from the business enterprise. No matter how stated and practiced, a period of time without grazing during the growing season allows the palatable species to gain in vigor and produce seed if climate permits, and lets the seedlings become established. If all parts of a range are to be grazed for production and ungrazed for improvement over a period of years, there must be some sort of planned rotation. Actual benefits from rotations have varied, and the above-stated objectives have not always been attained. Few studies and experiments have quantified this entire chain of events from better range to increased profits; yet considerable experience has established that scheduled rotational grazing benefits the range.

Vegetational Response

The most commonly stated benefit of rotated grazing is improved range condition. As nearly all range needs reclamation to some degree, few grazing plans have tried solely on excellent condition ranges. Favorable range responses have been expressed in different terms. In the United States, fewer acres were required per animals (Sarvis, 1923, 1941); the vegetation was maintained with more animals per unit area (Aldous, 1938; Anderson, 1940; Rogler, 1951); plant density increased and proportion of undesirable plants decreased (Hanson et al., 1931; Morris, 1932; Canfield, 1940; Clarke et al., 1943; Paulsen and Ares, 1962; Hickey and Garcia, 1964; Johnson, 1965); climax bunchgrasses increased (Hyder and Sawyer, 1951; Reynolds, 1959); dry weight of carbohydrates increased (Garrison, 1966); and vegetation deteriorated less during drought (Anderson, 1967b; Woolfolk, 1960). In other countries, favorable responses have been reported for the sweet, sour and mixed veld types in South Africa (Fig. 11-11) (Theron et al., 1959; Scott, 1967) and the *Triodia* type in the north of West Australia (Ealey and Suijdendorp, 1959).

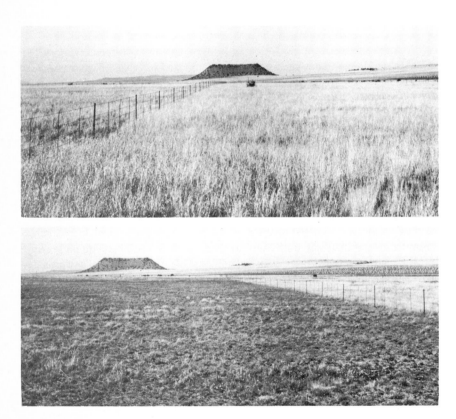

Figure 11-11   These two pastures in South Africa were grazed at the same stocking rate. Dry-season grazing (upper photo) promoted grasses, and wet-season grazing (lower photo) fostered nongrasses.

Ranges improved in many other studies, although the improvement was not reported. Proper before and after measurements may not have been taken, and the investigator may have been reluctant to report general observations. Another reason for cursory vegetational descriptions in grazing trials is that investigators hesitate to predict long-term changes from short-term studies. From an experimental test of grazing plans in Texas, Merrill and Young reported apparent range improvement in 1952. After two more years, Merrill (1954) found an increase in desirable vegetation but no apparent benefit to livestock production. By 1960, Keng and Merrill were able to say that range condition had improved 25 percent more on the deferred-rotation units than on units grazed continuously. After 11 years of the trial, stocking was increased from 32 to 43 animal units per 260 hectares, where it remained for 6 years, until prolonged drought necessitated reduction to the original number (Merrill et al., 1967). Changes in vegetation and production resulting from seasonal rotation of grazing are cumulative. Final evaluations cannot be made after only a few years of treatment.

Some studies do not show vegetational improvement or increased production from intermittent grazing as compared with continuous grazing. This result has been reported in the northern Great Plains (Black and Clark, 1942; Whitman et al., 1943; Hubbard, 1951; Campbell et al., 1962); in the mountains of Wyoming (Smith et al., 1967); in the mountains of eastern Oregon (Skovlin and Harris, 1970); in the sagebrush type (Hyder and Sawyer, 1951; Mueggler, 1950); in southern pine forest grazing (Biswell and Foster, 1947; Biswell, 1951); in cane range of the southeastern United States (Hughes et al., 1960); and in the Mediterranean annual grassland in California (Heady, 1961). Roe et al. (1959) found no significant difference in productivity between continuous and rotation grazing in eastern Australia. Greater range improvement for continuous grazing was reported by Fisher and Marion (1951) in the southern Great Plains. In southern New Mexico, perennial grasses fared best with yearlong grazing and least well under winter grazing (Martin, 1970). After eight years, a study in Texas concluded that *Bouteloua curtipendula* and other key species were affected more by intensity of grazing than by grazing plan (Mathis and Kothmann, 1968). At the Central Plains Experimental Range in Colorado, cattle on short-grass vegetation responded about the same whether they grazed seasonlong or early for three months and late for three months. However, concentration of animals caused early used pastures to suffer losses in herbage production and mechanical damage to plants and soil from trampling (Klipple, 1964).

Of 50 studies reviewed by Driscoll in 1967, 39 analyzed vegetation sufficiently to determine differential responses due to grazing plans. Five studies did not show differential responses due to any grazing schedule. Continuous grazing resulted in 3 instances of better range and 31 of poorer range in comparative tests with all other systems. This majority of tests in favor of seasonal grazing plans indicates that rotation of grazing can be an effective range improvement practice.

Failures suggest that rotational grazing has not been applied properly or should not be used at all in certain situations. Rotational grazing alone rarely suffices. Safe intensity of use and proper distribution of animals may be much more important than season of grazing.

Animal Responses

In the summary of 50 studies mentioned previously, Driscoll (1967) reported that 29 included livestock weight changes in their evaluations of grazing plans. Twelve favored continuous grazing, nine showed no difference among the plans tested, and eight favored some kind of rotational plan. Comparisons among these studies must be subjective, since none were sufficiently alike in vegetational type, design, season of use, degree of use, animals, and management to allow quantitative evaluations. Experiment station results summarized by Driscoll may not accurately state practical results from the use of grazing plans on ranches.

The plan (Fig. 11-6) used by Herbel and Anderson (1959) gave no livestock advantage to the deferred-rotation system, but widespread use of similar plans in the Flint Hills of Kansas indicates that practical values do exist. The rotation sequence on *Agropyron desertorum* (Table 11-1) averaged 1.8 kilograms more beef per hectare annually over an 11-year period than did continuous grazing for the same 60 days of grazing, but this difference was not significant (Frischknecht and Harris, 1968). The rest-rotation plan (Fig. 11-8) yielded more livestock gains from the seasonlong pasture than from the other two grazed pastures during drought (Woolfolk, 1960; Rader, 1961; Ratliff and Rader, 1962). These results are attributable to the overall rest-rotation plan because seasonlong grazing always follows a rest. Therefore forage reserves contributed to the advantage. Six years after drought, average livestock gains for a 13-year trial were about the same in all pasture treatments (U.S. Forest Service, 1968). Contrary to these results, the rest-rotation system has been used widely and successfully in range reclamation and is expected to show increased livestock production.

Highly significant experimental tests with grazing plans were those on the Sonora Experiment Station and the surrounding region of west and central Texas. The commonly used three-herd and four-pasture plan (Fig. 11-7) or a variation of it gave increases in livestock production after several years of tests (Keng and Merrill, 1960). Later work reported that average annual beef production per cow for seven years was 200, 211, and 223 kilograms for continuous, two-pasture, and four-pasture plans, respectively (Stewart and Leinweber, 1968). Calving percentages were higher and weaning weights averaged 9 to 14 kilograms in favor of the four-pasture plan (Waldrip and Marion, 1963; Waldrip and Parker, 1967; Mathis and Kothmann, 1968). The highest population of white-tailed deer occurred on units in this plan which were preiodically ungrazed and moderately grazed by cattle, sheep, and angora goats (Merrill et al., 1957).

For the Mediterranean-type annual grassland in California, Heady (1961) reported that 120-day weights of lambs averaged 35.6 kilograms on the continuously grazed treatment and 32.2 kilograms on the deferred-rotation pasture. Wool and lamb production was reported greater from continuous grazing than from rotation grazing in a New Zealand study (Suckling, 1965). Cattle grazing in a rotation schedule on subalpine summer range in Wyoming gained no more than those continuously using similar areas (Smith et al., 1967). A two-year rotation of grazing and no-grazing during the growing season in semidesert grass-shrub ranges in Arizona permitted a 50 percent increase in stocking after seven years (Martin, 1966). Wool production increased over 363 grams per head and sheep numbers were up by 65 percent after four years with a five-unit rotation at three-month intervals in rangelands of western Australia (Ealey and Suijdendorp, 1959). After 24 years of testing, a four-pasture deferred-rotation plan in South Africa averaged 23.3 kilograms of beef per hectare more than a rotational grazing plan and 27.9 kilograms more than a continuous grazing plan. The rotational plan included one pasture rested for a year and three grazed in rotation (Malherbe, 1963).

Animal responses to seasonal rotation plans and to continuous grazing have varied from highly significant results in favor of one plan to little difference at all. Reasons for these differences are discussed later in this chapter. On balance, the bulk of data and practical experience indicates an advantage, in many vegetational types, to grazing them in a rotational plan (Fig. 11-12). Annual grasslands and short-grass regions appear to be exceptions (Shiflet and Heady, 1971).

Responses in Economic Terms

Few grazing plans in experimental tests and practical use have been subjected to economic analysis. If specialized grazing schedules are to be adopted by ranch

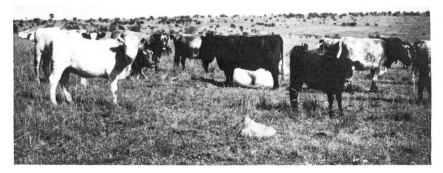

Figure 11-12 Shorthorns on "Tukulu" in South Africa. This 800-hectare ranch has been in a deferred-rotation plan of grazing since 1928. It has 28 pastures and 35 watering points.

operators, they must produce additional products or services that bring in income greater than the costs of installation not covered in improved capital values, maintenance, and management.

Current grazing capacity and its expected increase limit the intensity of development. Fence, for example as a per hectare cost, is less likely to justify small pastures than large ones where productivity is low. Ranchers in the southern Great Plains do not use deferred-rotation plans because they claim that the cost-benefit ratio is unfavorable (McIlvain and Shoop, 1969). In areas where labor costs and capital investments in fence and water development are high, seasonal grazing plans must yield high returns. In countries where labor costs are low, returns from grazing plans on many small range pastures are more likely to be profitable.

An analysis of 100 randomly selected ranches on the Edwards Plateau of Texas showed that 52 could install a three-herd and four-pasture plan without additional fencing and that 22 more could adopt a seasonal plan by building less than 2.2 kilometers of fence (Keng and Merrill, 1960). Costs of additional fencing and water developments should not be incurred until inventory and analysis demonstrate the need in an overall management program. Perhaps more ranches could institute grazing plans with little added cost. Better distribution of grazing and efficient handling of animals are other development values that may be important enough to justify improvement expenses. Although seasonal grazing plans require control of livestock with fences and water, these improvements do not require rotational grazing to be of value. Leithead (1960) reports a range improvement program (deferred grazing included) that increased net returns per hectare from ten cents to $2.05 in 11 years.

At Throckmorton in north central Texas, a three-herd and four-pasture plan yielded $1.60 greater annual return per hectare than did continuous grazing for a period of seven years (Stewart and Leinweber, 1968). In a later report, the added return had increased to $1.93 per hectare. Various seasonal grazing plans had little effect on total operational costs at the same stocking rate (Kothmann et al., 1971). On short-grass range at Barnhart, Texas, a three-herd and four-pasture plan averaged 83 cents more per hectare per year and a two-pasture switchback plan $1.09 more per hectare per year than did continuous grazing over a six-year period (Huss and Allen, 1969).

The rest-rotation grazing trial at Harvey Valley in northeastern California between 1954 and 1966 cost the Forest Service 28 percent and the permittee nine percent more than did seasonlong grazing on nearby allotments. Added costs amounted to 34 cents per AUM for a 30-year payoff period. The payoff period may be shorter now because range condition has improved, and a 10 percent increase in stocking rate was granted in 1967 (Ratliff et al., 1972).

Hubbard (1951) in western Canada wrote that expected benefits of the deferred-rotation plan would not be sufficient to offset the increased costs of fencing and water development. Along the Gulf Coast (Duvall and Whitaker,

1964), a rotation system of burning has resulted in a rotation system of grazing without the costs of increased fencing and water development since livestock favor newly burned areas. Although the burning entails some expense, it is required for maintainence of high-quality feed. Many practical successes with seasonal grazing plans—few of them analyzed in economic terms—indicate that they do yield favorable returns.

Other Benefits From Grazing Plans

Invariably, a benefit derived from seasonal grazing is better husbandry of the animals. A person with enough interest and concern about his range to initiate scheduled grazing also takes added interest in animal health, adequate feed quality, breeding, and daily care of animals. With smaller pastures, livestock are not so scattered and therefore are easier to see, gradually become tame, and are easier to catch than animals in large pastures. Pride in the whole operation increases. A well-managed grazing plan usually means a well-managed ranch.

Grazing plans serve as aids in the education of better managers. Planning a grazing schedule must, of necessity, consider the management of the whole ranch. Alternative range improvements must be studied and selected. Usually a whole range improvement program results. The popularity of grazing plans has aroused interest and activity in other range practices. Benefits from whole programs are sometimes inaccurately attributed to rotation plans.

Seasonal grazing schedules, which bunch animals into a few pastures and leave other pastures ungrazed for a time, aid establishment of rangeland improvements that require no interference from livestock. A rested pasture presents an ideal situation for brush control and seeding since the rest provides protection to new seedlings. Through much of the tropical and subtropical savannah areas, periodic burning reduces brush. A rest or deferred treatment promotes accumulation of sufficient fuel for that burning to be effective. In fact, any range improvement program that stipulates periodic burning for plant control also requires controlled grazing before and after the fire. Not all accumulations of herbage are desirable because they can increase hazards from wildfire. Sprouting of brush species after control may be discouraged with a rotation of goats.

Fire is used in coarse grasslands to remove the rough, standing dead material and to improve feed quality, as in Rhodesia (West, 1958), in Australia (Ealey and Suijdendorp, 1959), and in the marshes of the southeastern United States (Shiflet, 1966). In these situations, standing dead material accumulates with any type of grazing program. Rotational grazing prevents overuse of newly burned grasslands where animals congregate on the young, palatable plants.

More and more rangeland will be used to produce game animals for profit or strictly for their values to a sightseeing public, as on the National Bison Range in western Montana (Fig. 11-13). Seasonal plans that concentrate wild or semiwild

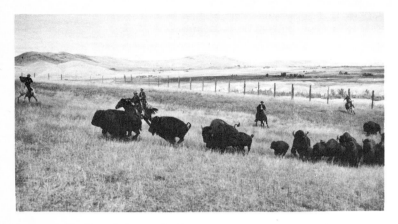

Figure 11-13 Bison being coralled for culling, health inspection, etc., and changed to a new pasture, National Bison Range. *(Photo by Fish and Wildlife Service.)*

animals in certain pastures make them easier to see, hunt, and harvest. Wild animal species in game farming can be kept separately and moved from one pasture to another in rotation. Separation facilitates harvesting, handling, and controls use by several species.

OPERATION OF SEASONAL GRAZING PLANS

Responses from seasonal grazing plans ranging from highly favorable to highly unfavorable defy adequate explanation. An individual failure may result from one mistake, but a single cause or even a few causes do not cover all failures. Plans require skill and continuous care on the part of the manager. One man may fail with a good plan for biological reasons, while another profits. The fact that one plan is successful on a particular ranch is no guarantee that it can be applied on the neighboring ranch and on different vegetational types. Ideal schedules are built and used for specific situations that include the whole enterprise and its management in the broadest sense. An effort to fit each plan to the individual ranch is essential, but criteria for doing so remain inadequate. The following sections attempt to analyze current practice, problems, and needs in the operation of grazing plans.

Uniformity of Area

Successful rotational plans, for the most part, have been those situated where every pasture had about the same set of conditions. In addition, having relatively level land facilitates an operation. North- and south-facing slopes where the vegetation is greatly different, say, forest and grassland, should be grazed as separate units. Steep slopes restrict livestock movement differentially according to season, cause variation in use pattern, and hinder application of rotational grazing. Probably, no pasture unit should include more than 200 meters of elevation because of the differential in growing season and range readiness. The preceding examples are illustrations of locational problems encountered with seasonal rotation of grazing. These problems should be met with combinations of different grazing plans.

Ideally, every pasture in a plan should be capable of being grazed during any part of the grazing season and as efficiently as any other pasture. This ideal situation requires similarity in topography, seasonal or altitudinal development of vegetation, slope aspect, approximate size and shape, water availability, accessiblity, safety of animals from poisonous plants and predators, and forage production. Few sets of pastures are ideal, but many can be improved with careful attention to fencing. Generally, as pastures are made smaller, their internal uniformity improves and their management becomes easier.

Change in Range Condition

Vegetational type, seasonal readiness, and range condition are important considerations in the design of pasture boundaries and grazing schedules. Not only should the pastures be alike at the beginning of the plan, but they also should remain alike. If they do not, the grazing schedule will need to be changed. Many specialized seasonal grazing plans are justified and started for range reclamation purposes. As range condition improves, the forage resource changes in botanical composition, seasonality, feed quality, and quantity. Presumably the stocking rate can increase, and likely the most efficient harvesting schedule will differ from the original reclamation plan. However, little published information is available on this point because few ranges have had full improvement coincidence with appropriate studies.

Rest Versus Yearly Grazing

A difference between plans that employ rest periods and those with deferred pastures is whether forage is harvested after plant maturity (Fig. 11-14). The principle question is: Does grazing deferred pastures after plant maturity produce greater benefits than leaving them ungrazed for the whole 12 months? Grazing, as an ageless process in the evolution of grassland ecosystems, probably left no area ungrazed for a complete cycle of seasons, so quite possibly, grasslands respond more rapidly with grazing after seed production than with no grazing at that time. Animals scatter seeds, plant them by trampling, reduce the dead standing material, and loosen soil crusts—conditions widely accepted as desirable because they promote the next forage crop and long-term range improvement.

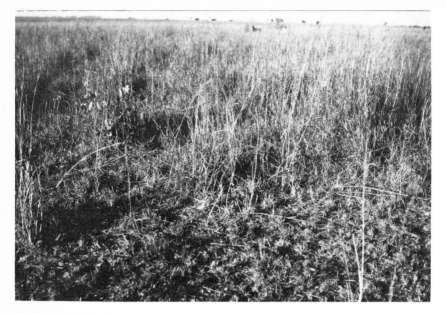

Figure 11-14 Mixed species that have extremes of palatability often show both heavy and light use, as in this example of Rhodesian grasslands, after the first dry-season grazing.

Rest-rotation grazing exploits the principle of a full year without grazing. Most other plans include shorter ungrazed periods, many not even qualifying as deferred grazing, and still improve the range. Except for specific purposes, such as providing fuel for prescribed burning, resting of range pastures seems an extravagant use of herbage.

Number of Pastures and Herds

The number of pastures in grazing plans varies from one used continuously to as many as 20 in the southern African short-duration grazing plan. Booysen (1969) showed that the proportion of time a pasture is ungrazed increases as the number of pastures increase. Thus, using two pastures gives one-half, using three gives two-thirds, and using four gives three-quarters of the rotation time without animals in each pasture. If a tenth pasture were added, each pasture would gain 1.12 percent in ungrazed time. Booysen suggested that using more than approximately six to eight pastures provides little additional relief from grazing. A two-herd plan requires twice as many pastures to attain the same proportion of ungrazed time as does a one-herd plan.

Successes and failures result from plans with a wide range of pasture numbers. This fact suggests that proportion of time livestock are absent is not a sensitive measure of effectiveness. For example, several studies have shown advantages for single-pasture plans (West, 1958; Smoliak, 1960; Heady, 1961; U.S. Forest Service, 1968; Murray and Klemmedson, 1968). The 3-herd and 4-pasture plan has shown great success with livestock grazing every pasture for a year or 75 percent of the rotation time in contrast to a 16-pasture short-duration plan that has livestock in any one pasture for 6.25 percent of the whole rotation. Vegetation probably responds to other factors, most likely the phenological timing of the relief from grazing and the intensity of utilization, rather than simply to pasture numbers. A major factor in determining number of pastures is that flexibility in operation improves and the need for constant care increases as more pastures are added.

Simplicity and Flexibility

All grazing plans should be simple. For ranchers to accept them, they must be understandable during the initial phases. Always, a simple operation results in fewer mistakes. Mostert and Donaldson (1959) wrote that farmers in South Africa have not widely accepted grazing plans because they cannot interpret and follow their specifications.

As Hedrick (1958) stated, the real success of any plan lies in its flexibility. Nearly all written plans and published descriptions show calendar dates when livestock are to be moved. Such specifications simplify the recipe but result in inflexibility. Seasonal development of vegetation varies by a month or more in nearly all range types. The key to livestock movement should be such conditions as enough soil moisture to permit regrowth and seed production by the key species or sufficiently dry soil to prevent trampling damage. Critical phenological stages for both grazing and relief from grazing are not well documented, but early use can be tolerated if relief is given later.

Experimental tests of grazing plans have tended to use fixed dates, or at least less flexibility than is common in rancher-used schedules. This inflexibility may contribute to the higher proportion of unfavorable results in experiments than in practice. Recognition by the manager that the phenology of plant growth requires flexibility in operation of grazing plans will help him to use rotation schedules successfully. Ranchers in South Africa reported that inflexibility in adjusting to fluctuating feed supplies causes most failures with grazing schedules (Roberts, 1970).

Phenology of Plant Damage and Response

Effective grazing plans need to include one or more periods of livestock absence at a time when relief from grazing does the most good. A period without grazing is not necessarily beneficial if plants do not grow because of cold or lack of moisture or if the period is too short.

Periods without grazing have different purposes when they occur at different stages in the growth cycle. The first critical period is the time plants are drawing on reserves, either immediately after winter dormancy or after any severe defoliation. Absence of grazing at those times fosters restoration of energy levels and enlargement of parts such as roots and leaves for absorbing nutrients and crowns for producing more stems. Seedling establishment also is promoted.

The second period begins when buds of grasses start to elevate and ends at seed maturity. It permits completion of seed production. The third period for perennials allows storage of energy that will be used during dormancy and initial growth thereafter.

These periods span the entire growth period. The timing and frequency of nongrazing, therefore, has value throughout the growing season and changes in relation to the type of response most needed. Vigorous plants on excellent range may require only proper use while depleted range needs several periods of protection from grazing.

The response of plant species to a single defoliation varies from stimulation of branching and increased production to near death. Growth may be little different through the growing season with light defoliations in one species but greatly reduced with clipping on a certain day or week in another species. Seasonal responses to defoliation in this context are unknown for many key range plant species, but they are known for some species. *Agropyron spicatum* is an example of one species with a short period during which harm by defoliation occurs (Heady, 1950). Severe defoliation at any time during the growing season and after seed was ripe reduced *Festuca idahoensis* (Hormay and Talbot, 1961). Other species that seem not to be damaged more at one time than another include *Phalaris tuberosa* and *Agropyron desertorum*.

If a grazing plan is to do the least damage to any species, it requires an ungrazed period during the times of greatest potential damage by grazing. But livestock must be somewhere every day; therefore one or more pastures will be grazed at the time of most harm. The grazing plan, then, should be constructed to emphasize the least damage during the time when grazing does the most harm. This may require the animals to be widely spread, perhaps evenly in all pastures or in all but one. Another approach requires that animals move at short intervals from one pasture to the next, before they graze any species closely.

One normally would conclude that the time when relief from grazing does the most good would be the time when grazing is most harmful. This is not necessarily true. Early-growing-season relief and later heavy grazing may be used to encourage early-growing species. Although grasses may be damaged by heavy grazing, sprouting brush species may need heavy use to reduce them. Increasingly, successful grazing plans will encompass both the harmful and beneficial effects of grazing and relief from grazing to produce the desired vegetational resource.

Criteria for Moving Animals

When livestock are moved in a grazing plan, the manager needs specifications or criteria for stopping grazing in one pasture and beginning it in another. Many managers use the condition of animals as the criterion, but using this criterion implies accepting the presumption that changes in range condition and in animals occur at the same time and rate, which they seldom do. Animals respond quickly to lack of feed and to lack of high-quality feed. Also, they may be gaining weight or maintaining condition on seeds and fruits when the vegetation itself is being harmed or, conversely, animals may be losing condition and the pasture may be receiving little harm. Animal weight losses during dry-season grazing on excellent range almost everywhere in the world amply show that animal condition is a poor indicator of trend in range condition. The lack of animal fill and the first signs of drop in animal condition indicate that the ideal time to move animals to another pasture has passed. An advantage of continuous grazing is that quality of the forage being eaten changes little from day to day. Rotations often result in wide variation in feed quality which causes digestive upsets in animals when they are placed in a fresh, succulent pasture.

Many grazing schedules operate with considerable dependence upon calendar dates. Examples include the opening and closing dates for grazing on national forests and public domain lands in the western United States and the short-duration grazing schemes in southern Africa, where a common recommendation has been to graze 20 pastures for 3 days each in a 60-day cycle that is repeated 6 times a year. More emphasis is placed on the 60 days than on the number of pastures although no pasture should be grazed longer than 2 weeks in any one cycle. While, for planning purposes, certain dependence on dates cannot be avoided, they should be considered only as guidelines. The same point in the growth curve of plants may vary by over a month or more among years. With constant animal numbers, three days or any fixed time per pasture could result in overuse during early growth and underuse later. Cycles of any fixed length would appear to have little justification when plant growth fails to occur before the rotation repeats, and more than one grazing cycle on dormant vegetation appears to be especially futile.

Ideally, the first factor in determining the time for livestock to leave a pasture should be the degree of herbage use. Criteria include stubble heights of palatable and unpalatable species, roughness in appearance of the range utilization, amounts of mulch, and hedging of shrubs.

Termination of grazing at the right time prevents damage to the pasture or the least harm by animals in large numbers on a small area. Chances of overuse are greater with high than with low stocking densities and with short terms of grazing. For example, a mistake of a day is four times more crucial when all the forage is to be harvested in a week than when grazing is spread over a month. Small pastures and rapid rotations require constant and informed attention. Several pastures may be grazed concurrently as a unit, so that daily grazing pressure is reduced during critical times.

When animals are to be moved, the manager must select a receiving pasture. Based on the assumption that every pasture has had new growth since it was last grazed, it would seem reasonable to graze the pasture that had the longest ungrazed period. During the first rotation in a growing season, all ungrazed pastures ahead in the rotation will have had the same time for new growth. Due to differences in site and range condition, the pasture with most growth or the one best suited for grazing may not be the one with the longest relief period. With numerous pastures in a plan, the one receiving the animals at each move should be the one that best combines livestock production and grazing without damage. The result is a different order of grazing in each rotation. For example, in a plan with ten pastures, all might be used for four days each during early growth, only six grazed on a weekly basis during the second rotation, and all ten grazed until the forage is properly harvested during the late growth and dry season. This flexibility permits the manager to favor any pasture he chooses at any time. Herein lies one of his principal tools for range improvement with a schedule of grazing. Removing livestock from a pasture at the right time reduces damage. Initiating grazing at the right time for each pasture fosters improvement in condition and productivity for all pastures in the plan.

The Ideal Length of Grazing Period

If one considers that other things are equal and that enough animals are available to graze a pasture properly in a day, a week, a month, or a season, what is the proper length of grazing period? Pasture workers have recommended as short a period as possible. Many dairy herds are operated with half a day or, at most, only a few days, of grazing in a pasture. Few authors have recommended grazing periods of less than two weeks in range situations except in southern Africa, where two weeks is a maximum in the multipasture plans being used here. The rationale for short grazing periods is, first, to gain utilization of poor-quality material (stems) along with high-quality feed (leaves) with short periods of heavy use. Second, animals are moved to ungrazed pastures before they have a chance to graze regrowth, on the proposition that plants are damaged if new growth is grazed as soon as it appears. Short rotations seem best for those forage species that recover rapidly after defoliation, produce more vegetative growth than reproductive stems, and mature slowly.

The ideal length of grazing period implies removal of the grazable herbage within a specified length of time that obtains most efficient use of the feed and at the same time does least damage to the vegetation. Whether the period is long or short, harvesting the forage from each plant requires several bites, except during the early growth period. If repeated bites in a short period of time are better than repeated bites in a long period remains to be determined. Probably the most important consideration is whether or not new culm apices are grazed.

The Ideal Time Span without Grazing

A recommendation for the length of period without grazing cannot be made with the certainty that the length is ideal. Relief from grazing permits plants to grow, to regain any vigor lost during grazing, to produce seed, to allow for seedling establishment, and to promote improvement in range condition. These functions may require different time periods. In actual practice, the length of period without grazing has been as short as three or four weeks or longer than a year. Many, but not all, schemes in southern Africa use short periods; in East Africa, which has two growing seasons per year, one season usually is a time without grazing. Some of the plans employed in the western United States call for no grazing during one year and a part of the next. One approach has been to shorten the grazed and ungrazed periods as much as possible. Another has been to lengthen both periods. These approaches have produced successes and failures.

Many key range plants extend their stems, flower, and produce seed in a short time. Such a growth period is the key time for relief from grazing. Longer periods, such as rests and growing-season deferments, always include the whole growth cycle. Successes with short relief periods for different purposes (vigor, seedling establishment) logically suggest that longer relief periods are not essential. Apparently, grazing during the dormant season does little harm. This idea is not universally accepted, however, and there is a trend toward increasing use of dormant-season relief periods.

NEEDED RESEARCH

Six propositions: (1) time of most harm by grazing; (2) time of most improvement without grazing; (3) criteria for leaving a pasture; (4) criteria for entering a pasture; (5) ideal timing, length, and frequency of grazing period; (6) ideal timing, length, and frequency of period without grazing, point to the main unanswered problems about grazing plans. These propositions phrased as questions should be studied as main effects and as interactions in experimentation with grazing plans. Such work will yield information on fundamentals that underlie grazing plans. If that knowledge were available for a vegetational type, the chances of designing a workable schedule for grazing it would improve. So much of the past work with grazing plans has been ineffective due to emphasis on a few of several hundred possible permutations of schedules rather than on determination of principles underlying the effects of seasonal grazing.

LITERATURE CITED

Acocks, J. P. H. 1966. Non-selective grazing as a means of veld reclamation. *Proc. Grassland Soc. S. Afr.* 1:33–39.

Aldous, A. E. 1938. Management of Kansas bluestem pastures. *J. Am. Soc. Agron.* 30:244–253.

Anderson, E. W. 1967a. Rotation of deferred grazing. *J. Range Mgmt.* 20:5–7.

————. 1967b. Grazing systems as methods of managing the range resources. *J. Range Mgmt.* 20:383–388.

Anderson, K. L. 1940. Deferred grazing of bluestem pastures. *Kan. Agr. Expt. Sta. Bull.* 291.

Biswell, H. H. 1951. Studies of rotation grazing in the Southeast. *J. Range Mgmt.* 4:52–55.

————, and J. E. Foster. 1947. Is rotational grazing on native range practical? *N.C. Agr. Expt. Sta. Bull.* 360.

Black, W. H., and V. I. Clark. 1942. Yearlong grazing of steers in the northern Great Plains. *U.S. Dept. Agr. Cir.* 642.

Booysen, P. de V. 1967. Grazing and grazing management terminology in southern Africa. *Proc. Grassland Soc. S. Afr.* 2:45–57.

————. 1969. An analysis of the fundamentals of grazing management systems. *Proc. Grassland Soc. S. Afr.* 4:84–91.

Campbell, J. B. 1961. Continuous versus repeated-seasonal grazing of grass-alfalfa mixtures at Swift Current, Saskatchewan. *J. Range Mgmt.* 14:72–77.

————. 1963. Grass-alfalfa versus grass-alone pastures grazed in a repeated-seasonal pattern. *J. Range Mgmt.* 16:78–81.

————, R. W. Lodge, A. Johnston, and S. Smoliak. 1962. Range management of grasslands and adjacent parklands in the Prairie Provinces. *Can. Dept. Agr. Res. Branch Pub.* 1132.

Canfield, R. H. 1940. Semideferred grazing as a restorative measure for black grama ranges. *S.W. For. and Range Expt. Sta. Note* 80.

Caputa, J. 1968. Influence of time of the first cut on regrowth of natural grassland. *Agr. Romande* 7:38–43.

Clarke, S. E., and E. W. Tisdale. 1936. Range pasture studies in southern Alberta and Saskatchewan. *Herb. Rev.* 4:51–64.

————, ————, and N. A. Skoglund. 1943. The effects of climate and grazing practices on short-grass prairie vegetation in southern Alberta and southwestern Saskatchewan. *Can. Dept. Agr. Tech. Bull.* 46.

Driscoll, R. S. 1967. Managing public rangelands: Effective livestock grazing practices and systems for national forests and national grasslands. *U.S. Dept. Agr.* AIB-315.

Duncan, D. A., and H. F. Heady. 1969. Grazing systems in the California annual type. *Abstracts of the 22nd Annual Meeting, American Society of Range Mgmt.*, pp. 23–24.

Duvall, V. L. 1969. Grazing systems for pine forest ranges in the South. *Abstracts of the 22nd Annual Meeting, American Society of Range Mgmt.*, p. 23.

————, and L. B. Whitaker. 1964. Rotation burning: A forage management system for longleaf pine-bluestem ranges. *J. Range Mgmt.* 17:322–326.

Ealey, E. H. M., and H. Suijdendorp. 1959. Pasture management and the euro problem in the North-West. *J. Agr. W. Aust.* 8:273–286.

Fisher, C. E., and P. T. Marion. 1951. Continuous and rotation grazing on buffalo and tobosa grassland. *J. Range Mgmt.* 4:48–51.

Frischknecht, N. C., and L. E. Harris. 1968. Grazing intensities and systems on crested wheatgrass in central Utah: Response of vegetation and cattle. *U.S. Dept. Agr. Tech. Bull.* 1388.

Garrison, G. A. 1966. A preliminary study of response of plant reserves to systems and intensities of grazing on mountain rangeland in northwest U.S.A. *Proceedings of the 10th International Grassland Congress,* pp. 937–940.

Goodloe, S. 1969. Short duration grazing in Rhodesia. *J. Range Mgmt.* 22:369–373.

Halls, L. K., R. H. Hughes, R. S. Rummell, and B. L. Southwell. 1964. Forage and cattle management in longleaf-slash pine forests. *U.S. Dept. Agr. Farmers' Bull.* 2199.

Hanson, H. C., L. D. Love, and M. S. Morris. 1931. Effects of different systems of grazing by cattle upon western wheatgrass type of range near Fort Collins, Colorado. *Colo. Agr. Expt. Sta. Bull.* 377.

Heady, H. F. 1950. Studies on bluebunch wheatgrass in Montana and height-weight relationships of certain range grasses. *Ecol. Monog.* 20:55–81.

———. 1961. Continuous vs. specialized grazing systems: A review and application to the California annual type. *J. Range Mgmt.* 14:182–193.

———. 1970. Grazing systems: Terms and definitions. *J. Range Mgmt.* 23:59–61.

———, R. T. Clark, and T. Lommasson. 1947. Range management and sheep production in the Bridger Mountains, Montana. *Mont. Agr. Expt. Sta Bull.* 444.

Hedrick, D. W. 1958. Proper utilization—a problem in evaluating the physiological response of plants to grazing use: A review. *J. Range Mgmt.* 11:34–43.

Herbel, C. H., and K. L. Anderson. 1959. Response of true prairie vegetation on major Flint Hills range sites to grazing treatment. *Ecol. Monog.* 29:171–186.

———, and A. B. Nelson. 1969. Grazing management on semidesert ranges in southern New Mexico. *Jornada Exp. Range Rep.* 1.

Hickey, W. C., and G. Garcia. 1964. Changes in perennial grass cover following conversion from yearlong to summer-deferred grazing in west central New Mexico. *U.S. Dept. Agr. Forest Service Research. Note* RM-33.

Hormay, A. L. 1970. Principles of rest-rotation grazing and multiple-use land management. *U.S. Dept. Agr. Forest Service Training Text* 4 (2200).

———, and M. W. Talbot. 1961. Rest-rotation grazing—A new management system for perrennial bunchgrass ranges. *U.S. Dept. Agr. Prod. Research Rep.* 51.

Howell, Denise. 1967. The rules of non-selective grazing. *S. Afr. Farmer's Weekly,* July 12, pp. 24–25.

Hubbard, W. A. 1951. Rotational grazing studies in western Canada. *J. Range Mgmt.* 4:25–29.

Hughes, R. H., E. U. Dillard, and J. B. Hilmon. 1960. Vegetation and cattle response under two systems of grazing cane range in North Carolina. *N.C. Agr. Expt. Sta. Bull.* 412.

Hugo, W. J. 1968. *The small stock industry in South Africa.* Dept. Agr. Tech. Services.

Hurtt, L. C. 1951. Managing northern Great Plains cattle ranges to minimize effects of drought. *U.S. Dept. Agr. Cir.* 865.

Huss, D. L., and J. V. Allen. 1969. Livestock production and profitability comparisons of various grazing systems, Texas Range Station. *Tex. Agr. Expt. Sta. Bull.* B-1089.

Hyder, D. N., and W. A. Sawyer. 1951. Rotation-deferred grazing as compared to seasonlong grazing on sagebrush-bunchgrass rages in Oregon. *J. Range Mgmt.* 4:30–34.

Jagtenberg, W. D. 1970. Predicting the best time to apply nitrogen to grassland in spring. *J. Br. Grassland Soc.* 25:266–271.

Jardine, J. T. 1915. Improvement and management of native pastures in the West. *U.S. Dept. Agr. Yearbook,* pp. 299–310.

———, and M. Anderson. 1919. Range management on the National Forests. *U.S. Dept. Agr. Bull.* 790.

Johnson, W. M. 1965. Rotation, rest-rotation, and season-long grazing on a mountain range in Wyoming. *U.S. Dept. Agr. Forest Service Research Paper.* RM-14.

Keng, E. B., and L. B. Merrill. 1960. Deferred rotation grazing does pay dividends. *Sheep and Goat Raiser* 40:12–14.

Klipple, G. E. 1964. Early- and late-season grazing versus season-long grazing of short-grass vegetation on the central Great Plains. *U.S. Dept. Agr. Forest Service Research Paper.* RM-11.

Kothmann, M. M., G. W. Mathis, and W. J. Waldrip. 1971. Cow-calf response to stocking rates and grazing systems on native range. *J. Range Mgmt.* 24:100–105.

Leithead, H. L. 1960. Grass management pays big dividends. *J. Range Mgmt.* 13:206–210.

Lodge, R. W. 1963. Complementary grazing systems for sandhills of the northern Great Plains. *J. Range Mgmt.* 16:240–244.

———. 1970. Complementary grazing systems for the northern Great Plains. *J. Range Mgmt.* 23:268–271.

———, S. Smoliak, and A. Johnston. 1972. Managing crested wheatgrass pastures. *Can. Dept. Agr. Pub.* 1473.

Malherbe, C. E. 1963. Sound systems of veld management give good results in the sourveld. *Farming in S. Afr.* 39(7):81–85.

Martin, S. C. 1966. The Santa Rita Experimental Range. *U.S. Dept. Agr. Forest Service Research Paper.* RM-22.

———. 1970. Vegetation changes on semi-desert range during 10 years of summer, winter, and year-long grazing by cattle. *Proceedings of the 11th International Grassland Congress,* pp. 23–26.

Mathis, G. W., and M. M. Kothmann. 1968. Response of native range grasses to systems of grazing and grazing intensity. *Tex. Agr. Expt. Sta. Consolidated Progr. Rep.* 2616-2626:21–23.

Matthews, L. H. 1954. The migration of mammals. *Smithsonian Inst. Pub.* 4190:277–284.

McIlvain, E. H., and M. C. Shoop. 1969. Grazing systems in the southern Great Plains. *Abstracts of the 22nd Annual Meeting, American Society of Range Management,* pp. 21–22.

Merrill, L. B. 1954. A variation of deferred rotation grazing for use under Southwest range conditions. *J. Range Mgmt.* 7:152–154.

———, P. O. Reardon, W. T. Hardy, C. L. Leinweber, and E. B. Keng. 1967. The influence of grazing management systems on vegetation composition and livestock reaction. In *Progress in range research, 17 western states, 1965,* pp. 141–142. U.S. Dept. Agr. Coop. State Res. Service.

————, J. G. Teer, and O. C. Wallmo. 1957. Reaction of deer populations to grazing practices. *Tex. Agr. Progr.* 3:10–12.

————, and V. A. Young. 1952. Range management studies on the Ranch Experiment Station. *Tex. Agr. Expt. Sta. Progr. Rep.* 1449.

Miller, H. W., A. L. Hafenrichter, and O. K. Hoglund. 1957. The influence of management methods on seedings of perennials in the annual range area. *J. Range Mgmt.* 10:62–66.

Morris, M. S. 1932. Can we improve our range? *Colo. Agr. Expt. Sta. Bull.* 313-A.

Mostert, J. W. C., and C. H. Donaldson. 1959. Rest periods for natural veld essential. *Farming in S. Afr.* 35(4):10–13.

Mueggler, W. F. 1950. Effects of spring and fall grazing by sheep on vegetation of the upper Snake River Plains. *J. Range Mgmt.* 3:308–315.

Murray, R. B., and J. O. Klemmedson. 1968. Cheatgrass range in southern Idaho: Seasonal cattle gains and grazing capacities. *J. Range Mgmt.* 21:308–313.

Paulsen, H. A., and F. N. Ares. 1962. Grazing values and management of black grama and tobosa grasslands and associated shrub ranges of the Southwest. *U.S. Dept. Agr. Tech. Bull.* 1270.

Rader, L. 1961. Grazing management pays on perennial grass range during drought. *Pacific Southwest For. and Range Expt. Sta. Research Note* 179.

Range Term Glossary Committee. 1964. *A glossary of terms used in range management.* Denver: American Society of Range Management.

Ratliff, R. D., and L. Rader. 1962. Drought hurts less with rest-rotation management. *Pacific Southwest For. and Range Expt. Sta. Research Note* 196.

————, J. N. Reppert, and R. J. McConnen. 1972. Rest-rotation at Harvey Valley—Range health, cattle gains, costs. *U.S. Dept. Agr. Forest Service Research Paper* PSW-77.

Reynolds, H. G. 1959. Managing grass-shrub cattle ranges in the Southwest. *U.S. Dept. Agr. Forest Service,* Agr. HB 162.

Roberts, B. R. 1970. The multi-camp controversy—A search for evidence. *S. Afr. Farmer's Weekly,* Jan. 14, pp. 30–31, 33, 35, 37.

Roe, R., W. H. Southcott, and Helen N. Turner. 1959. Grazing management of native pastures in the New England region of New South Wales. I. Pasture and sheep production with special reference to systems of grazing and internal parasites. *Aust. J. Agr. Res.* 10:530–554.

Rogler, G. A. 1951. A twenty-five year comparison of continuous and rotation grazing in the Northern Plains. *J. Range Mgmt.* 4:35–41.

Roux, P. W. 1968. Non-selective grazing. *S. Afr. Farmer's Weekly,* Dec. 4, pp. 32–33, 35, 37.

————, and T. E. Skinner. 1970. The group-camp system. *Farming in S. Afr.* 45(10):25–28.

Sampson, A. W. 1913. Range improvement by deferred and rotation grazing. *U.S. Dept. Agr. Bull.* 34.

————. 1914. Natural revegetation of range lands based upon growth requirements and life history of the vegetation. *J. Agr. Res.* 3:93–147.

————. 1951. A symposium on rotation grazing in North America. *J. Range Mgmt.* 4:19–24.

Sarvis, J. T. 1923. Effects of different systems and intensities of grazing upon native vegetation at the Northern Great Plains Field Station. *U.S. Dept. Agr. Bull.* 1170.

———. 1941. Grazing investigations on the northern Great Plains. *N. Dak. Agr. Expt. Sta. Bull.* 308.

Scott, J. D. 1967. Advances in pasture work in South Africa. Part I. Veld. *Herb. Abst.* 37:1–9.

Sharp, L. A. 1970. Suggested management programs for grazing crested wheatgrass. *Univ. of Idaho Col. of For. Wildl. and Range Sci. Bull.* 4.

Shiflet, T. N. 1966. Louisiana cattle drive enables ranchers to use forage in season. *Soil Cons.* 32:15–17.

———, and H. F. Heady. 1971. Specialized grazing systems: Their place in range management. *U.S. Dept. Agr.* SCS-TP-152.

Skoog, R. D. 1968. *Ecology of the caribou* (Rangifer tarandus granti) *in Alaska.* PhD. dissertation, Univ. of Calif.

Skovlin, J. M., and R. W. Harris. 1970. Management of conifer woodland grazing resources for cattle, deer, and elk. *Proceedings of the 11th International Grassland Congress,* pp. 75–78.

Smith, D. R., H. G. Fisser, N. Jefferies, and P. O. Stratton. 1967. Rotation grazing on Wyoming's Big Horn Mountains. *Wyo. Agr. Expt. Sta. Res. J.* 13.

Smith, J. G. 1895. Forage conditions of the prairie region. *U.S. Dept. Agr. Yearbook,* pp. 309–324.

Smoliak, S. 1960. Effects of deferred-rotation and continuous grazing on yearling steer gains and shortgrass prairie vegetation in southeastern Alberta. *J. Range Mgmt.* 13:239–243.

———. 1968. Grazing studies on native range, crested wheatgrass and Russian wildrye pastures. *J. Range Mgmt.* 21:47–50.

Stewart, J. R., and C. L. Leinweber. 1968. An economic evaluation of range improvement and grazing practices, Texas Experimental Ranch. *Tex. Agr. Expt. Sta. Consolidated Progr. Rep.* 2583-2609:25–27.

Suckling, F. E. T. 1965. *Hill pasture improvement.* N. Z. Dept. Sci. Ind. Res.

Talbot, L. M., and M. H. Talbot. 1963. The wildebeest in western Masailand, East Africa. *Wildl. Monog.* 12:1–88.

Theron, E. P., A. D. Venter, and R. I. Jones. 1959. Four-camp system not always solution to problem of selective grazing. *Farming in S. Afr.* 35(2):6–10.

U.S. Forest Service. 1968. 1967 forestry research. *Pacific Southwest For. and Range Expt. Sta. Annual Rep.*

Valentine, K. A. 1967. Seasonal suitablity, a grazing system for ranges of diverse vegetation types and condition classes. *J. Range Mgmt.* 20:395–397.

Waldrip, W. J., and P. T. Marion. 1963. Effect of winter feed and grazing systems on cow performance. *J. Ani. Sci.* 22:853.

———, and E. E. Parker. 1967. Beef cattle responses to different grazing rates, systems, and level of protein supplement. *Tex. Agr. Expt. Sta. Spur Tech. Rep.* 3.

West, O. 1958. Bush encroachment, veld burning and grazing management. *Rhodesia Agr. J.* 55:407–425.

Whitman, W., F. W. Christensen, and E. A. Helgeson. 1943. Pasture grasses and pasture mixtures for eastern North Dakota. *N. Dak. Agr. Expt. Sta. Bull.* 327.

Williams, R. M., and A. H. Post. 1945. Dry land pasture experiments at the Central Montana Branch Station, Moccasin, Montana. *Mont. Agr. Expt. Sta. Bull.* 431.

Wood, W. E., C. W. Zumwalt, and W. P. Dasman. 1960. Range analysis field guide. U.S. Forest Service, Calif. Region.

Woolfolk, E. J. 1960. Rest-rotation management minimizes effect of drought. *Pacific S.W. Forest and Range Expt. Sta. Research Note* 144.

Part Three

Management of Vegetation

Chapter 12

Modification
of Vegetation

Woody shrubs, noxious species, and poisonous plants cover much of the earth's land surface. In the United States, the estimated area of brush is 130 million hectares. *Artemisia* spp. occupy nearly 40 million hectares, and *Prosopis* in Texas alone inhabits 22 million hectares (Sampson and Schultz, 1957). Over 80 percent of Texas rangeland is brush-infested. Half of it has brush cover greater than 20 percent (Smith and Rechenthin, 1964). Large areas of brush occur in Mediterranean climates, Africa, Australia, and other continents.

Climax shrub vegetation has changed relatively little in recent decades. After being destroyed by fire or clearing, it returns rapidly to mature stand density. However, brush communities that are successional to climax forests gradually disappear as the trees overtop the shrubs. In still other situations, woody plants have increased in cover and have invaded grasslands because of overgrazing and changes in burning frequency. For example, *Prosopis* dominated about 5 percent of southern New Mexico ranges in 1858 and 50 percent in 1963 (Buffington and Herbel, 1965). Efforts to control brush and alter the stand compositions are more successful in the invaded and successional stands than in the climax.

THE PROBLEM

Losses of forage due to occupation of the land by weeds and brush (Fig. 12-1); losses of livestock due to plant poisoning and physical injury; and increased costs of management for livestock, game, and recreational services which are attributable to inaccessibility were estimated at $250 million annually on western United States rangelands in the early 1960s (U.S. Dept. Agr., 1965). The kinds of undesirable plants and the problems they cause are as diverse as the soils and climates they inhabit. Platt (1959a, 1959b) developed a list of the most important herbaceous range weeds and undesirable shrubs based on a questionnaire survey. The ten most important species and the millions of hectares occupied by each are as follows:

Herbaceous species	Area, million ha	Woody species	Area, million ha
1. *Salsola* spp.	41	*Gutierrezia* spp.	58
2. *Astragalus* spp.	18	*Prosopis* spp.	38
3. *Lupinus* spp.	13	*Artemisia* spp.	35
4. *Bromus tectorum*	10	*Opuntia* spp.	32
5. *Hymenoxys odorata*	6	*Juniperus* spp.	26
6. *Halogeton glomeratus*	4	*Larrea* sp.	19
7. *Zygadenus* spp.	3	*Quercus* spp.	16
8. *Xanthium* spp.	2	*Flourensia cernua*	5
9. *Delphinium* spp.	2	*Adenostoma fasciculatum*	3
10. *Oxytropis* spp.	1	*Chrysothamnus* spp.	2
Total of 33 species	107	Total of 31 species	243

Nationwide, the major genera of woody plants that create problems in livestock management are *Quercus, Juniperus, Artemisia, Opuntia, Chrysothamnus, Prosopis, Acacia, Adenostoma, Arctostaphylos,* and *Ceanothus.* These genera are widespread, but the individual species may be scattered locally. Some species quickly regenerate after removal of old plants. Some species are climax, others are successional, and still others may be either in different areas. Some live only a few years and vary in density as climatic cycles and environmental upsets occur. Others live for many years and may dominate their ecological systems to the detriment of other species. The effects of factors such as fire and grazing on these species have changed with the advent of domestic animals, but only in degree or intensity. Mechanical, chemical, biological, and burning procedures for controlling plants are used as replacements for impacts that originally maintained ecological balances.

The substitution of sometimes heavy-handed techniques for those that occur naturally contributes to differences of opinion concerning the types of needed

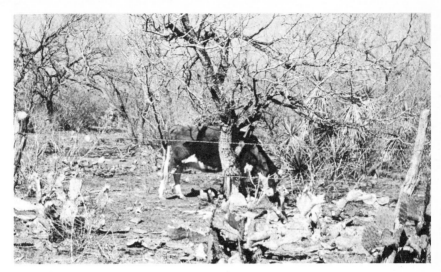

Figure 12-1 *Prosopsis, Yucca,* and *Opuntia* dominate the vegetation on this overgrazed range and retard the increase of desirable forage plants.

control. Some of the opinions are as follows. Is brush really a problem? Why not alter objectives and production procedures to take advantage of natural systems rather than alter the systems to meet objectives? For example, woody plants on rangeland provide many values. They are used for browse, fruits, charcoal, fuel wood, posts, shade for animals, gum arabic, oils, and wood stock for numerous purposes. Their deep root systems hold the soil from sliding, useful herbage grows in their shade, and many of them are ornamental because of their flowers, shape, and shade of green. The impacts of the plant-control procedure on other values, processes, and profitability in the rangeland system must also be considered. For example, *Cirsium* spp. and the poisonous *Rhus* spp. need to be controlled for visitor comfort. Grass dominance reduces the display of wild flowers. While controls of thistles and flowers have little direct monetary return on rangeland, they have value for people. Care for the wishes of the public promotes indirect returns.

Desirable forage species for livestock and game, and other desirable species for man's recreation, have been encouraged on many hundreds of thousands of acres of formerly unproductive rangelands. Modification of vegetational structure and botanical composition has been successful. Range improvements will continue whether their objective is restoration of depleted vegetation and soil or changes in vegetation for a different use. Whatever the type of range improvement, increasing care must be taken in its application.

THE ECOLOGY CRUSADE

The major elements in ecological systems are energy from the sun, food and its passage from one organism to another, water, oxygen and other components of the atmosphere, space, and a vast variety of organisms. The exchanges and interactions among these elements constitute the ecology of nature. Unfortunately, certain ecological fringe processes attract more attention than do the basic elements, probably because the economy of man is at stake. Oversupply of energy, stockpiling of energy, and too little capacity for storing minerals and energy overtax ecological processes to the point of breakdown. These are *pollution*. Population explosions cause overdemand and excessive competition, sometimes to the point of breakdown in food chains. The lockup kind of storage and the lockout kind of use, called *preservation,* are attempts to reduce impacts of pollution and excessive harvest due to overpopulation. More often than not, the attempt is destructive rather than beneficial, because ecological processes do not remain static for long. Those concerned with preservation must consider systems and processes as well as a target plant or animal.

Perhaps too many ecologists have spent too much time creating the perfect light bulb, all light and no heat, or all useful product and no losses. This approach is idealistic and seeks a final answer. An increase in efficiency may not be a final answer, but it is readily attainable and immediately practical.

One of the range manager's goals, as a practicing ecologist, is to combine the ecology of nature and the economy of man. This goal requires that he predict and evaluate the risks and possible benefits to the environment of his every influence. His understanding of basic ecological and economic processes is crucial. His second goal is to help society gain high production within an unimpaired environment for humanity. This requires that he choose wisely among the tradeoffs when no perfect ecological solution is in sight. He must not gamble with nature or with man's economy.

Let us apply these ideas to the pollution of rangeland with an oversupply of brush. Either complete or partial conversions may be the goal. A single use may require pure grassland, but the realities of incompletely attainable conversion, the advantages of diversity with mixed vegetational types and numerous animal species, and economic pressures for many rangeland products suggest that brush management, rather than brush eradication, is the practical goal. Many rangeland practices may be criticized because they have absolute goals. Ecological responsibility within an ever-changing complex of processes and demands for products requires flexibility in application of techniques.

Techniques that directly modify vegetation are aimed at reducing undesirable plants and thereby establishing desirable vegetation for forage production, soil protection, water production, wildlife habitat improvement, recreational services, and other uses as specific production goals require. Managing vegetation necessitates killing or suppressing plants by means of machines, chemicals, animals, and prescribed fire. Managing vegetation may include seeding species, adding minerals to the system, and increasing soil moisture by conservation practices. These three techniques, sometimes known collectively as *the biological range improvements,* exert considerable influence upon rangeland ecosystems; thus they are given central emphasis by people concerned over environmental impacts.

The public's recently expressed distrust for rangeland management by traditional users and for tinkering with rangeland ecosystems by scientists will lead to a greater wisdom in application of techniques (Day, 1972). The balance sought is a better life and a better environment for all who use rangelands directly or even indirectly. Controversies are beneficial because they promote caution. The wisdom with which a technique is used, as much as or more than the technique itself, determines its harmful and beneficial ecological effects. These problems are larger than chemicals, machines, and rangeland operations. They are a part of the fabric of mankind, but the technique of application often receives more attention than does the appropriateness of the application.

HOW MISTAKEN TACTICS HAVE CLOUDED ECOLOGICAL GOALS

Modification of range vegetation is a subtle art based on the manipulation of physical, biological, and chemical factors. Usually treatments aim at one or a few target species while most of the flora is ignored (Blaisdell and Mueggler, 1956; Heller, 1970; Parker, 1949). Pesticides and plant controls of all types are sometimes used indiscriminately, and they do have secondary effects. Mechanical brush control often destroys valuable grasses and shrubs. Machines, herbicides, fire, animals, and water conservation practices are widely used in attempts to obtain a yield revolution on rangeland comparable to that achieved with food crops on cultivated land (Barrons, 1973). These tactics aim to replace the natural assemblages of organisms with a few high-yield species of forage for domestic livestock.

Many writers protest against this approach to rangeland management. Conflicts of interest—arguments over the type of products rangelands should produce—suggest that rangelands should be managed on an ecological basis, that the aim should be to help or to guide ecological processes, that the consequences of seeding or fertilization should be considered as part of the total systems—not just as means of obtaining forage for livestock. Balanced use of resources means diversified plant and animal communities managed on an ecological basis rather than on the basis of obtaining pure stands, monocultures, and replacement of native communities.

How Catastrophe Stimulates Ecological Systems

Every ecological catastrophe stimulates natural ecosystems to new actions. Weeding a garden brings on a new crop, by succession chaparral soon replaces itself after a burn, and reproductive rates increase following catastrophe to many animal populations. An ecological error seldom is absolutely wrong, but rather favors some species and hinders others. In fact, ecological systems do not change much until a disaster occurs. Repairs come rapidly. For example, plant succession moves faster during early than during late stages, and reduction in grazing pressure immediately stimulates changes in vegetation. Few places are without fire, but plants soon regrow after a burn.

Reduction of top growth and elimination of some brush by chemical and mechanical means brings no more than temporary change in the vegetation. Soil sterility caused by phenoxy herbicides is short-lived. The selectivity of phenoxy herbicides leaves sufficient cover for erosion control (Barrons, 1969; Hunter and Stoble, 1972; Isensee et al., 1973; Mullison, 1972). These chemicals may cause long-term changes in the habitat (Klebenow, 1970), but the danger that cows will consume sprayed forage and their milk will be tainted lasts no more than a couple of weeks for 2,4-D and its commonly used relatives (Leng, 1972). To convert a forest to a meadow requires continuous application of saw or herbicides to keep the trees from invading and the forest from replacing itself. Superficially, it may seem that removal of part of the vegetation simplifies the system. In fact, removal is never complete and the attempts at removal stimulate the ecological processes and the return of stable systems. If the objective is a stable system, or a highly unstable one, for that matter, the intensity with which a practice is applied may be as important as the application itself.

Dosage Levels and Sites of Application

All range improvements involve decisions as to the intensity of application. Should an area be chained once or twice to kill brush adequately? What is the best recipe for application of herbicides? Improvements involve benefits and risks that vary biologically according to dosage levels. The questions to be answered are the following: How much benefit? For whose benefit? Who should decide? It is beneficial to nation and industry to be careful (Dominick, 1973).

Since the release of 2,4-D for general use in 1945, herbicides have become an indispensable tool in vegetational management. Chemicals are widely used to reduce woody species, poisonous plants, and competing herbaceous species. Although wildland managers have compiled an impressive safety record, accidents have occurred. Herbicides have been accused of simplifying plant and animal communities, causing nutrient loss and erosion, and reducing ecosystem productivity (Westing, 1972). Public concern following the disclosure of possible teratological effects from massive doses of 2,4,5-T fed to rats and mice and perhaps to humans during the Vietnamese war raised questions about the wisdom of continuing the use of 2,4,5-T for any purpose. The teratogenetic effects of 2,4,5-T may be due to a dangerous impurity known as Dioxin (2,3,7,8-Tetrachlorodibenzo-paradioxin), which decomposes rapidly and does not accumulate in the food chain (Johnson, 1971; Tschirley, 1972; Wilson, 1973). Its presence in 2,4,5-T is the fault of the manufacturer, not of the herbicide. This is not to invalidate concern for herbicides. Their use must become even more selective and application more precise than it is today.

Sprays, prescribed burns, mechanical treatments, and other practices are applied to defined sites. Careless application to unintended sites causes problems; for example, a few escaped fires have seriously jeopardized prescribed burning programs. Air currents make herbicides drift beyond the site of application. Certain regulations, some stipulated by law, are used to minimize both losses and damage caused by drift. Materials of low volatility used in air temperatures less than 24°C, relative humidities above 50 percent, and wind speeds below 10 kilometers per hour reduce possibilities of drift. Low flying speeds, heights less than 10 meters above the vegetation, and nozzles that produce large droplets are recommended for aerial applications. Spray thickeners, invert emulsions, foaming agents, and granular polymers that imbibe the sprays and swell to limited size are drift-reduction aids (Gratkowski and Stewart, 1973).

HOW TO AVOID REPEATING MISTAKES

Overgrazing and even other kinds of grazing by domestic livestock have been blamed for destruction of range vegetation and soil erosion. Senate Document 199 blamed much of the dust bowl problem in the 1930s on overgrazing with inadequate attention to the influences of weather. If grazing must be singled out, this should be done accurately and other causes of damage assessed properly. On rangelands, mining, logging, road building, right-of-way maintenance, cultivation and abandonment, off-road vehicles, recreational man, and climate cause changes and destruction (Arnold, 1963). These sources of problems need to be recognized and eliminated before range improvements are applied. Let us know the symptoms of all kinds of damage so that we may apply the correct remedies (Williams et al., 1973).

Mistakes or blind spots in ecological management of rangeland have been listed by Costello (1957): The complexity of all environments tends to be oversimplified, and poor interpretation and treatment of symptoms result. Producers and technicians alike look for quick results and become impatient with gradual improvement from management. We have glossed over many failures by stressing the successes and figuring averages. The time has come to emphasize range sites and to base range improvements upon biological units rather than upon physical and political land units. Range managers need to look at the effects of their range improvements with foresight. Unfortunately, mistakes tend to repeat themselves. Ecological squeezes occur over and over again. The parallels between grazing and recreational problems suggest that land-policy mistakes made in grazing management three or four decades ago are now being repeated in recreation (Heady and Vaux, 1969).

TOWARD FLEXIBILITY FOR THE FUTURE

Increasing population reduces available acreage for grazing, recreational services, and production of clean water. Because land becomes scarce when demands increase, range-vegetation management must be practiced with increasing intensity. Every tool must come into use. The era of extravagant use of natural resources is over. But at this time we do not know how much of each product society will require.

Chain reactions occur in rangeland ecosystems, and such interactions must be predicted. The trend in the use of chemicals will be toward the more selective, more effective, less expensive, and less persistent ones. Eventually chemical treatments must be minimized and made to fit the needs of man's environment, sociological desires, and economics. Some people now see agricultural chemicals as instruments of impending doom. We need the ecological knowledge necessary to manage and maintain a healthy biosphere (Tarrant et al., 1973) whether or not chemicals are used. Careful planning and use of ecological knowledge reduces public disputes and costly errors.

Vegetational management in this book follows the concept that any treatment is only one of a number of options available to the manager. However, due to limitations of linearity caused by one page following another, the techniques are described one at a time.

LITERATURE CITED

Arnold, J. F. 1963. Crusade for rangeland restoration. *Am. For.* 69(5):28–32.
Barrons, K. C. 1969. Some ecological benefits of woody plant control with herbicides. *Science* 165:465–468.
———. 1973. Some environmental benefits of herbicides. *Down to Earth* 29(1):30–32.
Blaisdell, J. P., and W. F. Mueggler. 1956. Effect of 2,4-D on forbs and shrubs associated with big sagebrush. *J. Range Mgmt.* 9:38–40.
Buffington, L. C., and C. H. Herbel. 1965. Vegetational changes on a semidesert grassland range from 1858 to 1963. *Ecol. Monog.* 35:139–164.
Costello, D. F. 1957. Application of ecology to range management. *Ecology* 38:49–53.

Day, B. E. 1972. Agricultural chemicals and range management. *Down to Earth* 27(4):11–13.

Dominick, D. D. 1973. Improving agriculture and the environment. *Weed Sci.* 21:379–381.

Gratkowski, H., and R. Stewart. 1973. Aerial spray adjuvants for herbicidal drift control. *U.S. Dept. Agr. Forest Service General Tech. Rep.* PNW-3.

Heady, H. F., and H. J. Vaux. 1969. Must history repeat? *J. Range Mgmt.* 22:209–210.

Heller, T. H. 1970. Herbicides. *J. Range Mgmt.* 23:378–379.

Hunter, J. H., and E. H. Stoble. 1972. Movement and persistence of picloram in soil. *Weed Sci.* 20:486–489.

Isensee, A. R., W. C. Shaw, W. A. Gentner, C. R. Swanson, B. C. Turner, and E. A. Woolson. 1973. Revegetation following massive application of selected herbicides. *Weed Sci.* 21:409–412.

Johnson, J. E. 1971. Safety in the development of herbicides. *Down to Earth* 27(1):1–7.

Klebenow, D. A. 1970. Sage grouse versus sagebrush control in Idaho. *J. Range Mgmt.* 23:396–400.

Leng, M. L. 1972. Residues in milk and meat and safety to livestock from the use of phenoxy herbicides in pasture and rangeland. *Down to Earth* 28(1):12–20.

Mullison, W. R. 1972. Ecological effects of herbicides. *Down to Earth* 28(2):4–24.

Parker, K. W. 1949. Control of noxious range plants in a range management program. *J. Range Mgmt.* 2:128–132.

Platt, K. B. 1959a. Plant control—Some possibilities and limitations. I. The challenge to management. *J. Range Mgmt.* 12:64–68.

———. 1959b. Plant control—Some possibilities and limitations. II. Vital statistics of range management. *J. Range Mgmt.* 12:194–200.

Sampson, A. W., and A. M. Schultz. 1957. *Control of brush and undesirable trees.* Rome:FAO, Forestry Division.

Smith, H. N., and C. A. Rechenthin. 1964. *Grassland restoration. The problem.* U.S. Dept. Agr. Soil Cons. Service.

Tarrant, R. F., H. J. Gratkowski, and W. E. Waters. 1973. The future role of chemicals in forestry. *U.S. Dept. Agr. Forest Service General Tech. Rep.* PNW-6.

Tschirley, F. H. 1972. The impact of government decisions and attitude on pest control. *Weed Sci.* 20:405–407.

U.S. Dept. Agr. 1965. Losses in agriculture. *Agr. Res. service Handbook* No. 291. 120 p.

Westing, A. H. 1972. Herbicides in war: Current status and future doubt. *Biol. Cons.* 4:322–327.

Williams, J. L., M. A. Ross, and T. T. Bauman. 1973. Looks can be deceiving—Herbicide injury? *Down to Earth* 29(1):11–14.

Wilson, J. G. 1973. Teratological potential of 2,4,5-T. *Down to Earth* 28(4):14–17.

Chapter 13

Mechanical Control
of Rangeland Plants

Modification of range vegetation by removal of certain plant species or individuals has been practiced since man has had domestic livestock. He learned centuries ago that certain chemicals, such as salt and arsenic, killed plants and that fire was a powerful tool in altering vegetation. Hand pulling and then hand tools were used for plant removal. Animal power and engines increased man's effectiveness in changing vegetation. Occasionally eradication has been the ideal objective of modification efforts, but control has been the practical result because species rarely are eliminated. Control has two major aspects. One is using land in a way that will maintain vegetation according to prescribed specifications, and the other is altering the vegetation to the type to be maintained. The practical problems of control are how to alter the percentage species composition and the height, succulence, and density of plants (Box and Powell, 1965). These practical problems require decisions on objectives, sites, methods, and specified time and intensity at which the methods should be applied. Sampson and Schultz (1957) put these decisions in the questions, ''Is control biologically and economically justified? What should be the choice of method and the intensity of its application?''

OBJECTIVES

Altering the plant cover on a range area has many purposes. For reasons of effectiveness and costs, mechanical techniques are largely limited to removal of woody plants. The most common objectives are to obtain cover and herbaceous forage, browse, and fruits for livestock and wild animals; flow of water in springs; accessible areas for hunting, viewing, and other recreational pursuits; opportunities for seeding and planting; erosion control; and decrease in the wildfire hazard to homes, parks, and people by fuel management.

SITES

One selects sites for brush control where success is likely or where the objective can be attained (Pechanec et al., 1954). Such sites usually are on relatively level land where soils are fertile and deep, as indicated by plant growth of exceptional density and height. These "best" sites have potential to be changed and to be properly used afterwards. They present little risk of increased erosion. Medium-textured soils greater than 50 centimeters in depth, with a pH range between 6 and 8, often characterize these sites. Slopes steeper than 30 percent limit use of machines in brush control.

The site has a major influence upon the intensity of management that can be attained. Steep slopes, rock outcrops, and irregular drainage patterns increase costs of controls. These factors restrict livestock movements and usually cause less forage to be produced than on bottomland sites. In general, lowland sites have the greatest potential for successful projects when both input costs and outputs are considered. Few areas with slopes greater than 30 percent should be considered for use by livestock. Mechanical brush control on steeper lands aims for other purposes such as wildfire control and fuel modification.

THE METHOD, TIME, AND INTENSITY OF APPLICATION

In choosing a technique for mechanical brush control, one must consider effectiveness on the target species; kill of nontarget, undesirable associated species; potential damage to desirable plants; suitability of the land for seeding and other follow-up treatments; reduction of regeneration by seed and sprout; matching of equipment and size of the problem; hazard from erosion; and cost. Undesirable vegetation almost everywhere has been treated with various techniques, so many of the brush-control-equipment problems have been answered locally through experience and trial and error practice. The popular methods of a region have survived practical tests. Usually, too, competent operators and specialized equipment or specifications for its construction are available locally. Choice of mechanical brush-control procedures starts with consideration of local experience.

Common practice points the way to the best timing and intensity of control. A few examples illustrate this concept. Undesirable plants should be mechanically removed before the seed crop is mature, so that the control operation does not scatter and plant the seed. Breaking and crushing of woody plants operates most effectively when materials are dry and brittle. Machines that remove woody roots and crowns operate with least energy and damage to equipment when the soil is moist, neither too dry nor too wet. In all situations, mechanical controls should be timed to be most effective in removing undesirable plants and least damaging to desirable rangeland values. Longhurst (1956) reports 100 percent sprouting of four *Quercus* spp. when trees were cut during the wet season but as low as 25 percent sprouting for one species when they were cut in the dry season. Another of the four species, *Quercus dumosa,* sprouted 100 percent when cut every month. Cutting at the termination of leaf growth was most detrimental to *Prosopis* near Lubbock, Texas (Wright and Stinson, 1970).

METHODS OF MECHANICAL BRUSH CONTROL

Machines used to control brush operate differently on various kinds of terrain and in different types and age classes of vegetation. Nonsprouting species do not require removal below ground level, light brush is easier to remove than heavy brush, slopes facing away from the sun may be difficult to prepare for burning, rocky soil restricts machines that remove roots, rock outcrops and steep slopes reduce maneuverability of equipment, and soil moisture alters drawbar energy requirements. Each of the following commonly used techniques has its own operational characteristics and effectiveness on different brush species.

Tractor with Dozer Blade

Straight or regular bulldozer blades and tractor tracks (crawler-type) effectively crush brush, thus aiding in clearing and piling woody materials in preparation for burning and other treatments. Effective bulldozing requires kinds of plants that easily pull from the ground, soil with few rocks larger than 3 or 4 decimeters in diameter, and smooth topography. Flexible woody stems bend before the blade. Rock outcroppings and large stones can be avoided with little trouble. Intense soil disturbance, piling of soil with the brush, and erosion signify that poor attention was paid to soil conservation and the needs of the next crop. Woody materials between the tractor tracks may be effectively crushed with a "sheep-foot" roller of the type used to pack soil in highway construction. One hectare per hour should be the average production rate for bulldozing to be worthwhile.

Tractor with Modified Blade

Front-end tractor blades for brush and tree removal vary greatly (Fig. 13-1). Two general types in common use are the brush rake and the short, often pointed blade for pushing individual trees. The rake, one type of bulldozer blade, may be short teeth attached to the lower edge of the bulldozer blade or a complete unit that replaces the blade. Generally the attachments with large blade surfaces pile more soil with the brush than do the blades with open teeth. A root plow or blade welded across the lower and leading tips of the rake teeth increases effectiveness in the

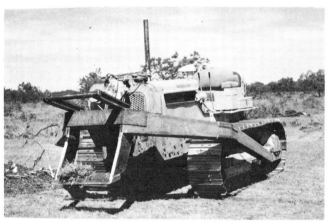

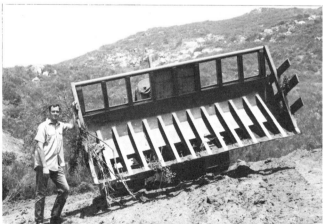

Figure 13-1   Upper photo shows a short blade used to uproot individual trees. Lower photo shows dozer attachments operating as a root plow and brush rake. *(Photo by San Diego County Department of Agriculture.)*

removal of light brush. When properly operated, none of the root rakes scrape off the topsoil and pile it with the woody debris. The operator can be selective as to which trees to leave. He can avoid rock outcrops and slopes where erosion might become a problem. As with any cultivator, the best work is done when the soil is moist. Soils that are too wet do not flow through the teeth, and dry soils take too much power. Rates of coverage average about an 0.5 hectare per hour and vary from 0.1 to 1.0 hectare.

Another major type of bulldozer blade is the tree-dozer, which is made to remove individual trees. The blade may be V-shaped or straight and is approximately 1.5 meters wide. It operates with a push bar that puts stress on the root system before the blade goes under the tree. This machine effectively removes single small trees such as *Juniperus* spp. in the United States and *Acacia* spp. in Australia with one pass. The regular dozer blade takes two passes, one to push the tree over and one to sever all the roots.

A pulled root plow blade may be attached to the tractor drawbar or built as a self-propelled brush eradicator. Some tractors are huge, pulling a 6-meter-long blade horizontally some 15 to 25 centimeters below the soil surface. Abernathy and Herbel (1973) described a machine that root plows, picks up the brush, forms large soil pits, firms the soil, plants seed, and replaces the brush, via an overhead conveyor, as a mulch on the planted area. Herbel et al. (1973) claimed successful control of *Larrea tridentata* and *Flourensia cernua* and good to excellent stands of seeded grasses on 50 percent of the sites treated with this equipment.

Disk

The brushland disk consists of heavy models of the disk-harrow and wheatland-plow, which have been used for many decades to prepare land for agricultural crops. Except with light brush such as young sagebrush, effective brush control requires machinery weighing more than 3 tons, with individual disk blades over a meter in diameter and gangs of disks at least 3 meters wide. Two gangs positioned at an angle to each other with the disk blades set to plow in opposite directions give a double disking with one pass of the equipment. More than one pass may be needed. Lighter-weight equipment rides over too much brush, and short gangs overturn too easily to be safe. Weight and cutting angle determine effectiveness more than does disk diameter. Properly operated brushland disks uproot, chop, and mulch even very heavy brush stands. They turn many roots, crowns, and root burls out of the soil, but, of course, some species are more difficult to remove than others. A "stump-jump" disk mounts pairs of disks separately so they can ride over obstacles without lifting the whole gang of disks (Fig. 13-2).

Disking leaves the soil in place but loosens it and may damage remnant perennial grasses. However, the debris acts as a mulch, and rainfall infiltration

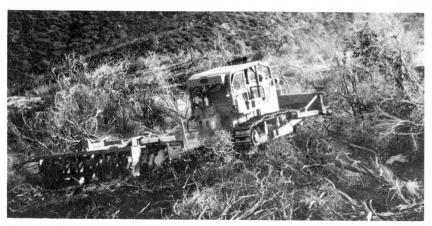

Figure 13-2 A scalloped disk reducing chaparral in southern California.

may be increased by disking. Contour disking has been effective in California chaparral, where only a scattering of surface rocks and trees occurs. Production rates vary between 0.1 and 1.0 hectares per hour.

Chaining or Cabling

A tractor dragging an anchor chain or a 1-decimeter-diameter group of wire ropes discarded by oil-drilling operations has been used as a brush-control method for at least 25 years. Unmodified chains and cables tend to be ineffective because they pass over fine and flexible woody stems without great damage to them and leave too many root crowns in the soil. However, this equipment is widely used because of low costs per hectare, effectiveness on some species, and adaptability to relatively difficult terrain.

Anchor chains range in weight from 60 to 135 kilograms per meter and come in 27-meter lengths. Two or three lengths commonly are used. The heaviest chains are the most effective, but they need to be cut into shorter lengths for ease in transporting. A tractor on each end of the chain maintains an average swath width about half the length of the chain. Pulling the chain in a J shape gives more drag on the bushes and less rolling over them. Where rolling materials might be dangerous to the tractor operator, the lead tractor should be the lower one.

After many trials, a modification to make the chain effective has become widely used. Its prototype is the Ely chain used by the Bureau of Land Management in Nevada and New Mexico (Aro, 1971). Crossbars of hard steel 2.5 by 10 by 45 centimeters are welded to every link or every third link so that adjacent bars are perpendicular to the chain and to each other. The bars cause the chain to roll and to do an improved job of crushing and pulling brush plants. The modified portion of the chain needs a swivel on each end and unmodified sections 6 to 8 meters in length between swivels and tractors (Fig. 13-3).

Two passes, in opposite directions, with the Ely chain prepare California chaparral for prescribed burning. One pass may be enough for certain burning conditions, but doing two provides additional flexibility in time of burning. The second pass tends to windrow and pile the brush more than the first. Chaining can be done on slopes as steep as 45 percent and in rocky terrain. Damage to road berms and drainage structures can occur. The modified chain may "walk" ineffectively over brush if the soil is hard. Areas covered vary between 0.5 and 3 hectares per hour.

Another modification of chaining has been used extensively on steep slopes in southern California. The modified chain, 20 to 45 meters in length and 30 to 90 kilograms per meter in weight, has a ball attached to one end. The opposite end is fastened to either a drawbar or a cable winch on the tractor. The ball is a spherical 1.5-meter-diameter buoy that is filled with water, gravel, or concrete and weighs 2.5 to 5 tons. Heavy chains and short chains need heavy balls for operation.

The tractor unit must remain on ridges and roads when ball and chain are used on extremely steep slopes. The ball drags the chain off the ridge and rolls as the chain follows the tractor in a wide loop. When used prior to prescribed burning, this technique is a valuable tool in the establishment of fuelbreaks. In operation, the chain often fails to ride over rocks, flat terrain, etc., which cause the ball to move upslope. Once the obstacle is passed, the ball swings downhill again, creating a considerable irregularity in the border between chained and unchained land. Problems arise where the chain digs too deeply, usually near the tractor, and where the ball leaves tracks that will erode.

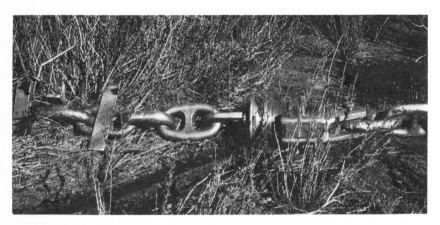

Figure 13-3   A modified anchor chain, showing crossbars and swivel.

Communication becomes difficult in chaining and requires three-way radio contact among the two tractor operators and the man overseeing the operation. If one tractor has trouble, the other needs to stop immediately.

Rolling Cutter

The rolling cutter developed as an enlarged version of the cotton-stalk cutter. It is a drum about 3 meters in length and 1 meter in diameter with the steel blades fastened on the outside and parallel to the axle through the drum (Fig. 13-4). As the cutter rolls, the heavy weight (2,500 to 4,000 kilograms per linear meter of the cutter) gives the blades a chopping action on the brush. Two cutters hooked in tandem but not aligned parallel with each other add a shearing action to the chop as each blade falls forward. The tandem cutter can be turned with ease only toward the side with the shortest hitch between the rollers. Slopes greater than 20 percent cause considerable sideslip. The cutting action crushes and compacts the woody material for prescribed burning, removes a few plants from the soil, and incorporates a part of the organic residue into the soil. Depressions in the soil made by the chopper blades should be on the contour to reduce runoff; therefore the equipment should work up and down the slopes.

Two passes at right angles to each other effectively reduced *Serenoa repens* in southern Florida (Lewis, 1970). Cutting and burning decreased the number of plants of *Acacia rigidula* in southern Texas but increased the number of stems per unit area (Dodd and Holtz, 1972).

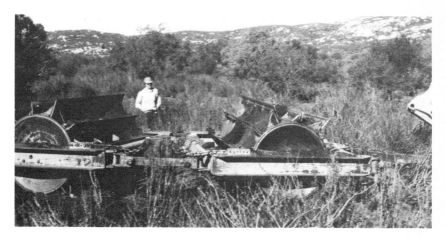

Figure 13-4   This photo shows a tandem pair of rolling cutters coupled closer together at one end than at the other, giving them a dragging action as well as a chopping effect.

Other Types of Brush-Control Equipment

Brush shredders or beaters are made with hammers or flails that operate from the power takeoff. Brittle woody material such as sagebrush may be mulched with shredders more readily than may the brush species of Texas and much of the chaparral in California. In normal operation, the machine does not remove plants from the soil or disturb the soil itself.

Railing is the crushing of brush with a railroad rail or other large beam that is dragged behind a tractor. It removes brittle shrubs and burned stems and covers broadcast seed.

Hand clearing was the first means of brush control and is the only means in situations where machinery becomes inefficient or damaging to other values. The common hand-clearing tools are chain saw, brush hook, axe, backpack-type power saw, and grubbing hoe. Hand clearing is the most selective of all brush-control methods and can be used to create the desired vegetational architecture. However, it is the most expensive method. Herbel et al. (1958) found grubbing effective on young, light stands of *Prosopis*. Arnold and Schroeder (1955) suggested hand grubbing of *Juniperus* spp. on the Fort Apache Indian Reservation as off-season work. Even if a small percentage of an area is cleared per year, total clearance can be accomplished in 10 to 20 years.

PLANT KILL

For sprouting species to be killed, root crowns and other organs with stem buds must be removed from the soil. *Opuntia* spp. must be removed from contact with the soil. Many species that do not sprout are killed by top removal below the lowest green limb. Methods (chaining, crushing, shredding, etc.) that remove only the tops of plants have little long-term effect on the sprouters. Root plows, root rakes, tree-dozers, etc., most effectively remove sprouters. However, wet soils may permit many sprouters to take root although they are disturbed. Chaining and using the rolling cutter with two or more passes remove part of the plants. Both sprouters and nonsprouters reproduce by seed, and brush seedlings often appear in abundance after the control operation. Except for land clearing for cultivated crops, very few examples exist of complete brush kills by mechanical means. Abandoned cropland taken from brushland soon returns to woody plants. Thick stands should be opened for specific purposes with the knowledge that kill will not be complete and that woody plants will return.

Effects of Plant-Kill Techniques

Aro (1971) found that dozing *Pinus* spp. and *Juniperus* spp. into windrows was the best mechanical approach in the southwestern United States, but that chaining was the most widely used and least effective. Treatments including using rolling cutter, scalping with a dozer blade, root plowing, root raking, and mowing resulted in different compositions of the brush stands in Texas. All methods reduced *Prosopis glandulosa*, but *Acacia farnesiana* increased with chopping and scalping. *Opuntia lindheimeri, O. fulgida, O. arbuscula, O. leptocaulis*, and *Aplopappus tenuisectus* greatly increased with chaining and root plowing (Box and Powell, 1965; Dodd, 1968; Schmutz et al., 1959). Successful and widespread mechanical controls are limited to a few species. Platt (1959) recommended no mechanical techniques for 23 herbaceous range weeds and for 16 of 25 woody species.

Herbage Increase after Brush Removal

Herbage for livestock greatly increases after removal of *Artemisia tridentata* and woody associates in the intermountain region. Hyder and Sneva (1956) found that grubbing the brush doubled the quantity of grass in central Oregon. There apparently was less increase in southern Idaho (Mueggler and Blaisdell, 1958), but the results may be due to the fact that there was less grass in the brush stand before treating and that railing did more damage to the grass than did grubbing. After mechanical treatment, seedlings of *Artemisia tridentata* gradually invade seeded and natural grasslands (Bleak and Miller, 1955; Frischknecht and Bleak, 1957).

Removal of *Juniperus osteosperma* by chaining increased forage production from 250 to 1,100 kilograms per hectare in northern Arizona (Clary, 1971). Bulldozing of pinyon-juniper on the Kaibab did not increase production of browse, which principally were *Cowania* spp. (McCulloch, 1966; 1971). Sparse stands of pinyon-juniper should not be removed from winter deer range.

Clearing of *Prosopis* and *Opuntia* spp. resulted in a threefold increase in native grass production and an eightfold increase in production from seeded grasses (Everson, 1951). In contrast, Pieper (1971) reported inconsistent grass increases after removal of *Opuntia imbricata*. He speculated that the cholla cactus may improve the environment for grasses and furnish no competition for water and nutrients.

Increases in tree-canopy density reduce yields of understory vegetation (Fig. 13-5), and vice versa. These results were shown for *Pinus ponderosa* in eastern Washington (McConnell and Smith, 1965; 1970) and in western South Dakota (Thompson and Gartner, 1971). An increase in tree dominance *(Pinus palustris* and *Pinus elliottii)* in the southern United States resulted in decreased understory production at rates between 7.3 and 11.7 kilograms per hectare for each 0.1 square meter of woody stem basal area (Grelen et al., 1972; Wolters, 1973).

DEBRIS ARRANGEMENTS

Mechanical treatments of brush leave the debris in different arrangements. Crushing produces coarse materials essentially in place but compacted close to the

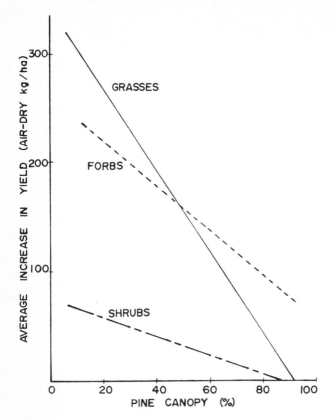

Figure 13-5 The relationship between *Pinus ponderosa* percent canopy cover and yield of understory plants *(McConnell and Smith, 1970)*.

ground surface. The rolling cutter makes small pieces still more compacted. Shredders, chippers, and rotary mowers make fine materials that closely compact on the soil surface. Mulching, as a general rule, increases infiltration and decreases erosion; therefore these treatments would be expected to improve soil conditions. Chaining of pinyon-juniper with the debris left in place increased soil moisture storage (Gifford and Shaw, 1973) and did not increase either runoff or sediment (Gifford et al., 1970; Gifford, 1973).

The second pass in chaining tends to arrange the debris in interrupted windrows. Scalping with a bulldozer blade and root raking usually result in piles or windrows, depending on job specification. Too frequently, an excellent job is equated with a complete cleanup in which the debris is neatly piled and burned. The needs for animal cover, protection for seedling grasses, and erosion control suggest that a variable degree of cleanup is a better overall management policy than is complete removal of debris.

SOIL DISTURBANCES

Resident grasses are healthiest and densest when soil disturbance is minimal (Powell and Box, 1967). Shredding, mowing, crushing, and hand cutting of brush have little direct effect on the soil beyond the impact of tractor wheels and tracks. Bulldozing of brush into piles and windrows tends to scalp the topsoil and to mix it with the woody debris. Scalping sometimes exposes topsoil and increases erosion hazard. Root raking takes the tops, crowns, and large roots and leaves the soil in a loosened condition. The soil may be compacted in the equipment tracks, and a bit of the residue may become mixed with the soil. Friable soil promotes infiltration, but under heavy rainfall its potential for erosion is increased (Fig. 13-6).

Equipment that is extremely heavy and difficult to handle has potential for local damage. Chaining will destroy the berm on roads, remove cover from road fills, and damage drainage structures. A chain pulled in a line behind one tractor will cut a soil trench that is a potential gully. When pits are dug, the soil is loosened and fine organic residues become buried; therefore the rolling cutter should be pulled across contours so that the pits are on the contour.

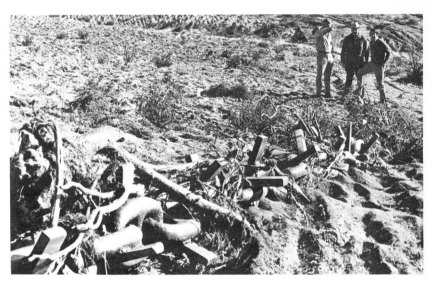

Figure 13-6 Chaining with the modified chain mixes some of the debris into the soil and leaves the soil surface roughened, which reduces erosion. *(Photo by San Diego County Department of Agriculture.)*

When care is taken to use the techniques properly, mechanical brush-control procedures increase erosion hazard temporarily, if at all. Infiltrometer tests on chained sites in Utah showed that soil bulk density, on which chaining has little effect, was the most important factor determining erosion (Williams et al., 1972). Runoff was correlated with soil cover more than mechanical treatment (Kincaid and Williams, 1966). If the soil does not become saturated during the rainy season, cover treatments may have little effect (Hill and Rice, 1963).

COSTS OF MECHANICAL BRUSH CONTROL

This section aims to review the costs of brush control alone and the factors altering these costs, not to analyze the whole land-management costs/returns system. Crushing of brush with a bulldozer is one of the least expensive treatments, costing $35 to $50 per hectare. It usually is followed by burning and perhaps seeding. Chaining costs about the same as crushing in light brush but may be 50 percent more expensive in heavy stands. The rolling cutter operation ranges in price from $50 to $80 per hectare, while root plowing and disking are more expensive, at $50 to $175 per hectare. Hand clearing runs as high as $3,500 per hectare. Earlier, Morrow et al. (1962) placed these techniques in the same cost relationship to each other but at a lower price per hectare.

On-site per hectare costs are functions of the type and size of equipment, labor, number of passes over the land to accomplish the objective, slope of the terrain, and roughness or rockiness of the soil. Hauling and moving expenses vary with weight and width of the equipment. Loads wider than highway specification require special handling.

Numerous small items should be included in the contract for mechanical brush control so that costs are minimized. Among others, these items include stipulation of both minimum and maximum horsepower, cleat size to provide adequate traction, and a limit on time out for repairs. Seasonal, weather, and fiscal year changes cause operating time to be short at best. Projects that require two or more types of equipment, such as crushing, chaining, and root raking, can provide enough flexibility to keep men and tractors working during breakdowns. Modifications of equipment and operational procedures should be specified in the contract.

The age and density of stand influence the proper timing of control. If costs of control increase more than benefits do as plants grow older, young stands should be treated. In most instances, older stands are optimal treatment areas when costs are fixed (Jameson, 1971).

APPEARANCE OF THE ALTERED LANDSCAPE

Success in brush control more often than not is evaluated by the appearance of the job rather than by measured results. The appearance that pleases one person does not necessarily satisfy another. The manager with domestic livestock looks for an increase in forage, water, and accessibility. The game manager wants cover, water, and food for the particular combination of shootable birds and big game in the area. The recreationist usually likes a variation in scene, few straight lines, water, accessibility, abundant life, etc. The ideal number of woody plants varies from none to perhaps 1,000 or more per hectare, according to different people.

Brush control can be done in a way that preserves or creates a landscape pleasing in appearance. Great variation in physical conditions and environmental concerns increasingly require more than one piece of equipment and more than one technique in a brush-control project. For example, a fuelbreak can be effective and can be made pleasing to the eye if the edges are irregular rather than straight, if islands of brush are left in the break, and if different brush densities are maintained along the edges. Cleared and uncleared land adjacent to each other and contrasting boundaries are to be minimized. Irregular applications require maneuverability in equipment and flexibility in operation. Although brush-clearing equipment is massive, it can be operated, with care, to preserve the appearance of an area.

A landscape mosaic has pleasing appearance and numerous values for domestic and wild animals. For sage grouse habitat, control of *Artemisia tridentata* should be done in strips and limited to areas under 100 hectares in size. Small brush areas and areas adjacent to booming grounds, streams, and *Populus* thickets should be left untreated. Sage grouse need mature stands of *Artemisia* for brooding and winter feeding, but during spring and summer the chicks must have a variety of young forbs and grasses that most commonly occur in disturbed areas. Complete conversion to grass for livestock should probably be restricted to the meadow sites (Schneegas, 1967). *Artemisia* provides food and cover for sage grouse, but they also need open areas (Martin, 1970).

LITERATURE CITED

Abernathy, G. H., and C. H. Herbel. 1973. Brush eradicating, basin pitting and seeding machine for arid to semiarid rangeland. *J. Range Mgmt.* 26:189–192.

Arnold, J. F., and W. L. Schroeder. 1955. Juniper control increases forage production on the Fort Apache Indian Reservation. *Rocky Mtn. For. and Range Expt. Sta. Paper* 18.

Aro, R. S. 1971. Evaluation of pinyon-juniper conversion to grassland. *J. Range Mgmt.* 24:188–197.

Bleak, A. T., and W. G. Miller. 1955. Sagebrush seedling production as related to time of mechanical eradication. *J. Range Mgmt.* 8:66–69.

Box, T. W., and J. Powell. 1965. Brush management techniques for improved forage values in south Texas. *Trans. N. Am. Wildl. and Nat. Res. Conf.* 30:285–296.

Clary, W. P. 1971. Effects of Utah juniper removal on herbage yields from Springerville soil. *J. Range Mgmt.* 24:373–378.

Dodd, J.D. 1968. Mechanical control of prickly pear and other woody species on the Rio Grande plains. *J. Range Mgmt.* 21:366–370.

————, and S. T. Holtz. 1972. Integration of burning with mechanical manipulation of south Texas grassland. *J. Range Mgmt.* 25:130–136.

Everson, A. C. 1951. Grass yields of three differently treated range areas. *J. Range Mgmt.* 4:93–94.

Frischknecht, N. C., and A. T. Bleak. 1957. Encroachment of big sagebrush on seeded range in northeastern Nevada. *J. Range Mgmt.* 10:165–170.

Gifford, G. F. 1973. Runoff and sediment yields from runoff plots on chained pinyon-juniper sites in Utah. *J. Range Mgmt.* 26:440–443.

————, and C.B. Shaw. 1973. Soil moisture patterns on two chained pinyon-juniper sites in Utah. *J. Range Mgmt.* 26:436–440.

————, G. Williams, and G. B. Coltharp. 1970. Infiltration and erosion studies on pinyon-juniper conversion sites in southern Utah. *J. Range Mgmt.* 23:402–406.

Grelen, H. E., L. B. Whitaker, and R. E. Lohrey. 1972. Herbage response to precommercial thinning on direct-seeded slash pine. *J. Range Mgmt.* 25:435–437.

Herbel, C. H., G. H. Abernathy, C. C. Yarbrough, and D. K. Gardner. 1973. Root plowing and seeding arid rangelands in the southwest. *J. Range Mgmt.* 26:193–197.

————, F. Ares, and J. Bridges. 1958. Hand-grubbing mesquite in the semidesert grassland. *J. Range Mgmt.* 11:267–270.

Hill, L. W., and R. M. Rice. 1963. Converting from brush to grass increases water yield in southern California. *J. Range Mgmt.* 16:300–305.

Hyder, D. N., and F. A. Sneva. 1956. Herbage response to sagebrush spraying. *J. Range Mgmt.* 9:34–38.

Jameson, D. A. 1971. Optimum stand selection for juniper control on southwestern woodland ranges. *J. Range Mgmt.* 24:94–99.

Kincaid, D. R., and G. Williams. 1966. Rainfall effects on soil surface characteristics following range improvement treatments. *J. Range Mgmt.* 19:346–351.

Lewis, C. E. 1970. Reponses to chopping and rock phosphate on south Florida ranges. *J. Range Mgmt.* 23:276–282.

Longhurst, W. M. 1956. Stump sprouting of oaks in response to seasonal cutting. *J. Range Mgmt.* 9:194–196.

Martin, N. S. 1970. Sagebrush control related to habitat and sage grouse occurrence. *J. Wildl. Mgmt.* 34:313–320.

McConnell, B. R., and J. G. Smith. 1965. Understory response three years after thinning pine. *J. Range Mgmt.* 18:129–132.

————, and ————. 1970. Response of understory vegetation to ponderosa pine thinning in eastern Washington. *J. Range Mgmt.* 23:208–212.

McCulloch, C. Y. 1966. Cliffrose browse yield on bulldozed pinyon-juniper areas in northern Arizona. *J. Range Mgmt.* 19:373–374.

————. 1971. Cliffrose reproduction after pinyon-juniper control. *J. Range Mgmt.* 24:468.

Morrow, J., C. W. True, Jr., and V. M. Harris. 1962. *An economic analysis of current brush control practices.* Robstown, Texas: Southwest Agr. Inst. and the M. G. and Johnnye D. Perry Foundation.

Mueggler, W. F., and J. P. Blaisdell. 1958. Effects on associated species of burning, rotobeating, spraying, and railing sagebrush. *J. Range Mgmt.* 11:61–66.

Pechanec, J. F., G. Stewart, A. P. Plummer, J. H. Robertson, and A. C. Hull, Jr. 1954. Controlling sagebrush on rangelands. *U.S. Dept. Agr. Farmers' Bull.* 2072.

Pieper, R. D. 1971. Blue grama vegetation responds inconsistently to cholla cactus control. *J. Range Mgmt.* 24:52–54.

Platt, K. B. 1959. Plant control—some possibilities and limitations. II. Vital statistics of range management. *J. Range Mgmt.* 12:194–200.

Powell, J., and T. W. Box. 1967. Mechanical control and fertilization as brush management practices affect forage production in south Texas. *J. Range Mgmt.* 20:227–236.

Sampson, A. W., and A. M. Schultz. 1957. *Control of brush and undesirable trees.* Rome:FAO.

Schmutz, E. M., D. R. Cable, and J. J. Warwick. 1959. Effects of shrub removal on the vegetation of a semidesert grass-shrub range. *J. Range Mgmt.* 12:34–37.

Schneegas, E. R. 1967. Sage grouse and sagebrush control. *Trans. N. Am. Wildl. and Nat. Res. Conf.* 32:270–274.

Thompson, W. W., and F. R. Gartner. 1971. Native forage response to clearing low quality ponderosa pine. *J. Range Mgmt.* 24:272–277.

Williams, G., G. F. Gifford, and G. B. Coltharp. 1972. Factors influencing infiltration and erosion on chained pinyon-juniper sites in Utah. *J. Range Mgmt.* 25:201–205.

Wolters, G. L. 1973. Southern pine overstories influence herbage quality. *J. Range Mgmt.* 26:423–426.

Wright, H. A., and K. J. Stinson. 1970. Response of mesquite to season of top removal. *J. Range Mgmt.* 23:127–128.

Chapter 14

Chemical Control
of Rangeland Plants

An extensive literature describes chemical control of many undesirable plants in all phases of agriculture. Numerous papers review various aspects of noxious range-plant control; several hundred report research results and practice, and an even larger number relate knowledge acquired through range-management practice. This chapter selects from that body of knowledge and makes no pretext of being complete in its coverage of herbicides. Recipes for specific chemical controls should be viewed as being locally determined by test and experience and for local use; hence no complete prescriptions are given in this chapter.

MAJOR CHEMICALS USED AS RANGELAND HERBICIDES

Only a few of a large number of available herbicides have been applied extensively on rangelands. For control of both herbaceous and woody plants, the following herbicides are selected for special emphasis. They best meet the requirements of an ideal herbicide: (1) selective action, (2) economical application, (3) ease in handling, (4) sure results, (5) nontoxicity to animals, and (6) noncumulative and nondamaging consequences in food chains. None of these chemicals is ideal in all respects.

2,4-D	(2,4-dichlorophenoxyacetic acid)
2,4,5-T	(2,4,5-trichlorophenoxyacetic acid)
Silvex	(2-(2,4,5-trichlorophenoxy) propionic acid)
Picloram	(4-amino-3,5,6-trichloropicolinic acid)
MCPA	(2-methyl-4-chlorophenoxyacetic acid)

2,4-D was the first selective herbicide to become widely used, and it continues as a popular chemical for weed and brush control. 2,4,5-T has become less widely used following recent controversies, but it remains a safe and effective herbicide for many purposes. The effectiveness of Silvex on broad-leaved herbaceous plants and a few woody plants requires that it be included. MCPA is probably the fourth of the phenoxy compounds in importance for rangeland treatment. Picloram has been effective on many species and may replace the phenoxy compounds for brush control. Use of it remains restricted to rights-of-way in the United States, but it is widely used on rangeland in Australia, Africa, and South America.

Acid forms of the phenoxy chemicals mentioned above are essentially insoluble in water; hence these herbicides are sold as esters or as watersoluble salts. They are usually in liquid form for dilution in water, light oils, or emulsions. Volatility is low for the salts and some of the esters, but all may drift when applied in fine spray droplets and when conditions are windy during application.

2,4-D is used to control broad-leaved herbaceous and woody species, and it is applied in foliage sprays or basal stem treatments. It may kill grass seedlings. Leaves readily absorb 2,4-D, and it moves out of the leaves with the sugars.

2,4,5-T, like 2,4-D, is a growth-regulator type of herbicide. It is handled and applied much like 2,4-D and, in fact, the two are mixed for increased effectiveness on a spectrum of species. Some woody species are tolerant to 2,4,5-T but susceptible to 2,4-D, some the opposite, some susceptible to both, and others resistant to both.

Silvex is a selective translocated foliar spray with characteristics similar to those of 2,4-D and 2,4,5-T. It is not so likely to drift during aerial spraying and is more effective on some species than are other herbicides. Silvex is less effective as a basal-bark and stump treatment than are the other phenoxys. Silvex is used to control several aquatic weeds. Heavy applications proved effective on *Opuntia* after it was crushed with a cultipacker (Thatcher et al., 1964).

Picloram is an organic compound readily absorbed by foliage and roots. It is selective on broad-leaved and woody species and does little harm to well-established grasses. Picloram shows great promise for control of noxious woody plants on rangelands throughout the world, but it is not cleared for use on rangelands and pastures in the United States. It is available in pure form or mixed with 2,4-D. The effectiveness of picloram on *Cirsium arvense* and *Convolvulus arvensis* suggests that it may replace other chemicals in the control of these weeds.

MCPA, another phenoxy herbicide, is similar to 2,4-D but is used more on broad-leaved herbaceous plants and less on woody species than are the other herbicides.

Other herbicides are used for specific situations. Many hundreds of these herbicides have been tested. Green (1973) estimated that 7,500 compounds are tested for each one that reaches commercial production. Chemical and biological testing of each successful herbicide takes six to eight years.

Application

To be effective, foliar sprays of systemic herbicides such as 2,4-D must be applied at a certain phenological growth stage. The stage varies among species, but most woody plants are susceptible after leaves and shoots have developed and before leaf cuticle has thickened. This is a short period during which carbohydrate reserves are replenished. Some of the criteria that determine this period are the following: (1) leaves nearly developed in *Prosopis,* (2) *Adenostoma fasciculatum* sprouts about 4 decimeters long, (3) soil moisture sufficient for additional growth, and (4) *Poa secunda* heading when *Artemisia tridentata* is most susceptible or in the bloom stage for *Chrysothamnus* spp.

Other techniques for chemical brush control may be used at different times. Stump treatments, application of chemicals in frills or bark girdles, and injection through the bark effectively kill most tree species when done anytime during the year. Spraying or pouring concentrated solutions on the trunks of trees should be avoided during dry and dormant periods. Soil treatments to kill woody plants must precede sufficient rainfall to carry the chemicals into the soil. Soil treatments should come earlier in the season than foliar sprays.

The equipment for spraying foliage may be hand-operated sprayers, booms with several nozzles, or aerial sprayers (Fig. 14-1). Mist blowers provide excellent coverage, but spray drifting may be a problem. Basal treatments, such as treating stumps, painting or wetting the lower trunks of woody stems, and pouring chemicals into frills and girdles are done with hand sprayers or squirt cans with long spouts. Tree injection is accomplished with tools that make a cut into the bark and inject a measured portion of chemical with each stroke. Treating soil around bushes and trees is usually done by sprinkling pellets or powder forms of the herbicides.

Hazards

Hazards of the five selected herbicides to livestock and wild animals are slight under directed and recommended use (Table 14-1). LD_{50} (the dosage that is 50

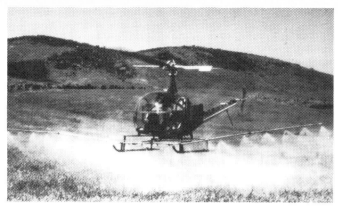

Figure 14-1 Aerial spraying of chapparral sprouts by helicopter in a brush conversion project in California. *(Photo by G. Burma.)*

percent lethal) for the phenoxy compounds appears to be no lower than 375–500 ppm in the diet of rats, and for picloram it is 8,200 ppm. No effect was found from feeding 1,000 ppm picloram to rats for 90 days (McCollister and Leng, 1969). Pecloram is low in toxicity to fish, birds, aquatic chain organisms, and soil microorganisms (Goring and Hamaker, 1971). Spraying of 2,4-D with and without picloram at ten times the normal rate of field application had no effect on chickens and pheasants before and after hatching (Somers et al., 1973). A mature cow showed no effect after 112 days on a diet containing 500 ppm of 2,4-D (Palmer and Radeleff, 1964). On a field with complete foliage cover, the total

Table 14-1 Chronic toxicity of three herbicides to several kinds of animals *(as summarized by Norris, 1971)*

	Concentration in diet, ppm	Duration of feeding, days	Effect
2,4-D			
Mule deer	2,400	30	Slight
Cattle	500	112	None
Sheep	1,000	481	None
2,4,5-T			
Cattle	1,250	15	None
Sheep	1,000	481	None
Picloram			
Sheep	1,100	30	None
Quail	500	Three generations	None

amount of 2,4-D eaten in this study would be the daily equivalent of the amount that would be taken in by a cow eating all the forage from 100 square meters of land that is freshly sprayed each day at the rate of 2.24 kilograms per hectare. Consumption rates might approach that amount, but spraying of herbicides more than once per year seldom occurs.

Phenoxy herbicides are classified as moderately to mildly toxic. Common table salt is rated mildly toxic to humans, with LD_{50} at 3,300 ppm (U.S. Dept. Agr., 1967).

The question still arises, "How safe is safe?" This question cannot be answered because standards change. For example, in 1950, safety evaluation required feeding to rats for 30 to 90 days. By 1971, safety tests required 90 days of feeding to rats and dogs; three generations of effects in rats; teratogenesis in rodents; effects on fish, shellfish, primates, humans, and birds; two-year carcinogenesis evaluation in hamsters; and evaluation of mutagenesis. Permitted analytical contents were lowered during 1950 to 1971 from 1 ppm in food crops to 0.01 to 0.05 ppm and as low as 0.005 ppm in milk (Johnson, 1971).

Safety involves stability, movement, and accumulation in man's environment; hazards of handling and residues; effects on nontarget organisms; and environmental impacts (Johnson, 1971). According to Mullison (1973), condemnation of herbicides and other chemical additives to the environment characterizes a fashionable position whether or not they are safe. To be hazardous, a chemical must have high toxicity and a high potential for exposure. To determine toxicity one must stipulate how much chemical is present under what conditions. Even the most toxic chemicals are not hazardous if there is no exposure. The likelihood of exposure to herbicides depends upon their chemical behavior, distribution, persistence, and movement in the environment and in food chains. The large doses of the major herbicides necessary to make them acutely toxic are not likely because the herbicides do not persist in the environment, lack biomagnification in food chains, and are excreted rapidly by animals. Sheep and cattle void 89 to 98 percent of 2,4-D, 2,4,5-T, and picloram within four days after consumption of single doses (Norris, 1971). Residues on grass forage immediately after spraying at the rate of 1.12 kilograms per hectare were about 100 ppm, which rapidly decreased to 30 to 50 ppm within two to four weeks (Morton et al., 1967; Getzendaner et al., 1969). Picloram is more persistent than the phenoxy herbicides but decreases to low levels within a year (Hoffman et al., 1972).

The decomposition and environmental dilution of herbicides include many processes. Biologically, herbicides are metabolized by *Aspergillus* (Altman and Dittmer, 1968). Chemically, they are reduced by oxidation and hydrolysis. Light destroys 2,4-D and picloram (Weber et al., 1973). Transfer through the air, through soil, and by runoff dilutes these chemicals to extremely low concentrations. Norris (1971) never found herbicide concentrations greater than 1 ppm and seldom found concentrations over 0.1 ppm in running water during seven years of monitoring spray application in the western United States. Picloram or mixtures of picloram with the phenoxy herbicides at 1,000 ppm had no detectable effects on four soil processes: ammonification, nitrification, sulfur oxidation, and organic matter decomposition (Tu and Bollen, 1969).

One of the most common hazards with spray applications of herbicides is that the material will drift to sensitive nontarget plants. Aerial application in winds less than 8 kilometers per hour and in air temperatures less than 32°C are recommended (U.S. Dept. Agr., 1969). Nozzle design should give large droplet size, with the nozzle pressure maintained below 70 grams per square centimeter. Spraying needs to be as close as possible to the target species. Liquid properties of high surface tension, high density, and high viscosity reduce drift (Yates, 1960).

Herbicides may enter water in lakes and streams via drift of materials and via direct application where water sources are within the boundaries of treated areas. Herbicides may enter water by surface flow and by leaching. Direct applications can be avoided, but the flow over and through the soil cannot be eliminated. However, the short persistence of most herbicides and the resistance of them to leaching reduce the potential for stream pollution. Hazards to fish are reduced if spraying over and near streams is avoided (Juntunen and Norris, 1972). Where proper precautions are taken, the hazard to fish is nil from the use of the five herbicides emphasized in this chapter.

When 2,4-D; 2,4,5-T; Silvex; picloram; and MCPA are applied according to recommended procedures, there is little hazard to man, animals, and food chains in their use. These chemicals are selective, potent, easy to handle, nonpoisonous, nonaccumulative, and noncorrosive (Klingman and Shaw, 1971). Their regulated use on rangelands needs to be continued.

RESPONSES OF RANGELAND SPECIES TO HERBICIDES

The genera and species selected for discussion here include major brush problems and undesirable broad-leaved plants on western and southern United States range-lands. The genera and species listed in Table 14-2 and others mentioned are broadly representative of many not mentioned. Herbicides are applied to areas of land and vegetation, but, more often than not, the results are reported for individual species. The following discussions are aimed at groups such as the *Artemisia* type, *Prosopis* brush fields, and the genus *Quercus*.

Control of *Artemisia*

Kearl (1965) estimated, on a basis of mail survey and interviews with researchers, that 200,000 hectares of the sagebrush type were sprayed in Wyoming during the

Table 14-2   Effectiveness of five herbicides on selected rangeland species[*]

Species	2,4-D	2,4,5-T	Silvex	Picloram	MCPA	Remarks
Acacia spp.	R[†]	I-R	...	S-I	...	
Adenostoma fasciculatum	S-I	S-I	R	S	I-R	On sprouts
Alnus spp.	S	S	S	...	S	2,4-D best
Arctostaphylos spp.	S-I	S-I	S-I	S-I	I-R	
Artemisia tridentata	S	S	S-I	S-I	R	2,4-D best
Chrysothamnus spp.	S-I	I-R	R	S	R	
Delphinium barbeyi	R	S	S	...	...	Mix Silvex and 2,4,5-T
Opuntia spp. (cholla)	...	I	S	S	...	
Opuntia spp. (pear)	...	I	S-I	I	...	
Prosopis juliflora	I-R	S-I	...	S-I	R	
Pteridium aquilinum	R	R	R	...	R	Use Amitrole
Quercus havardii	I-R	S-I	I-R	S-I	R	
Quercus spp.	I	S-I	I	S-I	R	Picloram best
Rhus spp. (poison oak)	S-I	S	S	S	I-R	
Rubus spp. (blackberry)	R	S	S-I	...	R	
Serenoa repens	...	...	S	...	...	
Ulmus spp.	R	I	S-I	S-I	R	

[*]The evaluation of effectiveness is a judgment based on many sources of information including Dunham (1965), Gantz and Laning (1963), Klingman and Shaw (1971), Leonard and Harvey (1965), Morton (1973), National Research Council (1968), Southwick (1973), U.S. Dept. Agr. (1967, 1969), and others.

[†]*S* indicates satisfactory kill (arbitrarily above 70 percent) with one application. *I* means inadequate kill. *S-I* designates satisfactory control following two or more applications or one treatment with heavy dosage. *R* suggests resistance to the chemical, and *I-R* indicates top kill with abundant resprouting.

period 1952–1964. Conversions of stands from brush to grass showed success at rates of 100 to 400 percent increased forage on 70 percent of the treated areas in Wyoming. In a few stands, clearing was complete; and 7 to 27 percent of the brush remained on 60 percent of the treated stands. Other intermountain states have controlled large areas of *Artemisia,* but estimates of area are not available. Presumably there was as much success in these states as in Wyoming. Clearly, spraying of sagebrush, mainly *Artemisia tridentata,* has successfully increased forage for livestock.

Spraying with 2 kilograms of 2,4-D per hectare has given 70 percent or better kill in Wyoming (Alley and Bohmont, 1958), in California (Cornelius and Graham, 1958), in Nevada (Eckert et al., 1972), in Oregon (Hyder, 1953), and in several other states (Shown et al., 1969). The principal times of spraying include when *Artemisia tridentata* twigs have reached half their growth (Hull and Vaughn, 1951; Hormay et al., 1962); immediately preceding anthesis of *Poa secunda* (Hull et al., 1952); and when new twig growth has reached 5 centimeters on *Chrysothamnus* (Mohan, 1973).

The effects of 2,4-D on other species associated with *Artemisia tridentata* have been erratic. Hyder (1972) reported 90 percent kill of *Delphinium geyeri;* Laycock (1967) found a two-thirds reduction of *Petradoria pumila. Chrysothamnus viscidiflorus* and *C. nauseosus* are less susceptible than *Artemisia tridentata,* and several workers recommend a mixture of 2,4-D and picloram for them (Paulsen and Miller, 1968; Eckert and Evans, 1968; Evans et al., 1973). However, 2,4-D may be effective if the *Chrysothamnus* plants have reached full leaf and the soil is wet (Mohan, 1973; Laycock and Phillips, 1968). *Purshia tridentata* mixed with *Artemisia* may be relatively undamaged if the dose of 2,4-D is less than 2.25 kilograms per hectare, favorable growing conditions occur after the spraying, and the *Purshia* plants are more than 30 centimeters tall (Hyder and Sneva, 1962b).

Spraying with 2,4-D reduced *Madia glomerata* and other broad-leaved herbs in *Artemisia* areas (Haas et al., 1962; Klomp and Hull, 1968) but did not decrease *Halogeton glomeratus,* which occurred in inverse proportions with *Agropyron desertorum* (Miller, 1956).

Artemisia tridentata invades sprayed and mechanically controlled stands. Mechanical controls after seed maturation speed the invasion, and seeding with *Agropyron* spp. slows it only somewhat. The life expectancy of controlled stands has been estimated to be between 15 and 20 years (Kearl, 1965; Johnson and Payne, 1968; Johnson, 1969; Sneva, 1972).

Reduction of *Artemisia* spp. and increase in grass have numerous effects in addition to providing more forage for livestock (Kearl, 1965). Moisture loss from deep soils is reduced (Tabler, 1968; Sturges, 1973), and wild animals may be favored with more grass and forbs, as are elk (Wilbert, 1963; Ward, 1973), antelope, and sage grouse if patches of *Artemisia* are left. The presence of more grass and less brush and forbs may favor mice and reduce the number of pocket gophers (Turner, 1969; Hull, 1971b). Tops of shrubs such as *Salix schouleriana* and *Amelanchier alnifolia* may be reduced and sprouts increased; thus game habitat may be improved (Mueggler, 1966).

Reduction of crown cover in dense *Artemisia* stands increases ranch values and returns per animal and may not require increased stocking rates to be profitable. Native grasses quickly take the place of the brush, even with continued moderate use of herbicides (Smith, 1969). The appearance of larger forage supplies on the sprayed areas permits improvement of untreated areas by reducing the grazing pressure on them. Improved distribution of animals follows brush control. Ranch values increase. *Artemisia* control on 5 to 15 percent of the best land promotes management of all the land.

Control of *Prosopis* and Associates

Reynolds and Tschirley (1957) estimated that *Prosopis juliflora,* including its three varieties in the southwestern United States, was a problem on 28 million hectares in Texas, New Mexico, and Arizona and that the area on which this species grows had doubled since the turn of the century. This species and many others associated with it are difficult to kill. If there are fewer than 125 large trees per hectare, the trees should receive an oil or herbicide treatment on the basal bud zone. Foliage sprays are applied by airplane to dense stands and to the bush type of growth. A mixture of 2,4,5-T and picloram appears to be the most satisfactory herbicide combination, but it gives low mortality of the bud zone. Defoliation gives the grasses and forbs an opportunity to grow for a few years until the brush cover returns. Two consecutive annual sprays with 2,4,5-T resulted in 58 percent mortality in southern Arizona (Cable and Tschirley, 1961). The best treatment of picloram and Dicamba in a Texas study attained 82 percent defoliation and 33 percent mortality (Meyer and Bovey, 1973). Reduction of *Prosopis* requires a variety of methods such as chaining or basal treatment of trees over 10-centimeters diameter, basal treatment on smaller plants with single stems, and foliage sprays on shrubs. Periodic fire may have a place in controlling *Prosopis* (Weddle and Wright, 1970; Ames, 1966).

In southern Texas, where numerous woody species are associated with *Prosopis,* spraying usually reduces the canopy for a few years. A mixture of picloram and 2,4,5-T as the best treatment, defoliated above 90 percent of *Aloysia lycioides,* about 50 percent of *Acacia farnesiana* and *Quercus virginiana,* and less than 25 percent of *Diospyros texana* and *Berberis trifoliata* (Bovey et al., 1970; Meyer and Bovey, 1973).

Sixty days after leaf emergence appears to be an average time for spraying *Prosopis* to attain greatest kill. Trees should have mature leaves and seed pods (Dahl et al., 1971). The soil should be moist and the soil temperature above 24°C at 25 centimeters below the surface (Sosebee et al., 1973). Niacin and other B vitamins, when added to 2,4,5-T and sprayed on *Prosopis* sprouts, increased root mortality (Sosebee, 1974).

Control of *Quercus* Species

The genus *Quercus* contains many species that occupy sizable rangeland areas. Most species sprout from the base when the tops are cut off or killed with herbicides. *Quercus* furnish browse for game, and the acorns are valuable food for many animals.

If *Quercus* control is desirable, each species must be approached as a separate problem. *Q. gambelii* in the intermountain region may be reduced with a spray mixture of 2,4,5-T and picloram (Marquiss, 1973) or picloram granules on the soil (Vallentine and Schwendiman, 1973). *Q. turbinella* is reduced but not killed with Silvex (Lillie et al., 1964). Sprouts and seedling trees soon dominate stands of *Q. stellata* and *Q. marilandica* after top kill in Arkansas and eastern Texas (Halls and Crawford, 1965). *Ulmus alata,* an associate of the *Quercus* species in Oklahoma and Arkansas, may be controlled by basal treatments with picloram (Kirby et al., 1967). In California, *Quercus douglasii* is controlled with 2,4,5-T (Leonard, 1956) and with picloram (Plumb, 1971) applied to the basal stems as a spray or in frills. *Quercus wislizenii, Q. dumosa,* and other California species are difficult to kill, although tops are reduced by chemical treatments (Emrick and Leonard, 1954; Plumb, 1968). No treatment fully prevents regrowth of *Q. havardii* on the sandy Rolling Plains of Texas. Perhaps no more than 70 percent reduction is ideal if erosion is to be prevented and wildlife values maintained. This degree of control may be attained with a mixture of Silvex and picloram (Scifres, 1972b).

Control of Herbaceous Range Weeds

Annual and perennial herbaceous plants on rangelands occupy many millions of hectares (see list in Chapter 12). Chemical control of annual forbs such as *Salsola* spp., *Halogeton glomeratus,* and *Madia glomerata* has not been successful, except on a small scale and in conjunction with other practices. Most annuals abound in pioneer successional stages, and problems with them disappear when range condition improves in response to managerial and cultural practices. For example, spraying reduces *Madia* and promotes establishment of seeded grasses in mountain meadows. However, the *Madia* would rapidly dominate without competition from the perennials (Hull and Cox, 1968; Hull, 1971a). *Hymenoxys odorata,* a poisonous annual species in Texas, retreats rapidly when management favors perennial vegetation.

Perennial range weeds are more permanent than the annuals and tend to occupy invaded areas for long periods. *Wyethia amplexicaulis* responds to 2,4-D, and control has increased forage production about fivefold in Utah (Tingey and Cook, 1955). Other plants of mountain meadows that have been reduced by spraying include *Geum rossii* (Smith and Alley, 1966), *Iris missouriensis* (Eckert et al., 1973), *Delphinium barbeyi* (Cronin and Neilson, 1972), *Helenium hoopesii* (Doran, 1951), and *Astragalus miser* var. *oblongifolius* (Williams, 1970). Thistles such as *Carduus nutans* and *Onopordum acanthium* are controlled by picloram (Hull and Evans, 1973; Hooper et al., 1970). *Zygadenus paniculatus* is highly sensitive to 2,4-D (Hyder and Sneva, 1962a).

Chemical control of herbaceous range weeds has been used most commonly in two situations. Mountain meadows that have become more or less permanently occupied by thick stands of weeds require plant control to begin rehabilitation. Often control is followed by seeding of perennial grasses and a seasonal livestock-management schedule. The second type of range-weed control situation aims to reduce poisonous plants.

Control of Other Species

The species of *Juniperus* on rangelands are difficult to control with chemicals, although they show moderate susceptibility to picloram (Beuhring et al., 1971; Scifres, 1972a). Mechanical controls and burning of *Juniperus* are more commonly used than are chemicals (Owensby et al., 1973). *Gutierrezia* spp. decrease with picloram but are less affected by 2,4-D and 2,4,5-T (Schmutz and Little, 1970; Gesink et al., 1973). Satisfactory reduction of sprouts of *Populus tremuloides* and associated shrubs in central Canada is difficult to obtain with chemicals and mechanical techniques (Bailey, 1972).

OVERALL EVALUATION

Herbicidal control of rangeland plants has been varyingly successful. *Artemisia* stands respond most consistently in terms of increased forage, but converted stands return slowly to the original brush cover. Reduction of woody plant canopy by spraying of hardwoods in Arkansas and mixed brush in southern Texas may last no longer than three to five years. Short of clearing for cultivation, brush control by any means has a finite life expectancy until the original stands return. Table 14-2 suggests the less than ideal results with herbicides on rangeland.

Herbicides are highly valuable tools in rangeland management. Always the objectives for application should be clearly stated. Herbicidal treatments must be parts of overall range programs. The causes of brush and weed problems need to be eliminated; otherwise controls will have little value, their effectiveness will be lost, and monetary losses will be incurred. Two examples suffice to show the need for overall management.

Meadows in the Sierra Nevada Mountains which have become choked with thick stands of *Ranunculus alismaefolius* should be treated with 2,4-D, which will also kill the *Artemisia tridentata*. If needed, gully plugs should be established to reduce erosion. Seeding of selected sites completes the rehabilitation. Livestock are managed so as not to overgraze and damage the rehabilitated cover.

Spraying of *Artemisia tridentata* in eastern Oregon and southern Idaho may be the only rehabilitation needed beyond good livestock management. If the brush has a scattered stand of perennial grasses, perhaps as little as 10 percent of what it should be, the death of the brush gives the grass a chance to gain vigor and increase in density. This program requires careful attention to livestock numbers, distribution, and seasonal grazing before and after *Artemisia* control.

LITERATURE CITED

Alley, H. P., and D. W. Bohmont. 1958. Big sagebrush control. *Wyo. Agr. Expt. Sta. Bull.* 354.

Altman, P. L., and D. S. Dittmer. 1968. *Metabolism.* Washington, D.C. Federation of American Societies for Experimental Biology.

Ames, C. R. 1966. Mesquite control on the Coronado National Forest. *J. Range Mgmt.* 19:148–150.

Bailey, A. W. 1972. Forage and woody sprout establishment on cleared, unbroken land in central Alberta. *J. Range Mgmt.* 25:119–122.

Bovey, R. W., J. R. Baur, and H. L. Morton. 1970. Control of huisache and associated woody species in south Texas. *J. Range Mgmt.* 23:47–50.

Buehring, N., P. W. Santelmann, and H. M. Elwell. 1971. Responses of red cedar to control procedures. *J. Range Mgmt.* 24:378–382.

Cable, D. R., and F. H. Tschirley. 1961. Responses of native and introduced grasses following aerial spraying of velvet mesquite in southern Arizona. *J. Range Mgmt.* 14:155–159.

Cornelius, D. R., and C. A. Graham. 1958. Sagebrush control with 2,4-D. *J. Range Mgmt.* 11:122–125.

Cronin, E. H., and D. B. Neilson. 1972. Controlling tall larkspur on snowdrift areas in the subalpine zone. *J. Range Mgmt.* 25:213–216.

Dahl, B. E., R. B. Wadley, M. R. George, and J. L. Talbot. 1971. Influence of site on mesquite mortality from 2,4,5-T. *J. Range Mgmt.* 24:210–215.

Doran, C. W. 1951. Control of orange sneezeweed with 2,4-D. *J. Range Mgmt.* 4:11–15.

Dunham, R. S. 1965. Herbicide manual for noncropland weeds. *U.S. Dept. Agr. Handbook* 269.

Eckert, R. E., Jr., A. D. Bruner, and G. J. Klomp. 1972. Response of understory species following herbicidal control of low sagebrush. *J. Range Mgmt.* 25:280–285.

———, ———, ———, and F. F. Peterson. 1973. Control of Rocky Mountain iris and vegetation response on mountain meadows. *J. Range Mgmt.* 26:352–355.

———, and R. A. Evans. 1968. Chemical control of low sagebrush and associated green rabbitbrush. *J. Range Mgmt.* 21:325–328.

Emrick, W. E., and O. A. Leonard. 1954. Delayed kill of interior live oak by fall treatment with 2,4-D and 2,4,5-T. *J. Range Mgmt.* 7:75–76.

Evans, R. A., J. A. Young, and P. T. Tueller. 1973. Current approaches to rabbitbrush control with herbicides. *Down to Earth* 29(2):1–4.

Gantz, R. L., and E. R. Laning, Jr. 1963. Tordon for the control of woody rangeland species in the western United States. *Down to Earth* 19(3):10–13.

Gesink, R. W., H. P. Alley, and G. A. Lee. 1973. Vegetative response to chemical control of broom snakeweed on a blue grama range. *J. Range Mgmt.* 26:139–143.

Getzendaner, M. E., J. L. Herman, and B. van Giessen. 1969. Residues of 4-amino-3,5, 6-trichloropicolinic acid in grass from applications of Tordon herbicides. *J. Agr. Food Chem.* 17:1251–1256.

Goring, C. A. I., and J. W. Hamaker. 1971. The degradation and movement of picloram in soil and water. *Down to Earth* 27(1):12–15.

Green, M. B. 1973. Are herbicides too expensive? *Weed Sci.* 21:374–378.

Haas, R. H., H. L. Morton, and P. J. Torell. 1962. Influence of soil salinity and 2,4-D treatments on establishment of desert wheatgrass and control of halogeton and other annual weeds. *J. Range Mgmt.* 15:205–210.

Halls, L. K., and H. S. Crawford. 1965. Vegetation response to an Ozark woodland spraying. *J. Range Mgmt.* 18:338–340.

Hoffman, G. O., M. G. Merkle, and R. H. Haas. 1972. Controlling mesquite with Tordon 225 mixture herbicide in the Texas backland prairie. *Down to Earth* 27(4):16–19.

Hooper, J. F., J. A. Young, and R. A. Evans. 1970. Economic evaluation of scotch thistle suppression. *Weed Sci.* 18:583–586.

Hormay, A. L., F. J. Alberico, and P. B. Lord. 1962. Experiences with 2,4-D spraying on the Lassen National Forest. *J. Range Mgmt.* 15:325–328.

Hull, A. C., Jr., 1971a. Spraying tarweed infestations on ranges newly seeded to grass. *J. Range Mgmt.* 24:145–147.

———. 1971b. Effect of spraying with 2,4-D upon abundance of pocket gophers in Franklin Basin, Idaho. *J. Range Mgmt.* 24:230–232.

———, and H. Cox, 1968. Spraying and seeding high elevation tarweed rangeland. *J. Range Mgmt.* 21:140–144.

———, and J. O. Evans. 1973. Musk thistle *(Carduus nutans):* An undesirable range plant. *J. Range Mgmt.* 26:383–385.

———, N. A. Kissinger, Jr., and W. T. Vaughn. 1952. Chemical control of big sagebrush in Wyoming. *J. Range Mgmt.* 5:398–402.

———, and W. T. Vaughn. 1951. Controlling big sagebrush with 2,4-D and other chemicals. *J. Range Mgmt.* 4:158–164.

Hyder, D. N. 1953. Controlling big sagebrush with growth regulators. *J. Range Mgmt.* 6:109–116.

———. 1972. Paraquat kills geyer larkspur. *J. Range Mgmt.* 25:460–464.

———, and F. A. Sneva. 1962a. Chemical control of foothill deathcamas. *J. Range Mgmt.* 15:25–27.

———, and ———. 1962b. Selective control of big sagebrush associated with bitterbrush. *J. Range Mgmt.* 15:211–215.

Johnson, J. E. 1971. Safety in the development of herbicides. *Down to Earth* 27(1):1–7.

Johnson, J. R., and G. F. Payne. 1968. Sagebrush reinvasion as affected by some environmental influences. *J. Range Mgmt.* 21:209–213.

Johnson, W. M. 1969. Life expectancy of a sagebrush control in central Wyoming. *J. Range Mgmt.* 22:177–182.

Juntunen, E. T., and L. A. Norris. 1972. Field application of herbicides—Avoiding danger to fish. *Ore. Agr. Expt. Sta. Special Report* 354.

Kearl, W. G. 1965. A survey of sagebrush control in Wyoming 1952–1964. *Wyo. Agr. Expt. Sta. M. C.* 217.

Kirby, B., P. Stryker, and P. Santelmann. 1967. Ground treatments for control of winged elm on rangeland. *J. Range Mgmt.* 20:158–160.

Klingman, D. L., and W. C. Shaw. 1971. Using phenoxy herbicides effectively. *U.S. Dept. Agr. Farmers' Bull.* 2183.

Klomp, G. J., and A. C. Hull, Jr. 1968. Effects of 2,4-D on emergence and seedling growth of range grasses. *J. Range Mgmt.* 21:67–70.

Laycock, W. A. 1967. Mortality of rock goldenrod in sagebrush stands sprayed with 2,4-D. *J. Range Mgmt.* 20:107–108.

———, and T. A. Phillips. 1968. Long-term effects of 2,4-D on lance leaf rabbitbrush and associated species. *J. Range Mgmt.* 21:90–93.

Leonard, O. A. 1956. Effect on blue oak *(Quercus douglasii)* of 2,4-D and 2,4,5-T concentrates applied to cuts in trunks. *J. Range Mgmt.* 9:15–19.

———, and W. H. Harvey. 1965. Chemical control of woody plants. *Calif. Agr. Expt. Sta Bull.* 812.

Lillie, D. T., G. E. Glendening, and C. P. Pase. 1964. Sprout growth of shrub live oak as influenced by season of burning and chemical treatments. *J. Range Mgmt.* 17:69–72.

Marquiss, R. W. 1973. Gambel oak studies in southwestern Colorado. *J. Range Mgmt.* 26:57–58.

McCollister, D. D., and M. L. Leng. 1969. Toxicology of picloram and safety evaluation of tordon herbicides. *Down to Earth* 25(2):5–10.

Meyer, R. E., and R. W. Bovey. 1973. Control of woody plants with herbicide mixtures. *Weed Sci.* 21:423–426.

Miller, R. K. 1956. Control of halogeton in Nevada by range seedlings and herbicides. *J. Range Mgmt.* 9:227–229.

Mohan, J. M. 1973. 14 years of rabbitbrush control in central Oregon. *J. Range Mgmt.* 26:448–451.

Morton, H. L. 1973. Weed and brush control for range improvement. *Crop Sci. Soc. Am. Special Pub.* No. 3, pp. 55–74.

———, E. D. Robinson, and R. E. Meyer. 1967. Persistence of 2,4-D, 2,4,5-T, and Dicamba in range forage grasses. *Weeds* 15:268–71.

Mueggler, W. F. 1966. Herbicide treatment of browse on a big-game winter range in northern Idaho. *J. Wildl. Mgmt.* 30:141–151.

Mullison, W. R. 1973. Herbicides—Are they safe? *Down to Earth* 29(3):7–11.

National Research Council. 1968. Principles of plant and animal pest control. II. Weed control. *National Academy of Sciences Publ. 1597.*

Norris, L. A. 1971. Chemical brush control: Assessing the hazard. *J. For.* 69:715–720.

Owensby, C. E., K. R. Blan, B. J. Eaton, and O. G. Russ. 1973. Evaluation of eastern red-cedar infestations in the northern Kansas Flint Hills. *J. Range Mgmt.* 26:256–260.

Palmer, J. S., and R. D. Radeleff. 1964. The toxicologic effects of certain fungicides and herbicides on sheep and cattle. *Ann. N.Y. Acad. Sci.* 3 (article 2):729–736.

Paulsen, H. A., Jr., and J. C. Miller. 1968. Control of parry rabbitbrush on mountain grasslands of western Colorado. *J. Range Mgmt.* 21:175–177.

Plumb, T. R. 1968. Control of brush regrowth in southern California with Tordon and phenoxy herbicide. *Down to Earth* 24(3):19–22.

————. 1971. Broadcast applications of herbicides to control scrub oak regrowth. *U.S. Dept. Agr. Forest Service Research Note* PSW-261.

Reynolds, H. G., and F. H. Tschirley. 1957. Mesquite control on southwestern rangeland. *U.S. Dept. Agr. Leaflet* 421.

Schmutz, E. M., and D. E. Little. 1970. Effects of 2,4,5-T and picloram on broom snakeweed in Arizona. *J. Range Mgmt.* 23:354–357.

Scifres, C. J. 1972a. Redberry juniper control with soil-applied herbicides. *J. Range Mgmt.* 25:308–310.

————. 1972b. Herbicide interactions in control of sand shinnery oak. *J. Range Mgmt.* 25:386–389.

Shown, L. M., R. F. Miller, and F. A. Branson. 1969. Sagebrush conversion to grassland as affected by precipitation, soil, and cultural practices. *J. Range Mgmt.* 22:303–311.

Smith, D. R. 1969. Is deferment always needed after chemical control of sagebrush? *J. Range Mgmt.* 22:261–263.

————, and H. P. Alley. 1966. Chemical control of alpine avens. *J. Range Mgmt.* 19:376–378.

Sneva, F. A. 1972. Grazing return following sagebrush control in eastern Oregon. *J. Range Mgmt.* 25:174–178.

Somers, J. D., E. T. Moran, Jr., and B. S. Reinhart. 1973. Effect of external application of 2,4-D and picloram to the fertile egg on hatching success and early chick performance. *Down to Earth* 29(3):15–17.

Sosebee, R. E. 1974. Herbicide plus various additives for follow-up control of shredded mesquite. *J. Range Mgmt.* 27:53–55.

————, B. E. Dahl, and J. P. Goen. 1973. Factors affecting mesquite control with Tordon 225 mixture. *J. Range Mgmt.* 26:369–371.

Southwick, L. 1973. Kuron Silvex herbicide continues to gain acceptance. *Down to Earth* 28:26–32.

Sturges, D. L. 1973. Soil moisture response to spraying big sagebrush the year of treatment. *J. Range Mgmt.* 26:444–447.

Tabler, R. D. 1968. Soil moisture response to spraying big sagebrush with 2,4-D. *J. Range Mgmt.* 21:12–15.

Thatcher, A. P., G. V. Davis, and H. P. Alley. 1964. Chemical control of plains pricklypear in southwestern Wyoming. *J. Range Mgmt.* 17:190–193.

Tingey, D. C., and C. W. Cook. 1955. Eradication of mule ear with herbicides. *Utah Agr. Expt. Sta. Bull.* 375.

Tu, C. M., and W. B. Bollen. 1969. Effect of Tordon herbicides on microbial activities in three Willamette Valley soils. *Down to Earth* 25(2):15–17.

Turner, G. T. 1969. Responses of mountain grassland vegetation to gopher control, reduced grazing, and herbicide. *J. Range Mgmt.* 22:377–383.

U.S. Dept. Agr., Agr. Research Service. 1969. Chemical control of brush and trees. *U.S. Dept. Agr. Farmers' Bull.* 2158.

U.S. Dept. Agr., Crops Research Division. 1967. Suggested guide for weed control 1967. *U.S. Dept. Agr. Handbook* 332.

Vallentine, J. F., and D. Schwendiman. 1973. Spot treatment for gambel oak control. *J. Range Mgmt.* 26:382–383.

Ward, A. L. 1973. Sagebrush control with herbicide has little effect on elk calving behavior. *U.S. Dept. Agr. Forest Service Research Note* RM-240.

Weber, J. B., T. J. Monaco, and A. D. Worsham. 1973. What happens to herbicides in the environment? *Down to Earth* 29(3):12–14.

Weddle, J. P., and H. A. Wright. 1970. An evaluation of five methods to retreat ,sprayed mesquite. *J. Range Mgmt.* 23:411–414.

Wilbert, D. E. 1963. Some effects of chemical sagebrush control on elk distribution. *J. Range Mgmt.* 16:74–78.

Williams, M. C. 1970. Detoxication of timber milkvetch by 2,4,5-T and Silvex. *J. Range Mgmt.* 23:400–402.

Yates, W. E. 1960. Minimizing spray drift hazards. *Down to Earth* 16(2):15–19.

Chapter 15

Fire as an Environmental Factor

This chapter develops the premise that fire is a part of natural systems, just as are plants, animals, moisture, and energy. Many writers have stated that fire causes grasslands. This particular vegetational type does burn frequently, but the presence of fire does not prove that grasslands need or are caused by fire. Most other vegetational types burn occasionally and some frequently, yet many do not become grasslands with repeated burning. The ponderosa pine type in Arizona has a record of burning every 7.3 years (Weaver, 1951), mixed pine in California burns about every 8 years (Show and Kotok, 1924), and the California coastal redwoods burn every 25 years (Fritz, 1931). Records such as these could support the hypothesis that fire causes forests. Where climate and vegetation favor burning, fire occurs frequently and species exhibit differing mechanisms for resisting damage from burning.

Fire does result in ecosystem changes, and man has altered these effects. He is learning to use fire as a modern tool in vegetational management (see Chapter 16). These two chapters include discussions on animal influences, because fire and grazing interact.

THE EVOLUTION OF TOLERANCE TO FIRE

The natural vegetation on which ruminant animals graze has developed over a period of time reckoned on the geological time scale. The period of domestic animals, estimated at 8,000 to 10,000 years (Whyte, 1961), is only the last moment on that scale. Grasses emerged as a distinct class of plants late in the Cretaceous, and by Miocene time they had attained dominance in areas of the world subsequently known as *grasslands* (Barnard and Frankel, 1964). Accompanying early Tertiary changes in vegetation, ancestral horses, swine, camels, hippopotamuses, peccaries, and many other grazing mammals developed. Cattle, bison, sheep, goats, deer, and antelope were present in the Miocene. In Australia, during these same periods, marsupials differentiated into many forms paralleling mammalian development on other continents. Thus, the evolution of grasslands on which herbivorous animals exploited a variety of niches was well-developed before the appearance of known evidence of man.

Widely accepted is the theory that both plants and animals proceeded through their structural changes in response to competition for a limited environment composed of space, water, energy, and minerals from the soil. Probably reciprocal evolutionary relationships developed between grazed plants and grazing animals. Structural features of the present grasses are adapted to reducing damage by grazing animals that have tooth structures and digestive tracts equipped to use coarse grass forage. Herbivorous animals were numerous in prehistoric times, so their grazing was intense. Their diets were selective. Grazing pressures probably varied both seasonally and over space. It seems reasonable to postulate that plants evolved in response to grazing and animals in response to differentiating plants.

Ecosystems that contain abundant forage resources as well as grazing animals are subject to burning. These ecological types include grasslands, shrublands, woodlands, and open forests. Dense temperate forests, tropical rain forests, and deserts, which seldom burn, have few large grazing animals. Thus fire must be considered as another factor in the coincident evolution of plants and animals.

Lightning is a common source of fire in natural vegetation. It is a weather phenomenon that is associated with both frontal and convectional movements of air. Starting of a fire by lightning depends on the presence of dry organic materials, either in dry climates or in wet climates with dry seasons. These climates have existed on earth for many millions of years, almost certainly from earlier than the beginnings of mammals and grasslands in the late Cretaceous.

Based on inference, prehistoric fires could have been prevalent. Arnold (1964) estimated that 1,800 lightning storms are occurring at any given moment on earth. Komarek (1967) believed that that estimate is conservative. He also gave evidence that lightning sets fires in grasslands and that fires originating in woodlands and forests, if unchecked, burn into adjacent grasslands. Fossil charcoal shows that fire destroyed vegetation in the Mesozoic era (Harris, 1958), long before man learned to use fire. Presumably, fire has been present and has been a factor in natural selection throughout the evolutionary history of higher plants and animals.

As each new mutant and recombination of factors in the gene pool was subjected to the sorting effects of fire, as well as the physical environmental factors and grazing, those individuals most fire-tolerant survived in greater proportion than the less well adapted. Fire was intermittent in its actions because of irregular time periods between its occurrences, and so was grazing. The physical factors, although constantly required for growth, were likely to be most selective at times of extremes, especially after fire and heavy grazing. Effects of catastrophes in climate, in overgrazing, and in fire differ in degree. All serve to select plant and animal species best adapted to each particular ecosystem.

If plant species have developed mechanisms for surviving fire and grazing, they may also depend on fire and grazing for successful regeneration. They may possess characteristics that enchance flammability (Mutch, 1970) and attractiveness to grazing animals. Fire-dependent vegetational communities burn more readily than do those that are fire-independent. Even when over-dry, litter from the monsoon forest of Australia does not burn as readily as that from a eucalyptus forest (Stocker, 1966). Elimination of grazing from many grasslands results in changed species composition, reduced soil cover, and less production. Shifts in physical environmental factors also result in vegetational changes. Minerals, water, energy, grazing, and fire have been part of the environment of individual plants and vegetation through geological time. They all are parts of the ecosystem in which one part is no more causative and natural than is another part. They all are needed.

Man, especially modern man with his domestic animals, is a relative newcomer to the environment of vegetation. He has changed the kinds of animal populations and the intensity of grazing by animals. He has changed the intensity and frequency of burning since he first learned to carry fire, perhaps a million years ago. The earliest evidence of fire used for warmth and cooking was associated with Peking man (*Homo erectus*) in Lower Pleistocene time about ½ million years ago (Howell, 1965). Humans have possessed fire and used it to enhance their lives for a period far longer than the age of modern man and his domestic animals. The current effects of fire and grazing differs only in degree from earlier influences. Whether the effects then (and now) were good or bad depended upon their values to man, not upon responses of vegetation and animals per se. The effects of fire were adjusted after many millions of years of burning and grazing without which much of the world's vegetation would be vastly different today.

FIRE TYPE AND FIRE SPECIES

The terms *fire type* and *fire species* refer to vegetation and species that are favored by burning. These are the types and species that are adapted to fire and may require burning in order to maintain their ecological position. They may be climax species such as those in grasslands and chaparral, which survive frequent fires by sprouting from unburned crowns. At the same time there would be climatic climaxes and even grazing climaxes. The fire types and fire species are stable with a combination of factors that include burning.

These terms are applied to successional stages that follow a fire, for example, *Pinus contorta* in the mountains of the western United States. A second fire kills this stand, as it does many subclimax tree stands. Pioneer successional stands of annuals such as *Epilobium angustifolium* in forests and *Emmenanthe penduliflora* in chaparral are called *fire species*. They need a fire for regeneration, but normal plant succession replaces them in a few years.

The terms should be restricted to those types that owe their origin to a particular fire and to the species that dominate the types. Characteristically the stands are pure and of even age. Whether fire is needed or tolerated in the climax types is not as clear-cut, and to call them *fire types* is confusing.

ADAPTATIONS OF PLANT SPECIES TO BURNING

Adaptations of grasses and forbs which permit them to resist, evade, or endure burning are similar to characteristics which suggest tolerance to grazing. Short basal internodes, vegetative growth by rhizomes and stolons, and basal meristems in linear leaves protect growing points. Annual habits, abundant seed crops, adaptations of fruits to rapid distribution and burial, and a short period for vigorous culm elongation and maturation foster survival during grazing and burning as well as in dry climates.

Many spring-aspect plants and early-maturing broad-leaved herbaceous species in grasslands are favored by fire, which removes smothering mulch. Woody plants have a different set of adaptations. Sprouting of adventitious buds high on the stems of certain trees, on stumps, from root crowns, and in buried lignotubers permits plants to live even though foilage and all above-ground live woody material has been removed. Thick, resistant bark protects many trees as they begin to mature, although when younger, they are highly susceptible to fire. In order of decreasing resistance to fire damage are mature trees of *Pinus ponderosa, P. lambertiana, Pseudotsuga menziesii, Libocedrus decurrens,* and *Abies concolor.* A number of subclimax pines (*Pinus contorta, P. attenuata*) are not especially resistant to fire but have closed cones that release seed only after a fire. Seeds of many species in the chaparral types require heat to break dormancy. Still other trees and shrubs produce seed at an early age before the plant material is dry enough to burn readily.

Perhaps the most effective combination of adaptations to burning is that of grasses that produce seed in a short time, die to the ground surface each year, have perenniating buds on live stems near or in the soil, can withstand repeated defoliations, and produce small seeds that tend to fall into soil cracks. These adaptations allow grasses to evade damage by fire, and at the same time, they produce fuel that tends to remove competing woody plants as its burns (Fig. 15-1). An abundance of species with protective characteristics suggests that many plants have been selected during their evolution because they can withstand defoliating influences. They may depend upon these same influences to reduce competition from other species.

EFFECTS OF FIRE ON SOIL

A fire in grassland, chaparral, forest, or any other natural vegetation reduces the litter and mulch, consumes most of the standing dead material, and can remove above-ground living materials. The degree to which soil cover is removed varies with the intensity of the fire. Following a fire and depending to a large degree upon the remaining cover, changes occur in soil temperatures, organic matter in the soil, ground-surface environmental conditions for plants, available nutrients, populations of soil micro- and macroorganisms, soil acidity, and erosion. Notwithstanding statements to the contrary, the mass of evidence indicates little permanent deterioration in these soil characteristics caused by burning.

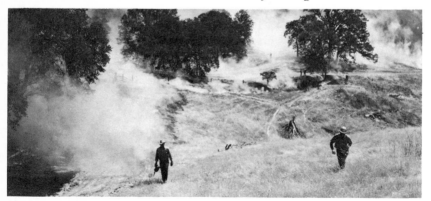

Figure 15-1   Fire has greater effect on woody vegetation than on grassland and is used to develop grassland.

Temperature

A thin cover of plants and litter rather than a thick cover results in more heat from the sun reaching the soil surfaces. A black surface after a fire readily absorbs heat. Maximum spring temperatures in the top 2.5 centimeters of soil were raised as much as 10°C, but minimum temperatures were not greatly altered following fire in the true prairie region of the central United States (Kucera and Ehrenreich, 1962). As green plants cover the soil, temperatures in the burned area become equal to those in adjacent unburned areas. An uncovered soil has greater temperature fluctuations than does a covered soil. The short period of higher soil temperatures, coincident with the beginning of growth, may be the cause of earlier growth of herbaceous plants on burned areas than on unburned areas.

Soil Organic Matter

Burning affects above- and below-ground organic matter, although the fire may not cause high soil temperatures. It alters amounts available for decomposition by reducing above-ground portions and often increases soil organic matter by killing plants. It changes the cycle of annual deposition of litter, at least during the first year after the fire. In forest types, the organic layer on the soil may be several inches thick; it may be left essentially unchanged or reduced to ash by fires of different intensities. There may be no natural accumulation of litter on the soil, as in many tropical grasslands or parts of the California annual grassland. In these grasslands, fire, which removes the standing dead, alters the habitat at the soil surface but has little influence on soil organic matter. However, Meiklejohn (1955) found that with burning of tall grasses in Kenya, fungi were reduced for one to two months, *Actinomyces* and bacteria had not recovered in three months, and *Clostridium* were not affected.

Grazing, as well as burning, alters the amount and position of litter. Normal litter cover in ungrazed grassland may take from one to six years to accumulate after a fire (Daubenmire, 1968). The relative influences of fire and grazing on litter have not been separated, but changes in botanical composition due to fire in the California annual grassland (Hervey, 1949) were nearly the same as those due to removal of litter by hand (Heady, 1956). Fire and hand removal of ungrazed herbage resulted in similar vegetational changes in South African grasslands (Scott, 1970).

Grasslands with a pine overstory in the southeastern United States frequently show increased soil organic matter after burning. Fires before the growing season in grasslands often have similar results. Moore (1960), working in Nigeria, found that 30 years of annual, early-dry-season burning increased soil organic matter but late-dry-season burns decreased it in comparison with complete protection. High soil temperatures that stimulate growth, a temporary abundance of annual pioneer plants, and decay of roots from plants killed by the fire are given as reasons for increased organic matter after fire (Daubenmire, 1968); however, results have been highly varied.

Soil Nutrients

Ashes left after a fire in vegetation are composed mainly of potassium, calcium, magnesium, and phosphorus as simple salts. The first three are basic in reaction. There is little direct loss of these due to burning except as they are released from organic binding and are moved by wind and water. Nitrogen and sulphur are volatilized and lost, especially where the fire is hot enough to leave white ash. If the ash is black, indicating a light burn, there is little loss of any mineral from the system. The major influences on soil nutrients appear to be a rapid release of minerals and generally a fractional increase in pH. Both influences are temporary and of little significance in grasslands where accumulations in wood or other perennial organs are slight. The ash from a forest fire may contain sufficient amounts of nitrogen to stimulate subsequent growth. Although nitrogen is lost in the smoke, reports do not always show a loss of nitrogen from grassland systems due to burning. Pioneer plants often include annual legumes that fix nitrogen. Higher soil temperatures during and after fires result in increased nitrification. Prescribed burning in the ponderosa pine type resulted in a nitrogen loss from the organic material on the soil and a nitrogen gain in the top inch of soil. The increase was attributed to leaching of the partially decomposed material left unburned (Klemmedson et al., 1962). After reviewing the results of work on changes in soil chemistry due to grassland fire, Daubenmire (1968) concluded that plant ash is too scant to change significantly mineral composition in most soils.

Soil Moisture

Burning of grasslands may reduce or increase soil moisture. Higher soil temperatures increase evaporation, and more plant growth increases transpiration. Without cover, runoff is high, but that situation may be eliminated quickly as new growth covers the ground. Soil moisture may be increased because there is less interception of rainfall by plants and litter (Burgy and Pomeroy, 1958), a higher proportion of pioneer and shallow-rooted species, and less total transpiring cover. Apparently, the infiltration rate remains unchanged or is decreased by burning (McMurphy and Anderson, 1965; Suman and Halls, 1955). Lack of soil cover and higher soil temperatures during the interim between the fire and establishment of a new cover appear to result in a drier soil surface after burning than before. Likely, the principal effect occurs in the altered moisture regime in the top few inches of soil.

Erosion

Fire has not accelerated erosion in the southeastern pine woodlands (Wahlenberg et al., 1939), tropical grasslands and savannas (Edwards, 1942), or shrub savanna in southern Africa (Banks, 1964). Wind erosion is likely to increase after burning in dry areas (Blaisdell, 1953). Water erosion will increase after burning if grazing is heavy and if slopes are steep (du Plessis and Mostert, 1965; O'Connor and Powell, 1963). The risk of erosion is highest after the fire but before a ground cover is reestablished. In southern California, where chaparral is on land steeper than the angle of repose, creep erosion occurs immediately after a fire, and erosion by water can be great during the first growing season if precipitation rates are intense. In most situations, accelerated erosion after a fire on relatively level land is of little consequence.

EFFECTS OF FIRE ON ANIMALS

Insect populations may be reduced or increased by burning. Many individuals are killed by fire, but enough escape to replenish populations. Of more importance is that certain species flourish on specific food plants that are abundant in different successional stages after a fire. Other insect species are abundant in relation to the amount of cover, which is influenced by fire.

Rodents generally escape all but the hottest fires because they take refuge in burrows. They are dependent on specific foods and cover, both influenced by burning. Vole populations crash when their habitat is burned, but white-footed mice may be little affected. Rodent populations return quickly when cover is reestablished.

Ground-nesting birds are vulnerable to loss of nests, cover, and foods. Because fire often affects both food and cover, bird populations respond to burning. For example, prescribed burning with hot fires in the southeastern United States promotes herbaceous legumes and quail, but the absence of burning and light burning reduce legumes and bobwhite quail (Martin and Cushwa, 1966).

Grassland fires have little effect on the larger animals, and most of these animals escape forest fires. Young sprout growth from surviving woody crowns generally is highly palatable and nutritious, so small burns or the edges of larger burns may be overused. Chaparral or shrubs that have grown beyond the reach of deer can be improved by burning of the tops so that sprouts and seedlings develop. The large animal species run to escape a fire, but they return to the new foods soon after a fire is out. Animals respond more to the changed habitat than to the fire itself.

EFFECTS OF FIRE ON PLANTS

Fire damage to individual plants depends upon the temperatures reached in live tissue, the length of time certain temperatures are maintained, and the physiological state of the plant at the time of burning. Growth stage, growth form, and size of plant influence the susceptibility of live tissue to heat damage. Lethal temperatures for meristematic tissue appear to vary between 45 °C and somewhat above 60 °C (Daubenmire, 1968). Many seeds have a much higher heat threshold and withstand temperatures over 100 °C. Seeds of *Erodium botrys* have been subjected to alternating temperatures of 100 °C and room temperature for four hours daily over a period of two weeks in order for dormancy to be broken.

Numerous studies have shown that stage of growth is an important determinant of fire damage. Invariably, a grassland fire occurring when some species are green and others are dry will damage the green species more than the dry ones. A fire that occurs after cool-season species begin to grow in the true prairie region will damage them but will do no harm to the warm-season species (Curtis and Partch, 1948). At the end of the growing season, fire has been used to reduce late-maturing *Taeniatherum caput-medusae* (McKell et al., 1962), an undesirable plant in the California annual grassland. The differential between the presence of sufficient mature annuals to carry a fire and the falling of *Taeniatherum* seed is about ten days. The objective of burning at that time is destruction of the seed crop. Once the seeds fall to the ground, a fire does little damage to them (Fig. 15-2).

The position of growing points on plants often determines temperatures attained in the tissue and severity of damage. Fire is more damaging to *Festuca idahoensis,* which has nodes and buds at or above the soil surface, than to

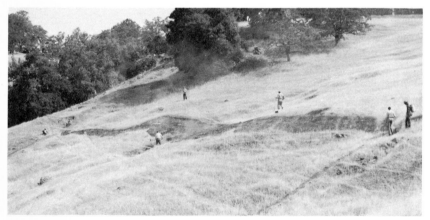

Figure 15-2   Grasslands are adapted to burning, and it results in temporary vegetational changes. *Taeniatherum caput-medusae* may be reduced but not eliminated by fire.

Agropyron spicatum, the buds of which are in the soil (Conrad and Poulton, 1966). Small bunches of a species usually sustain less damage than do large bunches because the small bunches contain less fuel within the bunch and near the basal nodes (Wright and Klemmedson, 1965).

New growth on burned areas may be different in chemical composition, moisture content, and growth stage from new growth on unburned areas, so burning attracts livestock and game. Generally, percentages of crude protein and ash are raised immediately after a fire (Killinger, 1948). Reasons for this response are not clear, but among the explanations are increased amount of available nutrients from the ash left by the fire, elimination of old stems that are using more food than they manufacture, and stimulation to new root growth due to heat treatment or warmer soil (Mes, 1958). Several authors showed that the moisture content of new herbage is higher in burned than in unburned areas (Mes, 1958; Halls et al., 1952; Sampson, 1944). New growth after fire frequently is a few days to as much as three weeks ahead of growth on unburned vegetation. Daubenmire (1968) discussed these relationships and mentioned exceptions to all of them. Two points seem clear: Grazing animals prefer burned areas; and any effects of burning on quality of forage and speed of growth are short-term, seldom lasting beyond the second year after a fire and usually disappearing during the first growing season.

Annuals have been reported to grow smaller the first season after a burn (Hervey, 1949). They are smaller also after hand removal of litter (Heady, 1956). Perennial grasses in the sagebrush-grass type in southeastern Idaho were shorter after a fire, but production was higher due to an increased number of culms (Blaisdell, 1953). As litter accumulates in tall-grass communities, basal area and size of parts decrease. Burning that reduces litter in these types generally stimulates growth, but on drier sites, frequent burning reduces cover and vigor of perennial grasses and may cause their replacement (West, 1965).

Decreased size of perennial-grass plants following a fire commonly is accompanied by increased flowering and seed production for one or two years. The species that respond in this manner are mainly warm-season species of the true prairie and of the tropical and subtropical grasslands. Short grasses and bunchgrasses of dry and cool grasslands tend to have fewer inflorescences after burning than do warm-season grasses (Daubenmire, 1968). Removal of litter without burning often has the same results as burning (Curtis and Partch, 1950).

Annuals depend upon seed that must survive during a fire. Heat generated by a grass fire may kill most seeds that have not fallen and those on a dry mulch surface. Seeds lying on bare soil, buried in soil cracks, and buried by the twisting action of awns survive in great numbers (Bentley and Fenner, 1958). Heat treatments, such as those that occur during burning, have increased germination of several species, including *Andropogon gerardi* and *Ambrosia artemisiifolia* (Curtis and Partch, 1948).

EFFECTS OF FIRE ON VEGETATION

A reduction in the number of fires that burned forests and grasslands in the United States during the twentieth century and a possible increase in the number of fires in other countries where populations have increased without efforts to reduce fires have given rise to much discussion on the values and ill effects of burning. There seems little doubt that species composition in the vegetation of many parts of the world has changed because burning has been increased or reduced. Increased woody plants and reduced grassland followed closely after fire reduction in southern Texas (Lehman, 1965). The Black Belt of western Alabama is believed to be the result of burning by Indians for cultivation and hunting (Rostlund, 1957). Protection from fire has resulted in dense, stagnant thickets of *Pinus ponderosa* in New Mexico (Weaver, 1964). Repeated burning produced the savannas of the Venezuelan Llanos (Aubréville, 1965). Humphrey (1953) argued that fire played a role in maintaining desert grasslands of the southwestern United States, and he concluded (1962) that reduction of fire increased woody plants at the expense of grasses. Biswell (1959) maintained that the *Pinus ponderosa* and mixed conifer types on the lower western slopes of the Sierra Nevada Mountains in California have thickened with excess tree regeneration and brush since burning was reduced.

A cursory search of the vast literature on fire leaves no doubt that change in burning patterns results in change in vegetation throughout the natural biomes. By selecting from among many studies and opinions, one can show that fire is destructive, that fire is a rejuvenative force required for the continued well-being of the landscape, and that fire is a useful management tool. The last view is becoming more prevalent and is common in recent literature.

Whether prescribed fire is used as a management tool depends, first, upon the chances of obtaining a specific land-management objective and, second, upon the prediction of a reasonable cost-return ratio. Three examples of the vast array of ecosystems and management objectives in which prescribed fire is used receive individual analysis in Chapter 16. Knowledge of expected changes in species composition and production is fundamental to the analysis.

Species Composition

Burning brings changes in the proportion of plant species present in an area. Greater density of *Pinus banksiana* in Minnesota (Grange, 1965) and *Pinus ponderosa* in Arizona (Weaver, 1964), fewer hardwoods and shrubs in the southern pine types (Stoddard, 1963), and more *Populus tremuloides* in the Lake States (Davis, 1959) are a few of many examples.

Fire in forest types that are not frequently burned reduces the proportion of climax woody species and sets the succession to begin at a seral stage. For example, burning of *Picea glauca* in well-drained northern forests results in successive dominance of moss, broad-leaved herbs, grass, hardwoods, and spruce again in about 20 years (Fig. 15-3). Removal of trees by burning in certain western United States mountains has resulted in an intermediate stage dominated by *Purshia* and *Artemisia* (Blaisdell, 1953). A second fire sets that succession back further by reducing the shrubs. Changes from dense woodland to savanna and then to grass with repeated burning in tropical and subtropical areas are further examples of the establishment of new types of vegetation from which plant succession proceeds anew until the next fire.

Those vegetational types closely attuned to burning also show changes, but they soon return to normal after a fire. The chaparral in California may appear to be destroyed by a fire because the aboveground parts of the shrubs have disappeared from the landscape (Horton and Kraebel, 1955). Soon, however, the shrubs sprout from root crowns and then dominate the site in four to six years. The shrubs sprout mainly from the original plants, but some develop from seed. It takes several fires at close intervals and heavy browsing for the chaparral to be reduced significantly.

Grasslands show slight changes in composition as a result of burning. The Mediterranean-type annual grassland has more broad-leaved annuals and fewer grasses for one year after burning than before burning (Hervey, 1949). *Andropogon scoparius* decreased and *Andropogon hallii* increased with burning

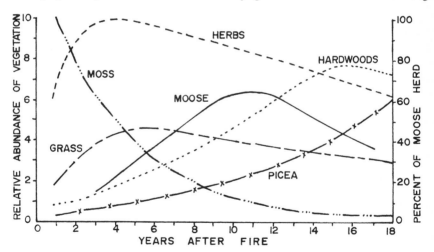

Figure 15-3 Vegetational succession following the 1947 wildlife on the Kenai National Moose Range, Alaska. From 10 to 12 years after the fire, over 50 percent of the moose herd was feeding in the burned area because abundant herbs, grass, and browse were available. As the *Picea glauca* and *P. mariana* increased, the other plants declined in quantity and moose feeding diminished. *(Adopted from Spencer and Hakala, 1964.)*

in western Oklahoma (McIlvain and Armstrong, 1966). In the South African veld, without burning, grasses give way to weeds (Scott, 1952), and the proportion of grass species changes considerably when the grasses are subjected to different burning regimes (Scott, 1967).

Change in the botanical composition of vegetation is related to the degree to which the vegetation is reduced from climax by burning. One forest may be set back to bare soil or to the very beginning of plant succession, but another may be converted to a shrub stage with a scattering of the climax dominants still alive. Fires frequently reduce the taller layers of vegetation and promote those near the ground. Grasslands and shrublands are favored when forest is destroyed. Shrublands, *Artemisia,* for example, can be removed almost completely in a single fire, and a grassland can result. Those shrub types that are successional to forest seldom are perpetuated by repeated fire. Grasslands are more permanent than shrublands under frequent burning.

The apparent permanence of species changes due to burning is related to the growth rates and generation times of dominant plants in the different successional stages. Evidence of a fire in the species composition of annual grassland may last for only a year or one generation of plants. Perennial grasslands recover in 1 to 3 years, but California chaparral takes about 10 to 15 years before evidence of a recent fire disappears. Dominance of *Epilobium* after burns suggests a fire within the last 5 years, but a *Pinus contorta* stand or any even-aged group of trees indicates a fire slightly older than the trees. Plant succession after a fire moves rapidly or slowly depending upon life-spans, so effects of burning may disappear quickly or last many years.

Production

The productivity of forage is increased or decreased by different burning situations, just as other results of burning vary. Burning increases the productivity of forage grasses in the southern United States forest types, as shown for pine types in Georgia (Greene, 1935), in Virginia (Cushwa and Redd, 1966), in *Arundinaria tecta* under pine in South Carolina (Hughes, 1957), for *Andropogon* spp. under pine in Louisiana (Duvall, 1962), and on the coastal plains of Florida (Hilmon and Lewis, 1962). In Florida, the coarse *Aristida stricta* is burned for improvement in the quality and palatability of livestock feed, although production per unit area is decreased. In several western United States rangeland types, grasses increase when *Artemisia* and other woody species are reduced by fire. These are examples of an increase in grass per unit area in direct relation to removal of competition by woody plants.

Grasslands themselves increase production following fire, as shown in the true prairie of the central United States (Kucera and Ehrenreich, 1962) and in tall grass of wet sites and regions in Africa (West, 1965). Burning usually lowers forage production in mixed prairie (Launchbaugh, 1964; 1972), California annual-type grassland (Hervey, 1949), other dry grasslands, *Molina caerulea* in the British Isles (Grant et al., 1963), and Arctic grasslands (Fridriksson, 1963).

Burning at different seasons has different effects on production in grasslands. Blydenstein (1963) found that burning at the beginning of the dry season reduced production of *Trachypogon* savanna in Venezuela about one-third. The production of grassland dominated by *Andropogon scoparius* in the Flint Hills of Kansas varied with time of annual spring burning (Anderson, 1964). In the Northern Territory of Australia, wet-season burning of the annual *Sorghum intrans* reduces it sufficiently that Townsville stylo can become established *(Stylosanthes humilis)* (Stocker and Sturtz, 1966).

FIRE AS A REGENERATIVE FORCE

When an area is burned, changes occur in animals, soil, and vegetation. For many organisms, a fire is a catastrophe, since conditions favoring their development are destroyed. They must retreat to unburned areas and await the return of suitable habitat. The waiting time may be short in a grassland or centuries long if mature climax trees are required.

For other organisms, burning brings conditions favoring their development. The Columbian black-tailed deer finds a higher quality and quantity of food in burned chaparral (Biswell et al., 1952). The Kirtland warbler in Michigan is limited to *Pinus banksiana* plantations with trees 5 to 15 feet in height and in blocks 80 acres and larger (Miller, 1963). The pine stands follow fires. The abundance of many animal species is related to x years following fire. Fire brings conditions that favor the development of some trees, also. Numerous tree species reproduce best where the seedbed is bare soil. Fire was one of the agencies, and perhaps the only one before man appeared, which could prepare the land for deer, for the Kirtland warbler, for regeneration of some tree species, and for many more animals and plants.

The succession of plants and animals following a fire, the dependence of so many animals upon the various successional stages, and even the restriction of animals to certain stages suggest that fire has been a relatively constant and continuously present ecological factor over geological time. Fire brings on renewed and increased activity by plants and animals. Without periodic destruction by fire, vegetation would have been essentially stable during the whole prehuman period. Conditions would not have existed continuously for the evolution of so many plant and animal species adapted to seral vegetational stages that are essentially nonexistent in climax vegetation. The complement to the destructive role of fire is the grazing and other activities of animals in swarm numbers, which can destroy climax vegetation.

Few large grazing species occur in the forest. Those that do occur there usually are in small numbers. Many more large grazing species inhabit grasslands, savannas, and open woodlands, which are the vegetational types with the greatest frequency of fire. Without implying cause and effect, one can see that nonforested vegetation, grazing animals, and fire are necessary for each other. If they are not necessary for each other, at least they exist together in perpetuating systems. Fire and succession in forests result in great fluctuations of herbivorous animals and changed habitat conditions. Fire should be looked upon as one of the forces that reduce large stores of organic materials to available nutrients. They stimulate regeneration first in plants and then in animals. This is a healthy process since it permits and supports a succession of different organisms and it fosters replacement of the old by the young. This process over thousands of generations has resulted in situations where burning is necessary for many species. A greater variety of landscape conditions and a larger number of species exist than would be the case if burning did not occur. Fire is a regenerative force that keeps a natural ecosystem healthy and even prevents the extinction of some species.

LITERATURE CITED

Anderson, K. L. 1964. Burning Flint Hills bluestem ranges. *Tall Timbers Fire Ecol. Conf.* 3:88–103.

Arnold, K. 1964. Project skyfire lightning research. *Tall Timbers Fire Ecol. Conf.* 3:120–130.

Aubréville, A. 1965. Les étranges savanes des llanos de l'Orenoque. *Adansonia* 5:3–13.

Banks, C. H. 1964. Further notes on the effect of autumnal veld burning on storm flow in the Abdolskloof Catchment, Jonkershoek. *For. in S. Afr.* 4:79–84.

Barnard, C., and L. H. Frankel. 1964. Grass, grazing animals, and man in historic perspective. In *Grasses and grassland,* ed. C. Barnard, pp. 1–12. London: MacMillan.

Bentley, J. R., and R. L. Fenner. 1958. Soil temperatures during burning related to postfire seedbeds on woodland range. *J. For.* 56:737–740.

Biswell, H. H. 1959. Man and fire in ponderosa pine in the Sierra Nevada of California. *Sierra Club Bull.* 44:44–53.

———, R. D. Taber, D. W. Hedrick, and A. M. Schultz. 1952. Management of chamise brushlands for game in the north coast region of California. *Calif. Fish and Game* 38:453–484.

Blaisdell, J. P. 1953. Ecological effects of planned burning of sagebrush-grass range on the upper Snake River plains. *U.S. Dept. Agr. Tech. Bull.* 1075.

Blydenstein, J. 1963. Cambios en la vegetación desqués de protección contra el fuego. Parte 1 y 2. *Soc. Venez. Cienc. Natl. Bol.* 23:233–244.

Burgy, R. H., and C. R. Pomeroy. 1958. Interception losses in grassy vegetation. *Trans. Am. Geophys. Union* 39:1095–1100.

Conrad, C. E., and C. E. Poulton. 1966. Effect of a wildfire on Idaho fescue and bluebunch wheatgrass. *J. Range Mgmt.* 19:138–141.

Curtis, J. T., and M. L. Partch. 1948. Effect of fire on the competition between bluegrass and certain prairie plants. *Am. Midl. Nat.* 39:437–443.

———, and ———. 1950. Some factors affecting flower production in *Andropogon gerardi. Ecology* 31:488–489.

Cushwa, C. T., and J. B. Redd. 1966. One prescribed burn and its effects on habitat of the Powhatan Game Management Area. *U.S. Forest Service Research Note* SE-61.

Daubenmire, R. 1968. Ecology of fire in grasslands. In *Advances in Ecological Research V*, pp. 209–266. London: Academic Press.

Davis, K. P. 1959. *Forest fire control and use.* New York: McGraw-Hill.

du Plessis, M. C. F., and J. W. C. Mostert. 1965. Run-off and soil losses at the Agricultural Research Institute, Glen. *S. Afr. J. Agr. Sci.* 8:1051–1060.

Duvall, V. L. 1962. Burning and grazing increase herbage on slender bluestem range. *J. Range Mgmt.* 15:14–16.

Edwards, D. C. 1942. Grass burning. *Emp. J. Expt. Agr.* 10:219–231.

Fridriksson, S. 1963. Effect of burning on the vegetation of moorlands (in Iceland). *Freyr Bunadarblad* 59:78–82.

Fritz, E. 1931. The role of fire in the redwood region. *J. For.* 29:939–950.

Grange, W. B. 1965. Fire and tree growth relationships to snowshoe rabbits. *Tall Timbers Fire Ecol. Conf.* 4:110–125.

Grant, S. A., R. F. Hunter, and C. Cross. 1963. The effects of muirburning *Molina*-dominant communities. *J. Br. Grassland Soc.* 18:249–257.

Greene, S. W. 1935. Effect of annual grass fires on organic matter and other constituents of virgin longleaf pine soils. *J. Agr. Res.* 50:809–822.

Halls, L. K., B. L. Southwell, and F. E. Knox. 1952. Burning and grazing in coastal plain forests. *Ga. Coastal Plain Expt. Sta. Bull.* 51.

Harris, T. M. 1958. Forest fire in the Mesozoic. *J. Ecol.* 46:447–453.

Heady, H. F. 1956. Changes in a California annual plant community induced by manipulation of natural mulch. *Ecology* 37:798–812.

Hervey, D. F. 1949. Reaction of a California annual-plant community to fire. *J. Range Mgmt.* 2:116–121.

Hilmon, J. B., and C. E. Lewis. 1962. Effect of burning on south Florida range. *Southeast Forest Expt. Sta. Paper* 146.

Horton, J. S., and C. J. Kraebel. 1955. Development of vegetation after fire in the chamise chaparral of southern California. *Ecology* 36:244–262.

Howell, F. C. 1965. *Early man.* New York: Time Inc.

Hughes, R. H. 1957. Response of cane to burning in the North Carolina coastal plain. *N.C. Agr. Expt. Sta. Bull.* 402.

Humphrey, R. R. 1953. The desert grassland, past and present. *J. Range Mgmt.* 6:159–164.

———. 1962. *Range ecology.* New York: Ronald Press.

Killinger, G. B. 1948. Effect of burning and fertilization of wire grass on pasture establishment. *J. Am. Soc. Agron.* 40:381–384.

Klemmedson, J. O., A. M. Schultz, H. Jenny, and H. H. Biswell. 1962. Effect of prescribed burning of forest litter on total soil nitrogen. *Soil Sci. Soc. Am. Proc.* 26:200–202.

Komarek, E. V., Sr. 1967. The nature of lightning fires. *Tall Timbers Fire Ecol. Conf.* 7:5–41.

Kucera, C. L., and J. H. Ehrenreich. 1962. Some effects of annual burning on central Missouri prairie. *Ecology* 43:334–336.

Launchbaugh, J. L. 1964. Effect of early spring burning on yields of native vegetation. *J. Range Mgmt.* 17:5–6.

———. 1972. Effect of fire on shortgrass and mixed prairie species. *Tall Timbers Fire Ecol. Conf.* 12:129–151.

Lehman, V. W. 1965. Fire in the range of Attwater's prairie chicken. *Tall Timbers Fire Ecol. Conf.* 4:127–143.

Martin, R. E., and C. T. Cushwa. 1966. Effects of heat and moisture on leguminous seed. *Tall Timbers Fire Ecol. Conf.* 5:159–175.

McIlvain, E. H., and C. G. Armstrong. 1966. A summary of fire and forage research on shinnery oak rangelands. *Tall Timbers Fire Ecol. Conf.* 5:127–129.

McKell, C. M., A. M. Wilson, and B. L. Kay. 1962. Effective burning of rangelands infested with medusahead. *Weeds* 10:125–131.

McMurphy, W. E., and K. L. Anderson. 1965. Burning Flint Hills range. *J. Range Mgmt.* 18:265–269.

Meiklejohn, Jane. 1955. The effect of bush burning on the microflora of a Kenya upland soil. *J. Soil Sci.* 6:111–118.

Mes, Margaretha G. 1958. The influence of veld burning or mowing on the water, nitrogen and ash content of grasses. *S. Afr. J. Sci.* 54:83–86.

Miller, H. A. 1963. Use of fire in wildlife management. *Tall Timbers Fire Ecol. Conf.* 2:18–30.

Moore, A. W. 1960. The influence of annual burning on a soil in the derived savanna zone of Nigeria. *Trans. 7th Internatl. Cong. Soil Sci.* 4:257–264.

Mutch, R. W. 1970. Wildland fires and ecosystems—A hypothesis. *Ecology* 51:1046–1051.

O'Connor, K. F., and A. J. Powell. 1963. Studies in the management of snow-tussock grassland. I. The effects of burning, cutting and fertilizer on narrow-leaved snow tussock (*Chinochloa rigida* (Raoul) Zotov) at a mid-altitude site in Canterbury, New Zealand. *N.Z. J. Agr. Res.* 6:354–367.

Rostlund, E. 1957. The myth of a natural prairie belt in Alabama: An interpretation of historical records. *Annals Assoc. Am. Geog.* 47:392–411.

Sampson, A. W. 1944. Plant succession on burned chaparral lands in northern California. *Calif. Agr. Expt. Sta. Bull.* 685.

Scott, J. D. 1952. A contribution to the study of the problems of the Drakensberg Conservation Area. *S. Afr. Dept. Agr. Sci. Bull.* 324.

———. 1967. Advances in pasture work in South Africa: Pt. 1. Veld. *Herb. Abst.* 37:1–9.

———. 1970. Pros and cons of eliminating veld burning. *Proc. Grassland Soc. S. Afr.* 5:23–26.

Show, S. B., and E. I. Kotok. 1924. The role of fire in the California pine forests. *U.S. Dept. Agr. Dept. Bull.* 1294.

Spencer, D. L., and J. B. Hakala. 1964. Moose and fire on the Kenai. *Tall Timbers Fire Ecol. Conf.* 3:10–33.

Stocker, G. C. 1966. Effects of fires on vegetation in the Northern Territory. *Aust. For.* 30:223–230.

————, and J. D. Sturtz. 1966. The use of fire to establish Townsville lucerne in the Northern Territory. *Aust. J. Expt. Agr. and Ani. Husb.* 6:277–279.

Stoddard, H. L., Sr. 1963. Bird habitat and fire. *Tall Timbers Fire Ecol. Conf.* 2:163–175.

Suman, R. F., and L. K. Halls. 1955. Burning and grazing affect physical properties of Coastal Plain forest soils. *Southeast Forest Expt. Sta. Research Note* 75.

Wahlenberg, W. G., S. W. Greene, and H. R. Reed. 1939. Effects of fire and cattle grazing on longleaf pine lands, as studied at McNeill, Miss. *U.S. Dept. Agr. Tech. Bull.* 683.

Weaver, H. 1951. Observed effects of prescribed burning on perennial grasses in the ponderosa pine forests. *J. For.* 49:267–271.

————. 1964. Fire and management problems in ponderosa pine. *Tall Timbers Fire Ecol. Conf.* 3:60–79.

West, O. 1965. *Fire in vegetation and its use in pasture management.* Commonwealth Bur. Pasture and Field Crops. Mimeo.

Whyte, R. O. 1961. Evolution of land use in south-western Asia. In *History of land use in arid regions,* ed. L. D. Stamp, UNESCO No. 17:57–118.

Wright, H. A., and J. O. Klemmedson. 1965. Effects of fire on bunchgrasses of the sagebrush-grass region in southern Idaho. *Ecology* 46:680–688.

Chapter 16

The Use of Fire in Rangeland Management

To use fire as a tool in rangeland management, one must employ it skillfully and confine it to predetermined areas. One should manage intensity of heat and rate of spread to attain stipulated objectives. This is *prescribed burning* or, as it is sometimes called, *controlled burning* (U.S. Forest Service, 1956). In contrast with activities aimed at prompt discovery and suppression of wildfire, prescribed burning concentrates on setting of fire in a manner that will accomplish desired purposes. Understanding of fire behavior, precaution in the use of fire, and firing procedures have accumulated from experience with wildfires and intentionally set ones.

FIRE BEHAVIOR

Knowledge of fire behavior is essential to successful use of fire in rangeland management. As a fire proceeds across a landscape, it responds to differences in weather, topography, and fuel. Fire control requires that unexpected increases in fire intensity and rate of spread be held to a minimum. Fire storms or blowups should be avoided unless they are a part of the planned burning program.

Combustion is an oxidation reaction that requires the proper combination of heat, oxygen, and fuel. Ignition will not occur until the three factors permit combustion. Variations in the rate of burning are controlled by the balance among them. Smoldering indicates a combination of heat, oxygen, and fuel that permits slow oxidation. As combustible conditions improve, flaming occurs; and under extremely favorable conditions, flaming may involve leaping flames, loud noises, and rapid air movements. In fire-management operations, control of heat, oxygen, and fuel regulates combustion.

Water, as moisture in fuel, acts in three ways. First, it has a cooling effect, because heat converts water to steam, thus reducing intensity of burning. For this reason, water used to stop a fire should be directed at the fuel in front of the flame rather than on the flame itself. Partial combustion and increased smoke indicate that less heat is being liberated than was being liberated before water was applied. Second, moisture present in the air as steam or humidity reduces radiation, thus slowing drying of fuels near the flames. Third, cooling reduces release of volatile oils, thus retarding combustion. Volatile oils in fuels have an effect opposite to that of water since they promote rapid combustion (Pompe and Vines, 1966).

Control of oxygen often is accomplished by the smothering of the flames with soil, water spray, and chemical fogs. These substances reduce the oxygen content of the air reaching the flames to less than approximately 15 percent. Combustion ceases when the oxygen content becomes that low. Beating a light grass fire with wet sacks or special swatters removes oxygen from the fire for an instant. Reignition depends on the amount of heat retained in the fuel. Any fire line from which combustible materials have been removed is an example of fuel control.

Fire continues across a landscape only with heat transfer sufficient to ignite new fuels, which is accomplished by heat conduction, convection, radiation, or a combination of all three methods. Conduction is of little consequence in managed burning because wildland fuels are poor conductors of heat. Convection, or direct movement of hot air masses, is associated with weather phenomena and with the fact that warm air rises. Radiation, the rays of energy sent out from the fire, plays a major role in fire behavior. Burning piles of debris radiate heat toward each other. Flames from a fire on a slope radiate more heat to new fuels on the uphill side than to fuels on the downhill side because the uphill side is closer to the heat source. Radiant heat received by an object decreases as the square of the distance from the fire. An object 10 meters away from a fire receives 0.01 as much heat as one 1 meter away. Thus fire behavior, including ignition, combustion, and spread, is closely dependent upon oxygen, heat, and organic materials. These elements are supplied in amounts that vary because of differences in weather, topography, and fuel characteristics.

Weather

Precipitation, air temperature, relative humidity, and wind velocity are the major weather variables that relate to prescribed burning. The seasonal precipitation pattern determines the length and severity of the dry season. Mediterranean climates often have a dry period lasting six months or longer. During this period, wildfires are frequent and prescribed burning possible. Areas with monthly rain or a short growing season due to cool temperatures are not so susceptible to wildfires. However, prescribed burning a few days after a rain can be of value in reducing unwanted standing debris without damaging the base of living plants or exposing mineral soil. The day of the burn should be selected so that organic materials on the soil surface will not burn because they are still wet. Biswell and Schultz (1956) found that dead brush and other debris in the ponderosa pine type in northwestern California could be burned on approximately 50 days during the 6-month wet season.

Precipitation influences the amount of herbaceous material produced, the time of its curing, and its moisture content. Dampening of light fuels quickly reduces combustion, but they dry rapidly. A grass cover may be unburnable immediately after a light shower or after dew in early morning and may become an extremely combustible fuel a few hours later. Conversely, heavy fuels, such as logs, stumps, and limbs, wet slowly and dry slowly. Although regions with continuous green vegetation may have little wildfire, most vegetational types are subject to prescribed burning if proper fuel conditions are selected.

Air temperature, as most factors, has direct and indirect effects. Less heat is required to raise fuel temperature to the ignition point when air temperature is high than when it is low. This relationship has a direct effect on initial ignition and continued combustion as a fire spreads. High air temperature has an indirect effect since it decreases moisture in air and fuel, thereby favoring burning conditions.

Relative humidity is the measure of air dryness. Other conditions being equal, humidity decreases with increase in temperature. The drier the air, the drier the fuels and the more likely prescribed fires will burn out of control. While no exact guidelines can be given, probably prescribed fires in light fuels (grasslands) should not be attempted when the relative humidity is below 25 percent and the temperature is above 24° or 27°C. If fuels are dry and heavy with loose mixtures of twigs and combustible leaves, relative humidity should be above 35 percent and temperature below 24°C during prescribed burning. In most regions, these conditions fluctuate more or less predictably according to time of day and season of year. These three weather conditions, along with wind conditions, determine whether prescribed burning should be done in morning, afternoon, or night.

Wind causes a flame front to move ahead, crown, and jump to new locations. Moving air brings oxygen to the flames and removes carbon dioxide, increasing combustion rate. It also moves hot air masses ahead of the flame and close to the ground, where radiant heat dries and preheats new fuels; thus ignition is made easier or even spontaneous ahead of the advancing flame front. Combustion runs with high winds; long fingers of burned areas result. As the fire point is pushed forward, the sides tend to be drawn inward. Of 12,790 fires in the northern Rocky Mountain region from 1936 to 1944, the average size at control was 3,500 acres if wind velocity was greater than 62 kilometers per hour but only 8 acres if wind velocity was less than 13 kilometers per hour (Barrows, 1951).

Winds tend to increase in velocity upslope during the day and downslope at night. Dust devils or whirlwinds and clouds of the cumulus or lenticular type foretell unstable air, gusty winds, and danger with fire. Awareness of wind conditions at the time of ignition and prediction of winds until a prescribed burn is completed are necessary to successful use of fire as a tool. Seldom should a fire be set if the wind velocity will be greater than 10 to 12 kilometers per hour. At those speeds, trees of pole size in open stands sway gently, wind is distinctly felt on the face, loose paper moves, small flags flutter but are not continuously extended, and grasslands show continuous wave motion.

Fuel moisture, more than any other single factor, reflects precipitation, air temperature, relative humidity, and wind velocity. It has been used extensively in fire danger-rating systems. Precautions to prevent wildfires and even admission to forests and brush fields are determined by fire danger ratings. In fine fuels, dryness and fire danger change rapidly. When fire danger ratings begin to indicate that care is needed to prevent wildfires, prescribed burning should not be attempted.

Topography

Roughness of the land surface influences weather generally and causes day-to-day variation in weather, and hence in fire behavior. In the Northern Hemisphere, southern and southwestern slopes have the highest rate of fire spread and more than their portion of wildfires, probably because they are warmer and dryer than are other slopes. The opposite usually is true in the Southern Hemisphere. Mountaintops tend to be cooler and moister than the lowlands by day but warmer and drier by night. Fires that are set or start at the bottoms of slopes tend to burn rapidly to ridge tops, partly in response to differences in wind velocity, temperature, and relative humidity and partly because fuels on the upslope side of the flames are closer to the heat source and receive more radiant heat than do fuels on the downslope side. In the northern Rocky Mountains, 10 percent of the windfires that started at the bottoms of slopes reached 4 hectares in size, but only 1.5 percent of those started at the tops of slopes became that large.

As steepness of slope increases, rate of fire spread increases. Narrow, steep-sided canyons tend to act as chimneys that enclose heat, so fires burn rapidly with the upward air movements. Elevation influences the growing season and fire season. Grasslands and shrublands at low elevations may be subject to burning for six months or longer, while alpine grasslands a few kilometers away may not get dry enough to burn.

Slope may be used to advantage in prescribed burning. Fires set at the bottom may burn to the ridgetop and go out under fuel conditions that would prevent burning on level ground. Fires set on ridges burn slowly downslope. However, burning material may roll and cause spotting ahead of the flame front. In forest areas, a ground fire moving downslope against a wind can develop into a racing upslope crown fire with slight increase in wind. At night, downslope winds can fan a ground fire out of control.

Fuel

The third major element that controls fire behavior is fuel. The moisture content of fuel was discussed as a weather factor. Fuels themselves have several characteristics, such as volume or size, continuity, and compactness. Small materials with a high ratio of surface area to volume burn readily. For example, a sheet of paper burns easily, but a book may be difficult to ignite. Twigs, needles, and grass leaves ignite quickly and completely oxidize in a short time, while logs and large limbs may only char on the outside. A mixture of large and small materials is the most flammable fuel in terms of size. The small materials ignite easily and promote rapid fire advance, while the larger pieces increase heat release and burn-out time.

The horizontal and vertical continuity of fuel influences fire behavior. Patchy fuels will burn irregularly, leaving unburned islands. A young coniferous forest that has abundant herbaceous fuel, dead overtopped shrubs, and lower limbs draped with pine needles is subject to rapid and severe burning. Chaparral and *Artemisia* with an herbaceous ground cover provide combinations of material size and continuity of fuel which burn rapidly.

Compact material does not burn as readily as fuels that are loosely structured. Mulch on the soil surface has little influence on rate of fire spread, but it may contain a smoldering fire for long periods. It may flame if drafts bring oxygen, or go out with lack of oxygen. Other conditions being equal, fire spreads most rapidly in grasslands and second most rapidly in logging slash with fine woody materials and a mixture of dry herbaceous plants. Brush fields and forests with abundant dead materials are intermediate. Timber stands with little or no ground fuels burn least rapidly, if at all.

CHARACTERISTICS OF FIRE WHICH INFLUENCE ITS ECOLOGICAL EFFECTS

Few precise descriptions exist of weather-topography-fuel combinations that resulted in a particular fire behavior and caused certain ecological effects. Some studies are based on observations of changes in vegetation and animals following one or more fires but give little regard to the fire itself. Other studies use fire as a treatment in plots to study the influence of burning frequency and timing on organisms. They commonly do not include measurements of weather and fuel or descriptions of fire behavior. Most studies concerned with fire behavior include minimal information on its ecological effects. Without combined work on all these aspects of fire behavior, burning will remain a tool in the hands of experienced persons but a danger for the novice, who is being given minimum information.

This lack of predictive information on fire behavior and criteria for prescribed burning has its causes. As noted previously, different atmospheric and fuel conditions contribute to varying fire behavior. Not only are many conditions involved, but also they change in magnitude over short distances as a fire travels, and in time. Adequate characterizations of free-burning fires are lacking because acceptable instruments for measuring wildland fires are expensive to build and operate. Variations of fire behavior in vegetation result from extremely complex interactions of differing factors (Lindenmuth and Davis, 1973).

Heat intensity and heat duration probably are the principal ecological influences of fire on plants and animals. For a fire moving through vegetation on a single front, intensity has been expressed as Btu released per second per meter of fire front (1 Btu equals 252 calories). This index varies directly with the energy per kilogram of fuel, the weight of fuel in kilograms per square meter, and the rate of forward spread in meters per second (Byram, 1959). Intensity expressed this way was shown to vary from 1.5 to 9000 Btu/second/meter in forest and 1.5 to 2000 Btu/second/meter in grassland in Australia (McArthur and Cheney, 1966). Calculation of the intensity index is relatively easy because fuel quantity and rate of fire spread can be measured, and the number of Btu per kilogram of fuel is relatively constant (approximately 187,000). In the Australian study, fire did little damage to trees when intensity ratings were low. Boles and crowns of *Eucalyptus* were damaged, and regenerating trees as large as 5 meters high were killed if the rating was high.

Fire intensity varies with both quantity of fuel consumed and rate of spread. McArthur and Cheney (1966) found that as the quantity doubled, the rate also doubled, and, as a result, intensity increased fourfold. For example, fuel consumed increased four times between 6.4 and 23.2 tons per hectare and intensity increased by a factor of almost 8 (Table 16-1). Fast-moving fires usually consumed more fuel than did slow fires. The available quantity of fuel that will burn is a function of the moisture profile in the vegetation, as indicated for four time periods after rain (Table 16-1). If another line were added to Table 16-1 in which intensity was 6560 Btu/second/meter, a crown fire would be indicated, adding about 7.4 more tons of fuel per hectare and resulting in a wall of flames 20 to 25 meters in height. If such a fire traveled at 0.6 meters per second, the intensity would be 100,000 Btu/second/meter of fire front.

Table 16-1   Fire intensity in a *Pinus radiata* stand in Australia as influenced by fuel moisture *(McArthur and Cheney, 1966)*

Treatment, days after rain	Total fuel, tons/ha	Fuel consumed, tons/ha	Rate of spread, m/min	Flame height, m	Intensity, Btu/sec/m
1	42.2	6.9	1.5	0.3	220
2	42.2	6.4	1.5	0.6	275
14	42.2	23.2	2.9	1.2	1770
30	42.2	34.1	4.0	2.7	3675

Fire duration—burn-out or residence time—also influences fire effects. It is directly related to heat yield and fuel quantity and indirectly related to rate of combustion. In the Australian study mentioned above, the rate of combustion was faster when fuel moisture content, particle size, and compactness of fuels were less. Under similar burning conditions, *Eucalyptus* leaves and twigs had a combustion rate of 233 Btu/second/square meter; *Pinus radiata,* 350; wheat stubble, 860; and a dry grass-clover area, 1600. The faster rates were accompanied by longer burning times. Twenty-five tons of *Eucalyptus* material per hectare burned at the rate of 353 seconds per square meter, while 5 tons of grass per hectare burned in 10.3 seconds. Heat penetration into soil, through bark, and into living tissue increases as fire duration increases.

Damaging effects of fire on living organisms are related to fire intensity and burn-out time, which have been characterized by studies of stationary fire under controlled conditions. Fires in ecological settings are moving fires that seldom have the characteristics of laboratory fires. Continuously accurate prediction of effects from prescribed burning requires knowledge of the correlation between fire characteristics and biological consequences. An adequate system for analyzing these relationships is not available for rangeland burning. One needs to be developed.

OBJECTIVES IN THE USE OF FIRE

Primitive man used fire as a tool with which to manipulate vegetation and animal populations for his benefits. Modern man has developed public attitudes and has built a fire-fighting organization aimed at eliminating and controlling fire on wildlands. This organization is highly effective, but it has not achieved full control of fire.

Increasingly, land managers are making use of prescribed fire as a tool. As might be expected, the objectives of these persons vary widely as to kinds of conditions they hope to develop, to maintain, or to prevent with fire.

To Reduce Undesirable Plants

Perhaps the most common purpose of prescribed fire in natural vegetation, is removal of undesirable plants. Land managers may use fire to remove hardwood regeneration in pine forests of the southern United States, to remove chaparral in California, and to thin stands of *Pinus ponderosa* in Arizona and New Mexico. Land managers may burn brush to reduce mature growth in preparation for herbicidal treatment on sprouts. In Africa, prescribed burning of grasslands prevents invasion of woody plants and makes more grasslands. Prescribed burning of *Pinus palustris* seedlings during the grass stage in their development is the field method used to remove needles infected with brown-spot needle blight (*Scirrhia acicola*) and to control the disease (Lightle, 1960). Land clearing, whether it is for the purposes of shifting cultivation or developing modern types of agriculture, nearly always requires fire. Normally, water output or runoff is increased when vegetation is reduced. Therefore reduction of undesirable species suggests benefits from more desirable species, additional water, or better recreational situations.

To Favor Certain Plant Species

Plants that are not climatic climax dominants and those which require bare soil for seedling establishment often are encouraged by burning. The regeneration of shade-intolerant and weakly tolerant tree species is facilitated by prescribed burning either before or after logging. In addition to trees, the seral species include many that produce abundant forage, browse, nuts, berries, seeds, and tubers that favor various animal species (Stoddard, 1963). Burning of marshes along the southeastern United States Gulf Coast reduces *Spartina* and encourages legumes and annuals, thereby increasing waterfowl food (Givens, 1962). Prescribed fire is used to prepare sites for and to encourage regeneration of many desirable plant species.

To Produce Ash for Fertilization

Woody material spread evenly over a small field and then burned produces ash that can be hand mixed into the soil. Subsequent crops on this land are improved for two or three years. This rotation of woody vegetation, burning, and cropping is known in the tropics as *shifting cultivation* because a new area of freshly cut brush is used for each new field.

After a wildfire in chaparral and forests in the western United States, favorable sites usually are seeded to grasses and legumes for forage. Where the ash is white and thick, both plant establishment and growth show a response to the residual minerals for a year or two. Black ash indicates incomplete combustion and contains few available minerals. It results in new stands lower in vigor than those growing in white ash. Any increase in available minerals due to burning is temporary because fire cannot add minerals to the system. It releases those minerals already present but unavailably bound in organic compounds. Advantage is taken of the minerals released by a rangeland fire, but this release seldom is a major objective in prescribed burning.

To Produce More Forage for Livestock

The ability of prescribed rangeland fire to increase quantity of livestock feed depends almost entirely upon changes in botanical composition of the vegetation, such as development of grasslands in place of woody vegetation. Shrubs that furnish browse for domestic animals and game often grow beyond the reach of animals. Burning can be used to maintain shrubs in a usable size by killing the taller growth, stimulating sprouts, and fostering seedling establishment that renews browse production without greatly altering botanical composition.

Burning appears to reduce the quantity of forage produced in the grasslands of central North America (Aldous, 1934; Elwell et al., 1941; Hopkins et al., 1948; Robocker and Miller, 1955; Hanks and Anderson, 1957) and on annual grassland in California (Hervey, 1949). Conversely, Wahlenberg et al. (1939) reported increased forage after ten years of burning stands of pine and bluestem in Mississippi. Forage yields of *Sorghum plumosum* and *Themeda australis* in northern Australia were reduced by burning (Smith, 1960). However, Ehrenreich and Aikman (1963) found a slight increase in tall-grass production the first year after a fire and concluded that an occasional burn did no serious damage. In a 15-year study in the Flint Hills of Kansas, Owensby and Anderson (1967) found that late-spring burning reduced yield little but early- and midspring fires did reduce yield. Burning of grassland appears to reduce herbage production in more situations than it increases production.

To Increase Quality of Livestock Feed

The increase in animal production following burning of coarse grasses probably is due to the improved quality of the feed rather than to an increase in quantity of feed. Smith (1960) in Australia found that the crude protein percentage in the herbage was increased after burning although the total herbage per hectare decreased. Similar results were obtained in Louisiana by Grelen and Epps (1967), who found that spring burns gave better-quality feed than did winter burns. Several studies in longleaf pine-bluestem and pine-wiregrass ranges in the southeastern United States showed that burning improves quality, palatability, and availability of forage, all three improvements resulting in increased livestock production (Duvall, 1962; Lewis, 1964; Halls et al., 1964; Southwell and Hughes, 1965).

Where grasses are tall and coarse, it may be necessary to burn them to reduce accumulations of poor-quality and undecomposed old growth. Burning will make the new growth available earlier in the growing season. Burning of *Spartina patens* and *Distichlis spicata* improved the quality of forage by removing old growth and making new growth readily available (Williams, 1955; Lynch, 1941). Where the mature growth of grass is palatable and of reasonable quality, burning does more harm by reducing quantity of growth than the good that is gained by increased quality. Most studies in the coarse-grass areas of the southeastern United States and in tropical grasslands have shown increased livestock production with burning. In *Andropogon scoparius* prairies, this benefit appears in a few studies when timing of the fire is carefully controlled. Further west in the mixed prairie, burning is not a common practice and has received little study, nor has burning been found advantageous in the bunchgrass and annual-grass types of the western United States.

To Control Distribution of Animals

Domestic and game animals prefer to graze on recently burned areas. They may be attracted to more palatable feed, to more easily available feed, or to both. Often they overgraze burned areas, especially when these areas are small in relation to the number of animals attracted. However, this behavioral characteristic of animals may be used to advantage in certain situations. Duvall and Whitaker (1963, 1964) found that burning every three years increased forage production on cutover pine rangelands in Louisiana that were dominated by *Andropogon tener*. Forage utilization was heavy on the new burn, moderate on the two-year-old burn, and light on the three-year-old burn. Animals followed the burn, so rotation of burning resulted in rotation of grazing without the cost of extra fencing.

A system of burning 10 to 15 percent of a management unit each year in the chaparral of California has been suggested for deer-management objectives. Unburned areas provide cover, and burning results in nutritious sprouts for two to three years. The proportion of the area burned each year is determined as a fraction of 1 over the years it takes the chaparral to reach burnable conditions and to become too dense for efficient deer use (Biswell et al., 1952).

To Control Undesirable Animals

Control of tsetse flies, other insects, ticks, and reptiles has been attempted with burning. In tsetse fly reduction schemes in Africa, the real purpose is to change the fly's habitat from brush-grass or woodland to grassland, in which it cannot live. The fire itself kills few flies and is only one of many methods used to combat them. Success depends upon the completeness of vegetational conversion and its maintenance as grassland.

Burning destroys ticks that are on the herbage at the time of the fire, but those on hosts and in sheltered positions escape the heat. A high reproductive potential makes effects of fire on tick populations temporary. So many individual ticks and other animals too escape the heat of fire that direct control with fire has doubtful value. The use of prescribed fire to control animal populations through change of habitat is more promising.

To Encourage Certain Animal Species

Burning encourages many species of animals by changing the vegetation. Numerous animal species are best adapted to seral vegetational stages and to mosaics of dense and open vegetation which provide shelter and food. As the following examples show, favorable conditions for certain species may be developed with judicious use of fire. Red grouse in Scotland thrive best in the second successional stage after a fire, which is maintained by burning every three to seven years (Peterle, 1958). In Michigan and Wisconsin, grassland with less than 25 percent woody cover is needed for the prairie chicken (Amman, 1957). Sharptail grouse require less than 40 percent woody cover in scattered clumps (Miller, 1963). Ruffed grouse are best adapted to woody cover with a scattering of openings about 1/10 hectare in size where grass, herbs, and brush are dominant. The habitats for these three grouse species may be maintained by general burning, selective burning, and spot burning. The eastern wild turkey does well with 1-hectare forest openings where insects are abundant (Wheeler, 1948). Black-tailed deer along the Pacific Coast increase severalfold when forest is converted to brush (Dasmann and Dasmann, 1963) (Fig. 16-1). Moose thrived with burning and logging in northern North America because these activities encouraged *Salix* spp., *Betula* spp. and *Populus* spp. There are few moose in hemlock forest (Leopold and Darling, 1953). Keeping *Salix, Betula,* and *Populus* within reach of these animals requires a fire at 15- to 20-year intervals (Spencer and Chaletain, 1953). Prescribed fire is a useful tool in the development and maintenance of optimum wildlife habitat, including food, cover, and ideal conditions for animal harvesting.

To Reduce Hazards from Wildfires

As undecomposed organic materials accumulate, the danger of damaging wildfire increases. Potential fuels may be in the form of large debris deposits left after logging; thick litter, dead shrubs, and young trees making a continuous fuel supply from soil to tree crowns; large areas of mature chaparral; or grasslands with abundant litter. Wildfires have greater chances of burning unchecked and doing considerable damage to life, property, and natural resources when fuels are abundant. Land managers have used prescribed burning to reduce the fuel supply

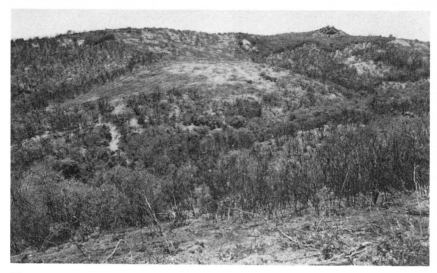

Figure 16-1   Chaparral may reach a height and a density that discourage deer. This photo shows spot burning to open the cover and to produce sprouts for deer browse.

and thereby to reduce the chances of large catastrophic wildfires. Since 1905, the U.S. Forest Service has recommended burning to eliminate logging slash. The Service began using burning as a hazard-reduction practice in about 1930 (Thompson, 1962). Contruction of fuelbreaks started in California chaparral types in the late 1950s (Bentley and White, 1961). Much research has been done into the benefits of hazard reduction by burning in the southern pine types (Lotti, 1962), in the ponderosa pine type in California (Biswell, 1963), and in the southwestern United States (Weaver, 1967).

To Facilitate Management and Occupancy

The reduced cover produced by burning facilitates movement and visibility for the traveler. Using burning to reduce cover gave primitive man a measure of protection from dangerous animals and places where grazing animals concentrated. Primitive man used fire to drive game. Modern hunters prefer relatively open vegetation. Their use of land and hunting success are directly related to accessibility. Few modern hunters hunt, camp, and hike in dense brush and forest when openings and edges are available. Fires, at least among primitive peoples, were set for purposes of excitement and warfare. These same objectives may be in the minds of those who set fires today in order to see the fires burn, to get jobs fighting fire, and for spite.

Access is important to the modern land manager and administrator. Livestock control is difficult in dense vegetation. Openness in the forest understory facilitates timber inventories and sales. Viewing natural landscapes requires openings. It is common for burning to be done in the southern United States to ease the collection of gum naval stores and to protect tapped trees from wildfires during the pitch-collecting season. Various reasons exist for maintaining open vegetation with prescribed fire.

PRESCRIBED BURNING

The prescription or plan for burning a particular land area includes four main types of activities. The first is a planning phase, the second concentrates on preparation for the fire, the third concerns the fire itself, and the fourth is postburn management. In practice the second, third, and fourth steps include continual updating of plans.

Planning for a Prescribed Fire

Planning for a prescribed fire begins when the manager realizes that a certain area of land might be improved for his purposes if it were burned. Evaluation of alternative methods such as bulldozing and use of chemicals should have indicated that fire would do a better job at less cost than other methods. Burning to remove an excess of dry grass in tall-grass vegetational types and thick brush in chaparral types may be the only feasible technique. It is an effective method of reducing regenerating brush in developed grasslands, but spraying with herbicides may be as effective, less damaging to certain grasses, and no more costly. Costs of burning include labor, rental of equipment, supplies, food purchase and preparation, liability insurance for men and property, any loss of forage that must be left as fuel, and depreciation on equipment. These costs may total five or six times more per hectare on a 20-hectare chaparral burn in California than on one 200 to 250 hectare in size. Conversely, costs per hectare tend to increase with fires larger than 500 hectare because the danger of escape increases, and thus more men and machines are required to control the fire (Sampson and Burcham, 1954).

The exact area to be burned requires careful consideration in two respects. First, soil and vegetation must be such that they will produce a profitable return; the area, in other words, must be both worthy and capable of being improved. Second, the area must be of a size and shape that will permit burning in a day with reasonable expectations of successful burning and complete fire control.

Prescribed burning requires cooperation among many organizations. The necessary skills and experience to be a good "fire boss" reside in only a few people. The tools for fuel preparation and fire control may be different and may belong to different organizations. For example, a private landowner may have adequate machinery to build fire lines but is not likely to have adequate fire-suppression equipment. Rangeland ownerships are usually mixed, so neighbors, those responsible for public lands, police forces, and fire-fighting organizations will need to be kept informed from the beginning day of planning until the fire is out. The labor and equipment in service on the actual fire often include volunteers and persons working on an exchange basis. Where prescribed burning has succeeded, there has been continuous cooperation among all concerned.

An example of successful cooperation for prescribed burning is the effort organized by county brush-range-improvement associations in California. These county groups pool available talents in many aspects of the program. They schedule the burns so that equipment and men are available; they appoint the fire boss for each burn; and after on-site inspection, they give the landowner instructions to make sure the burn is successful. Included in the instructions are items such as fire line location, distance to clear debris from fire lines, preburns or night burns to widen fire lines where danger of escape is great, winter cleanup of brush piles and logs, and date in the spring to discontinue grazing so that grass will carry the fire. A common adage about prescribed burning is that preparation gives a successful burn, planning promotes adequate preparation, and cooperation permits adequate planning.

Preparation of the Site

Construction of a fire line that completely encloses the proposed burn is of first importance. *Fire lines,* sometimes called *firebreaks, fire lanes,* or *control lines, are strips of land devoid of burnable materials.* Roads are utilized for this purpose, and other fire lines are constructed by scraping of land with a bulldozer blade, road grader, disk or other power equipment, and by hand. The strip width of bare soil that is scraped depends on the width of the machinery and conditions of fuel and topography. One pass with a bulldozer blade is about the maximum width. Other strips, hand prepared in light fuels, may be as narrow as 0.3 meter. A width greater than 3 meters is of little value because conditions that cause fire to spot will cause it to jump much farther than 3 meters. If a fire line 3 meters in width will not permit fire control, prescribed burning should not be attempted.

Two hand-prepared lines about 0.6 meter wide, 15 to 25 meters apart, with the area between them burned when danger of fire escape is extremely low make a highly effective firebreak in grassland. This system has been used in preventing burning of isolated tree thickets in wide expanses of grassland that were burned later.

A fire line may be a part of a *fuelbreak system,* which is *a strip perhaps as much as 400 meters in width, in which fuel has been changed to facilitate fire suppression.* Examples of fuelbreaks include reduced tree cover and snags in woodlands and strips of chaparral on ridges converted to grassland. The reduced fuel provides soil cover against erosion and still permits fire fighting in dangerous fuel situations. Removal of snags within 60 meters of a fire line, burning-out of danger spots at night, and winter cleanup of debris are methods of preparing a fuelbreak system around a proposed prescribed burn.

Placement of the fire line in an advantageous relationship to topography, access, fuels, and predictable wind changes reduces danger of fire escape. The fire line is placed so that the fire crew can reduce spotting, have control if the direction of fire spread changes, and be prepared if the speed of fire travel increases. The most common location for a fire line is a ridgetop. Irregular and gusty air currents, including whirlwinds, may carry embers across a ridgetop fire line, but the fire must spread downhill after crossing the ridge. A rule of thumb for reducing fire spread is that most trees, snags, and brush cover that extend above the ridgetop level on either side of the fire line should be removed. Resulting brush piles near the fire line should be removed ahead of the prescribed fire. Obviously, sharp angles in the fire line and narrow fingers to be either burned or unburned should be avoided. Fire lines should not be placed at the bottom of a valley, but 10 to 30 meters up the slope of the side within the planned burn. There is great danger of spotting onto the adjacent slope. Attempts to burn a part of a narrow, steep-sided valley should be avoided. Saddles are danger points where air currents converge and move to cross slopes. Firebreaks need extra width on saddles.

Fire lines may be needed within the prescribed burn for control of rate of burning in projected hot spots, exclusion of areas from the overall fire, and facilitation of a firing plan. For these lines to be properly located, the sequence of firing must be selected early in the planning process.

Closely associated with preparation of internal fire lines is manipulation of fuel. Undesirable trees, such as *Pinus sabiniana* in the California chaparral, should be felled several months ahead of the fire so that they will be consumed and will not contribute to dangerous fire spread during burning or hinder land use after the fire. Chaparral or heavy brush may need crushing to reduce moisture content to a point that permits burning. Alternate strips of crushed and uncrushed brush (strips the width of one or two bulldozer blades) will provide sufficient dry fuel to burn the more moist live material at times when green material alone would not burn. The advantages of fuel preparation are more complete consumption of large woody materials, reduced fuel moisture content so that burning may occur when danger of escape is minimal, and rearrangement of fuels to facilitate ignition.

One-Day Preignition to Fire-Out

The day ahead of the prescribed burn is one for final check on preparations. These include notification to police, fire-fighting organizations, and neighbors for three purposes. The first is to warn them of impending fire, the second is to invite observers, and the third is to determine who will be helping with particular equipment at appointed places and times. Invitations to press, radio, and television personnel for them to report the objectives and progress of the fire will help gain public acceptance of prescribed fire. Other preignition activities include obtaining necessary permits and taking due regard of air-pollution regulations. The latter are changing rapidly.

Although the day of the burn may have been selected a year or more before ignition in order for men and equipment to be properly scheduled, the final decision to set the fire is left to the last minute. Excellent weather forecasts are prerequisite to successful prescribed burning. Predictions of wind direction and velocity, air stability, temperatures, and relative humidity are essential. These need to be available to the fire boss on the day before the fire, on the day of the fire before it is set, and afterwards if changes are likely to occur.

The time of day that the fire is set may result from local experience which has shown the time when sufficient heat will be generated to obtain the desired objectives. The cooler, more humid parts of the day can be the times for best containing a fire. A plan of ignition during late morning after dew has dried and burning of the whole area by mid-afternoon often meets these specifications. Logs, stumps, limbs, and other large fuels will continue to burn, but fire escape from them is unlikely because lighter ground fuels are gone. Late afternoon, when air turbulence tends to increase, should be a time of patrol and containment rather than one of fighting escaped flames. Prescribed burning at night usually takes advantage of the highest humidity and least wind for extremely hazardous fuels, but night burning may reduce communications and visual appraisal of burning progress. This is especially true in mountainous areas. Night burning is most successful on flat lands. The actual day and hour of ignition, then, is determined largely by tactics for managing the fire. The season in which the day of ignition occurs is related more to fire effects than to fire control and was discussed in the previous chapter.

Many designs for igniting wildland burns have been used. The simplest is a single line of fire that is set to burn either with the wind as a headfire or against it as a backfire. It may be set to burn slowly downhill or rapidly uphill. In general, a safe backfire requires light, continuous ground fuels such as grass or low, dead, woody plants draped with pine needles. If a backfire increases dead material by killing woody vegetation, dangerous conditions can increase for headfires.

Another design is ignition of the entire perimeter of the prescribed area. Normally, fire is first set on the lee or uphill side and is allowed to widen the firebreak before the windward or downhill side is set. As the perimetric flames burn toward the center, heat builds up and a very hot fire develops. In such a fire, the time of spread is less than that of the single-line type of burn, but heat intensity varies over the area from a relatively cool fire that consumes little woody material, near the edge, to one that burns all organic material, near the center.

Whatever ignition design is used, the original fire sets should be 15 to 30 meters inside the outside fire line, where they will burn in two directions. Sparks, burning embers, and heat are drawn into the prescribed area since that is the center of heat intensity; therefore the chances of fire jumping the line at ignition time are reduced. The principle that one fire tends to draw another toward it, in this case across an already burned strip, is used in developing a slow-burning fire that widens the firebreak.

The same principle is used in developing intense heat and rapid burning where fuel exists between the fires. Many designs take advantage of this principle. In one design, a new line of fire is set repeatedly a few yards ahead of an advancing wall of flame. As the center of one strip burns out, another strip is set (Fig. 16-2). Still another design calls for ignition in the center of a prescribed area at the same time as or just before the perimeter is set. If danger of escape is high, most of the perimeter is set first and the center lighted only when a safe firebreak has been burned (Fig. 16-3). A more intense type of set is one in which the perimeter is set at about the same time as ignition occurs at more or less regularly spaced locations over the entire area to be burned (Fig. 16-4).

The latter designs are known as *types of area ignition.* An extensive example of area ignition is used in the Karri and Jarrah (*Eucalyptus* spp.) forests in western Australia. Spot fires are set by incendiaries that are dropped from an airplane. The grid pattern spaces the spot fires so that each burns about 2 hectares. Ideally, each fire spreads slowly during the day, joins other fires toward evening, and goes out at

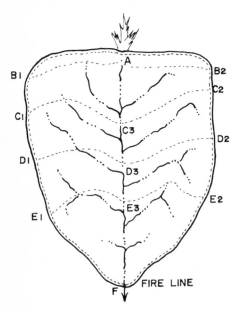

Figure 16-2 Firing in successive strips permits greater control with somewhat less intensive burning than the types shown in Figures 16-3 and 16-4. The first fire set is at A, and crews move toward B_1 and B_2, setting fires as they go. After a sufficient firebreak has developed, the crews set fire to C_1 and C_2 and, at the same time, two other crews begin setting fires from C_3 toward C_1 and C_2. When that block is burned out, the crews move to the next area and repeat the process. This design is well suited for relatively flat lands where internal fire lanes permit fire control, access, and safety of personnel.

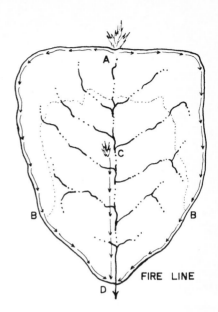

Figure 16-3 This is an example of center firing after the perimeter is set in order to promote intense heat from rapid burning. The first fire is set at A, and the flame front is gradually extended, as safety allows, to points B on either side of the watershed. When the flame front is at points B, it approximates the dotted line. Crews are held at points B while another crew begins setting fire at C and along the drainage toward point D. When the crew reaches point D, but not until then, crews at B proceed to point D. Shortly, the whole watershed will seem to be aflame as the fires burn together.

night. Prescribed fires as large as 12,000 hectares have been burned in a day with this procedure. Incendiaries should be dropped first on the ridges and later on lower slopes so that the fire cannot spread rapidly (CSIRO, 1970).

Electrical circuits and fuse lighters provide effective simultaneous, multiple ignition points in places where rapid escape of men is limited by topography or

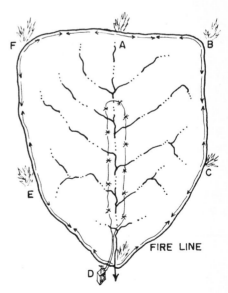

Figure 16-4 This illustrates area ignition in which all fires are set as rapidly as possible. A circuit of preset incendiaries near the bottom of the watershed ignites fire by electric shock at points marked*. When smoke appears from these points, personnel stationed along the perimetric fire line begin setting fires in each direction from lettered locations. Flames envelope the whole watershed and burn the fuel rapidly. After the fire is set, personnel patrol the fire line.

thick vegetation. Circuits fired in sequence provide control of fire progression. Ignition by electrical means reduces labor requirements, providing more men for perimetric control. The principal disadvantage is that the circuits must be placed on the ground ahead of the prescribed day. Even a few hours is time enough for damage by animals and falling limbs or set-off by accident at the wrong time.

A recommended circuit (Schimke, Dell, and Ward, 1969) consists of the following parts: No. 14 or 18 bare aluminum wire, because this wire tends to melt in the fire; a fire lighter that is like a blasting cap that burns instead of explodes; and an ignition fuse that transmits fire to a charge made of diesel-gel, napalm, or balled waxed paper. The required number of these devices should be set in a series circuit, although a bad connection may cause failure of the whole circuit. Paralled circuits require more wire and labor than do series circuits and are subject to shorting-out if the wires touch. The best power source is a generator-type blasting machine, but batteries or other type generators may be used. The resistance of each circuit determines the voltage required.

Men and equipment on a prescribed burn are used to set fires, patrol the fire lines, control escapes, and mop up danger spots, including burning any islands missed by the main fire. For safety, men should be stationed on a fire line and should work in pairs or threes. Their tools should include rakes such as the McLeod and a backpack pump with water. Power equipment, such as a bulldozer and pumper truck, should be nearby. If the line has been prepared properly, men will not need equipment for cutting live trees and snags or brush. However, such equipment should be on hand in case a fire escape occurs. An escape may call for heavy equipment and dropping of fire retardants from aircraft. Common equipment for firing includes the flame thrower, oil-drip torches, and incendiaries of various types. Each crew, no matter if it consists of only two men, needs to be in radio communication with the fire boss. He is the one who keeps the firing on schedule and moves men to control hot spots. The purpose of the mop-up period is extinguishing or speeding the burning process so that all of the fire is out as soon as possible. Burning logs and other materials often roll as limbs or other supports are consumed, so fire in any material that might roll across the fire line needs to be put out quickly. Tactics from fire-set to fire-out cannot be described to cover all situations. An experienced fire boss and others on the crew who have worked in prescribed burning are necessary for successful use of fire as a tool in land management.

Postburn Management

A single fire, although it may result in desired effects, seldom attains a land-management objective. Expectations that it will lead to disappointment. Burning is only a part of a management program. Other aspects of management need to be included. Treatments before a fire contribute to the intensity of the fire. Grazing reduces fuel supply. Herbicidal treatment and bulldozing increase fire intensity by killing plants that then dry and become more combustible. Treatments after a burn contribute to the results. Heavy grazing reduces establishment of native and introduced plant species. Soil deterioration may occur immediately following a burn when cover is thin or absent. Herbicidal treatments of sprouts reduce undesirable trees and brush. In fact, a land manager may use burning to obtain sprouts and seedlings that are more susceptible to herbicides than is old growth, as is practiced in control of *Adenostema fasciculatum*. Seeding must follow prescribed burning of woody vegetation if productive grasses and legumes are to be obtained quickly. Prescribed burning, then, is one land-management tool to be used on a continuing basis, when necessary, along with other practices, to promote desired vegetational composition and production.

RELUCTANCE TO USE PRESCRIBED FIRE

Justification exists for a cautious attitude toward using prescribed burning as a management tool. Catastrophic wildland fire destroys homes, resources, and lives every year, although large fire-control organizations exist. Years of educational efforts regarding destruction by fire and ways to prevent fire have resulted in a general view that all fire is bad.

Laws to regulate or to prevent fire on western United States lands started with forest fire statutes in California and Oregon in 1850. Early problems caused by fires included loss of forage for livestock accompanying wagon trains crossing the plains, reduced forage for bison, destruction of roads by erosion in blackened areas, the disaster of the Peshtigo forest fire in 1871, and other Northwest forest fires in 1910. Each major catastrophe resulted in new laws and appropriations aimed at fire prevention and control. The principal thrust of these laws and appropriations was building larger and larger fire-fighting organizations.

Most people fear fire to a certain degree. A fear of prescribed fire escaping stems from inability to predict fire behavior. Times of floods and severe erosion develop a fear of land destruction after a fire. A view that prescribed burning is good might weaken support for wildfire control. Other arguments against prescribed burning center on lack of knowledge of its effects, dangers of air pollution, unfavorable cost-benefit relationships, and unknown tradeoffs with alternative practices. During the last decade, arguments against prescribed fire have decreased and its use has increased. Individual situations vary from a need to burn annually or even more often to infrequent use of prescribed fire. A few examples illustrate the problems and possibilities of fire use. Different areas have their individual problems, but in most, the ecology is sufficiently known so that decisions to burn or not are economically based.

EXAMPLES IN THE USE OF PRESCRIBED FIRE

Prescribed burning, or at least the use of fire to attain an objective in rangeland management, has many facets. Three broad vegetational types are selected for brief discussion because they span a wide spectrum of situations in which range managers are involved with prescribed fire. Also, brushlands, grasslands, and open forests, wherever they are found, have much in common.

California Chaparral

After 70,000 hectares of chaparral brushland burned in the 1970 Laguna fire, San Diego County in southern California still had 85 percent of its remaining chaparral in highly flammable condition. The Laguna fire was one of 15 large fires that occurred in chaparral between September 25 and October 3, 1970. These fires burned more than 200,000 hectares, destroyed 1,000 structures, and caused the loss of 14 lives. About 2.7 million hectares of mixed chaparral and coastal sage in southern California are highly susceptible to catastrophic fire. An additional 1.0 million hectares of brush in the Sierra Nevada–southern Cascade region differ from those brushlands in botanical composition, slope gradients, wind velocities, soil conditions, and erosion hazard; but they also are subject to wildfires under conditions that restrict control. Less than 3 percent of the wildfires in this broad chaparral region exceed 40 hectares in size, but it seems unlikely that all fires will be controlled at that small size.

Flash runoffs carrying large amounts of debris often originate on steep slopes made bare by fire in the chaparral of southern California. The costs of removing deposited mud and rocks in the cities below burned watersheds averaged about $2.75 per cubic meter in the 1970 fire. Debris removal and land repairs cost more than $250 per hectare for the 11,000 hectare Malibu fire in 1970. Thus the problems in chaparral are the raging wildfires and subsequent floods. Watershed damage does not follow all fires in southern California and follows only a few in other areas of the chaparral types. However, erosion control must be considered in any ventures with chaparral manipulations.

Many objectives have been proposed for justifing manipulation of the botanical composition of brush fields and the condition of the brush itself. These objectives include reduction of plant stature from mature chaparral shrubs to sprouts and seedlings, opening of the woody canopy, and increasing of the ground cover with grasses and legumes.

Type conversions for livestock forage have been the principal objective in the burning of the California chaparral and closely associated oak woodland (Fig. 16-5). Prescribed burning in the Brush Range Improvement Program from 1945 through 1969 was conducted on 974,518 hectares of which 289,333 were reburns and 295,624 were seeded to grasses and legumes. About 75 percent of these burns were conducted during the middle to late dry season, July through September (Raymond, 1970). Much of the chaparral in southern California is on slopes too steep to be grazed by livestock, so little effort has been made to produce forage in that area.

Manipulations of chaparral to improve habitat for game, principally deer and quail, and for the hunter aim to develop a mixture of vegetational types. These types include nutritious young brush sprouts, escape cover, open areas, and yearlong feed. In coastal California, patches of annual grass make good winter deer feed, while acorns are staples in the late-summer diet. Sprouts are better feed than is old growth because they are easily available and have higher nutritional quality. Young brush and a mixture of brush, woodland, and grass cover types are better situations for animal and hunter than are pure stands, especially old stands. Few chaparral manipulations have been made for planned commercial game production alone. Normally, the needs of game have been considered only when the main objective was development of another product.

Recreational pursuits in chaparral are hunting, hiking, camping, nature study of plant and animal communities, and other activities that are closely related to the landscape. To serve these activities best, the vegetation needs to be a combination

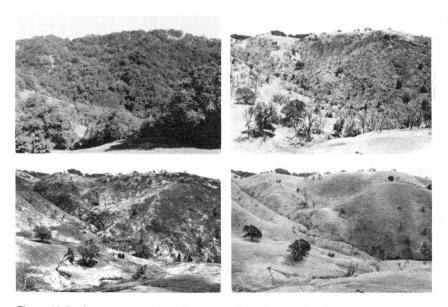

Figure 16-5   An untreated oak woodland (upper left). The same location five years after the trees were killed by girdling and 2, 4-D, (upper right) just previous to burning (lower left). The watershed had an excellent cover of grasses the following year (lower right).

of types, such as chaparral on the slopes, grasslands on the flats, and stringers of woodland along the streams or on other sites that will support trees. A variety of vistas is needed. Large, uniform expanses of chaparral make poor vistas but usually contain a wide variety of soil types that could support different plant and animal communities. Efforts to develop a vegetational architecture for recreationists other than hunters have been scanty.

Where the soil is deep, grasslands yield more water than does chaparral, other conditions being equal. Removal of woody plants from stream sides will reduce water loss through transpiration and increase water flow. Destruction of the woody cover and conversion to grass increases water output from the slopes. Usually, surface erosion will be less, or at least no more, with grass cover than with woody cover, but conversions for erosion-control purposes should be in small areas, on soils at least 50 centimeters deep, and generally on slopes of less than 35 percent. Where land slips might occur, a partial cover of woody plants should remain.

Fire-hazard reduction is another objective used in justifying reducing chaparral and increasing grass. These changes can cut the fuel load per hectare from 85 or more tons to less than 5 tons. Grassland fires are of lower intensity than those in chaparral, but fire may travel more rapidly in grass. The advantage of grass lies in the fact that less fuel permits more effective fighting of wildfire.

Only partial success can be claimed for chaparral conversion to grassland. Improvements in forage production have occurred, but highly flammable chaparral still covers wide expanses of land. The effectiveness of all control procedures has varied from site to site. The work of maintaining a grassland increases as slopes increase or as the soils become less fertile. Chaparral tends to return quickly. The most controversial tool in this complex of objectives, biological potentials, and physical conditions is prescribed burning.

While most prescribed burns in the California Brush Range Improvement Program were successfully held within the lines, escapes burned 75,623 hectares (7.76 percent of the total area burned) during the 25-year program. In a few instances, the resulting liability and costs of suppressing escapes were assessed to landowners, which dampened enthusiasm for prescribed burning. To date, most of the prescribed burning has been on private land where the owner believed he could obtain a profitable return from livestock grazing. Public-land administrators have not always had that incentive and have had to fight the escapes on private land. The danger of erosion during the time between brush control and growth of a grass cover may be too great for fire to be risked except on small, selected areas. Prescribed burning may add to air pollution, but not as much as do wildfires because timing and size of the fire are controlled. Before prescribed burning can become a common and predictable tool for managing the California chaparral to increase its variety of products and to reduce hazards of raging wildfires, large-scale, objective evaluations of many factors are needed.

Grasslands

All grasslands are burned, except the extremely dry desert grasslands, which have too little fuel to carry a fire. Tropical grassland with two dry seasons may be burned twice a year. In general, mountain bunchgrass areas, temperate grasslands, Mediterranean annual grasslands, and some desert grasslands, although subjected to wildfires that retard woody species, seldom are burned on a prescribed basis as a management technique. The main purpose of burning in these grasslands is reduction of shrubs. In contrast, grasslands in moister areas, such as the true prairie of central North America and tropical or subtropical tall grasslands that are dominated by species in the tribe *Andropogoneae,* frequently are burned for reduction of mature dry grass material that is unpalatable and of low nutritive value as well as for maintenance of relatively shrub-free conditions.

The role of burning in the 100-year grazing history of bluestem (*Andropogon* spp.) ranges in the Flint Hills of Kansas illustrates continuing arguments over the practice. Beginning in the 1880s, cattle were moved from Texas in April, fattened on the Kansas pastures, then shipped to market in the late summer or fall. Steers gained more on burned range, so leases usually contained a clause demanding spring burning (Anderson, 1964). As early as 1923 Hensel and in 1934 Aldous reported reduced yield and changes in botanical composition due to early-spring burning. After many experiments, the advantages of burning appear to be an increase in *Andropogon gerardi*, a decrease in *Poa pratensis,* changes in other species, and greater beef gains (Table 16-2). The disadvantages include an increase in *Rhus glabra* and a reduction in water infiltration rate, soil moisture, and herbage yield. During the studies, late-spring (May 1) burning emerged as the treatment least detrimental to the range and most productive of beef.

Burning of bluestem ranges in the Kansas Flint Hills is likely to continue, although changes from seasonal grazing by steers to yearlong range use by breeding herds may alter the annual burning practice. Yearlong grazing with cows and continued livestock trampling could reduce the standing dead material to a degree that burning would become unnecessary. Anderson (1964) suggests that if one must burn, to minimize possible harmful effects, one should burn in late spring, after soil and plant crowns are wet with rain. The fire should be set when a breeze will move it briskly. Grazing immediately after the burn and close grazing should be avoided.

Spring burning has stimulated dry-matter production and flowering with no serious harm throughout the true prairie of central North America (Old, 1969). Clipping has given responses similar to those from burning, which indicates that the major effect is due to removal of litter rather than to direct heat of the fire (Hulbert, 1969). Soils with reduced litter showed increased temperature, more microbial activity, and more available plant nutrients than those soils covered with dense litter. A second effect that increases productivity of tall grass is the reduction

Table 16-2 Long-term results of burning bluestem pastures
in the Flint Hills of Kansas *(Some data from treatments
started by Aldous, 1934)*

Time of burning	Soil moisture, cm/m*	Decreasers, %†	Yield, kg/ha‡	Steer gains, kg§
December 1	28.4	67.7	2,194	...
March 20	31.0	70.2	2,260	108
April 10	31.2	75.3	2,407	115
May 1	32.4	87.1	2,629	118
Unburned	33.5	68.5	2,919	106

*Centimeters of water per meter of soil on Aldous' ungrazed
plots for 1960–1961 (McMurphy and Anderson, 1965).

†Decreasers were mainly *Andropogon gerardi, A. scoparius,
Sorghastrum nutans,* and *Koeleria cristata* in 1957–1961 on Aldous'
ungrazed plots (McMurphy and Anderson, 1965).

‡Thirty-year average kilograms per hectare on the ordinary upland bluestem type (Anderson, 1964).

§Average kilograms per head gain, May 1–October 15, for 1950–
1963 inclusive (Anderson, 1964).

of cool-season species, namely, *Poa pratensis* and perhaps *Bromus inermis.*
Evidently, these species are more likely to be growing rapidly than are the native
warm-season species; hence they are damaged by spring burning.

African grasslands south of the Sahara which are dominated by tall species
respond to burning approximately as do those in North America. Experimental
work on the effects of grassland burning in Africa began with plots near Pretoria in
South Africa (Phillips, 1919). Protection from fire permits buildup of litter and
accumulation of unpalatable materials which leads to elimination of palatable
species, such as *Themeda triandra.* Burning, grazing, and mowing singly and in
combination maintain a desirable grassland (West, 1965). Burning of the sweet-
veld in South Africa is widely condemned, but the sourveld may be improved with
an occasional fire after the first spring rain and in conjunction with sound livestock
management (Scott, 1967). Burning, to be most effective for maintenance of good
range condition, should occur as late as possible in the dormant season but before
the desirable grasses begin to grow. Burning may be annual in areas of high rainfall
with exceptionally tall grasses, but should be less frequent in regions with lower
rainfall. The season and the frequency of burning that maintan the grassland also
result in the most effective control of woody vegetation. The timing of prescribed
burning of grassland dominated by tall grass is the most important consideration.

The principal purpose for prescribed burning of other grassland types is
reduction of undesirable plants. Mixed prairie in the western plains usually is not
burned because fire reduces the cover and the productivity of the palatable grasses

(Hopkins et al., 1948). Dominants in the semidesert grassland, such as *Bouteloua eriopoda* and *Hilaria jamesii,* produced less in the year following fire but were back to preburn levels in two or three years (Jameson, 1962). *Haplopappus tenuisectus* was easily killed by fire, but this species, *Aristida glabrata, Bouteloua rothrockii,* and other perennial grasses on the Santa Rita Experimental Range showed little effect of fire after two years (Cable, 1967). *Bouteloua gracilis* in New Mexico changed little due to wild fire, although herbage production was reduced for a year (Dwyer and Pieper, 1967). Detrimental effects of fire in these grasslands are loss of forage in the fire and reduced herbage the next season. The Mediterranean annual type in California responded in the same manner (Hervey, 1949).

In northeastern Oregon, *Agropyron spicatum* was more resistant to burning than was *Festuca idahoensis* (Conrad and Poulton, 1966). Four other grass species of the Palouse Prairie type in southern Idaho were subjected to three intensities of burning, at three points in the growth cycle, on two sizes of plants. *Poa secunda* was not affected by the treatments. *Sitanion hystrix* was damaged in July. *Stipa thurberiana* and *Stipa comata* were damaged severely by burning in June and July. (Wright and Klemmedson, 1965). Variation in production of the bunchgrass species due to burning was reported by Blaisdell (1953) in southern Idaho. All grasses were injured, the bunch type more than the rhizomatous species, but all recovered. Sprouting shrubs were favored, and the nonsprouting *Artemisia* gradually returned. The bunchgrass type should not be burned except possibly where *Artemisia tridentata* is to be killed and *Bromus tectorum* is the main fuel that carries the fire. Seeding should follow this practice.

Pinelands

Prescribed burns in pinelands have one or more objectives: slash removal, seedbed preparation, disease control, hardwood control, wildfire-hazard reduction, game production, and forage for livestock. Many pinelands in Florida, elsewhere on the southeastern coastal plains, and, to a limited extent, in the Piedmont bordering the inner coastal plain of the southeastern United States are burned annually so that production of cattle forage is enhanced, wildfire is reduced, and timber is promoted. They were so treated in the late 1800s, but a period of no prescribed fires and intense controversy about burning occurred from about 1900 to the 1940s. The monographic book on bobwhite quail (Stoddard, 1931) was a major influence that signaled the return to prescribed burning in managing southern pinelands.

The southeastern United States is a large area with numerous range sites, species of pine, and species of forage plants. Generalizations on the use of and specifications for prescribed burning are misleading because of these infinitely numerous combinations of vegetation, objectives, fuel, and weather conditions. A person who uses fire as a management tool in the southeastern pineland needs to learn the "tricks of the trade" from the masters in his area. Indeed, this is true for the use of fire anywhere. Brief descriptions for several different extensive vegetational types illustrate southeastern conditions (Hilmon and Hughes, 1965a).

In *Pinus taeda–Pinus echinata,* young stands are burned with slow-burning back fires so that fuel accumulations are reduced. The soil is wet and surface fuels damp. Immature stands are less susceptible to damage than are mature stands, so head fires or fires angling into the wind are used to reduce hardwood and shrubs, which are more common here than in the longleaf pine type. Summer fire in mature stands removes litter and shrubby plants in preparation for natural seeding after timber harvest. Hardwood control is mostly by winter burns (Lotti, 1962).

Pinus palustris requires prescribed burning to reduce disease, lessen competition, decrease danger of wildfire, and increase forage production. *Andropogon divergens* constitutes the major forage resource for livestock, and there may be little brush except in areas of *Serenoa repens* in Florida. Longleaf pine needles and grass constitute a highly flammable fuel that may be burned soon after a rain and before other pinelands will burn. This suggests burning the longleaf pine type first and the other pines, mainly *Pinus elliottii,* on a later day. The principle of burning from highly flammable fuel to an area with less danger eases fire control in most prescribed burning programs.

Seedlings of *Pinus palustris* need protection the first year, but during the grass stage in their life cycle, frequent burning is needed to reduce brown spot disease. When the stem begins to elongate, longleaf seedlings should not be burned until they are at least 1.3 meters tall. Afterwards, burning is done at three- to five- year intervals as needed to reduce hardwoods and promote forages. Young longleaf will be damaged by fire if the terminal bud is showing new growth, which restricts fires in this type to the winter season. Burning early in the fall tends to reduce the *Andropogons* and increase native legumes, especially where fire has been withheld for several years. Species of legumes that increase are in the genera *Cassia, Desmodium,* and *Lespedeza.* Annual burning can double the legume plants per hectare (Wahlenberg et al., 1939). Burning every two or three years is better than burning annually in the pine-bluestem type and may be used to facilitate grazing rotations. Grelen and Epps (1967) suggest, on a basis of measurement in Louisiana, that burning portions of the range in winter, spring, and summer will prolong the period of adequate protein in the forage. A burning program increases forage production and quality of feed for birds, large game, and livestock.

Mature slash pine with an understory of wiregrasses, *Aristida stricta,* and *Sporobolus curtessii* is burned annually in the northern part of its range, where frost cures the herbage. The wiregrasses sprout quickly after a fire and are palatable for a few months. Species of *Andropogon, Panicum,* and *Eragrostis* tend to increase with repeated fires in this type. Further south in Florida, the grasses stay green through the first winter after a fire, so prescribed burning should be done every two or three years. Burns conducted in March to May consistently have resulted in more forage and seed. *Ilex glabra* and *Serenoa repens* may be held in check but not eliminated by burning. They are most susceptible to summer fires (Hilmon and Hughes, 1965b). Seedlings of slash pine should be protected from fire until they are ten years old or 4 to 5 meters tall.

Marsh burning along the coastal plains is practiced on nearly all the waterfowl refuges and on areas used by livestock. Food supplies for birds and forage for livestock are increased as the dry, unpalatable litter is removed. Because the growing season of many Gulf Coast marsh grasses extends into the winter, a fall burn provides new growth for winter grazing (Givens, 1962). Marshlands in Africa, Central America, and South America burn frequently, even over standing water (Budowski, 1966).

Arundinaria tecta is a common associate of *Pinus serotina* on wetlands in the lower coastal plains of the Carolinas and Virginia. The stands of grass gradually deteriorate with protection from fire. Because stems live for three to four years and dead stems persist for several years, new growth is retarded. Canebreaks may lose half their production over a ten-year period. Fire results in renewed vigor and forage of increased nutritional qualities, less wildfire hazard, and more accessible range (Hughes, 1966). Canelands should be burned at five- to ten-year intervals. If sufficient land is available, a burning rotation gives fresh feed each year and a fire on all lands at recommended intervals.

Second-growth *Pinus ponderosa* in several western states often occurs in thick, stagnated stands. As these become older, fire hazards increase because there are dead trees, woody debris, and a cover of pine needles. If a shrub stage precedes dominance by the regenerating pine, the woody debris in the understory can amount to many tons per hectare. Prescribed fire has been used in the ponderosa pine types in Washington and Arizona (Weaver, 1964) and in the mixed pine type at middle elevations in the Sierra Nevada Mountains of California (Biswell, 1963; Biswell et al., 1973) to reduce fire hazard, relieve competition on dominant trees, and thin regenerating stands. While development of forage production for livestock may not be an important objective of these prescribed fires, they are intimately associated with rangeland problems. Mature trees of *Pinus ponderosa* often occur as an open stand with important forage and browse in the understory that is used in the spring and summer by livestock and as winter range by game. Development of open stands in second-growth timber enhances these uses as well as recreational values. Prescribed burning in the ponderosa pine type usually is a reclamation practice to reduce accumulated debris. Large fuel loads necessitate burning in winter and spring when the soil is wet and in safe weather conditions. Two or more fires may be needed to accomplish the desired objectives.

Prescribed burning in *Pinus* spp.–*Juniperus* spp. stands is an infrequent practice and is aimed principally at controlling undesirable brush and trees.

Associated grassland types usually are palatable when cured, so burning destroys forage and may reduce growth of desirable grasses for a year or more. As these woodlands provide important deer habitats, fire reduces the trees and improves forage and browse for wild animals. McCulloch (1969) suggested that crown fires, which move rapidly and result in little heat accumulation in the soil or damage to herbaceous perennials, are the most acceptable type of fire.

Whether one is considering a prescribed fire in chaparral, grasslands, or pinelands, timing is a prime factor. Pines, except *P. palustris,* are highly susceptible to fire until they are about 4 meters tall, so frequency of burning of pinelands varies with the age of the pine. Different species of chaparral and grasses respond differently to fire on a seasonal basis. For example, wiregrasses in Florida produce abundant seed if burned in May, but little seed in response to winter fires. Fuel moisture changes hourly. Weather is critical, because a fire can escape if wind increases or can become too hot if dead calm develops. A fire to prepare a seedbed may need to be very hot and leave a soil covering of white ash, while another to reduce fire hazard would aim to leave mulch unburned. Timing with respect to soil moisture often determines the severity of fire and the degree of change that a fire inflicts upon the ecosystem. Prescribed burning is an art requiring the integration of many factors.

LITERATURE CITED

Aldous, A. E. 1934. Effect of burning of Kansas bluestem pastures. *Kan. Agr. Expt. Sta. Tech. Bull.* 38.

Amman, G. A. 1957. *The prairie grouse of Michigan.* Mich. Dept. Cons.

Anderson, K. L. 1964. Burning Flint Hills bluestem pastures. *Tall Timbers Fire Ecol. Conf.* 3:88–103.

Barrows, J. S. 1951. Fire behavior in northern Rocky Mountain Forests. *N. Rocky Mtn. For. and Range Expt. Sta. Paper* 29.

Bentley, J. R., and V. E. White. 1961. The fuel-break system for the San Dimas Experimental Forest. *Pacific Southwest Forest and Range Expt. Sta. Misc. Paper* 63.

Biswell, H. H. 1963. Research in wildland fire ecology in California. *Tall Timbers Fire Eco. Conf.* 2:62–97.

———, H. R. Kallander, R. Komarek, R. J. Vogl, and H. Weaver. 1973. Ponderosa fire management. *Tall Timbers Res. Sta. Misc. Pub.* 2.

———, and A. M. Schultz. 1956. Reduction of wildfire hazard. *Calif. Agr.* 10:4–5.

———, R. D. Taber, D. W. Hedrick, and A. M. Schultz. 1952. Management of chamise brushlands for game in the north coast region of California. *Calif. Fish and Game.* 38:453–484.

Blaisdell, J. P. 1953. Ecological effects of planned burning of sagebrush–grass range on the upper Snake River plains. *U.S. Dept. Agr. Tech. Bull.* 1075.

Budowski, G. 1966. Fire in tropical American lowland areas. *Tall Timbers Fire Ecol. Conf.* 5:5–22.

Byram, G. M. 1959. Combustion of forest fuels. In *Forest fire: Control and use*, ed. K. P. Davis, pp. 61–89. New York: McGraw-Hill.

Cable, D. R. 1967. Fire effects on semidesert grasses and shrubs. *J. Range Mgmt.* 20:170–176.

Conrad, C. E., and C. E. Poulton. 1966. Effect of a wildfire on Idaho fescue and bluebunch wheatgrass. *J. Range Mgmt.* 19:138–141.

CSIRO. 1970. The bushfire problem in Australia. *Rural research in CSIRO.* 69:8–13.

Dasmann, W. P., and R. F. Dasmann. 1963. Abundance and scarcity in California deer. *Calif. Fish and Game.* 49:4–15.

Duvall, V. L. 1962. Burning and grazing increase herbage on slender bluestem range. *J. Range Mgmt.* 15:14–16.

———, and L. B. Whitaker. 1963. Supplemental feeding increases beef production on bluestem-longleaf ranges. *La. Agr. Expt. Sta. Bull.* 564.

———, and ———. 1964. Rotation burning: A forage management system for longleaf pine-bluestem ranges. *J. Range Mgmt.* 17:322–326.

Dwyer, D. D., and R. D. Pieper. 1967. Fire effects on blue grama-pinyon-juniper rangeland in New Mexico. *J. Range Mgmt.* 20:359–362.

Ehrenreich, J. H., and J. M. Aikman. 1963. An ecological study of the effect of certain management practices on native prairie in Iowa. *Ecol. Monog. 33:113*–130.

Elwell, H. M., H. A. Daniel, and F. A. Fenton. 1941. The effects of burning pasture and woodland vegetation. *Okla. Agr. Expt. Sta. Bull.* 247.

Givens, L. S. 1962. Use of fire on southeastern wildlife refuges. *Tall Timbers Fire Ecol. Conf.* 1:121–126.

Grelen, H. E., and E. A. Epps, Jr. 1967. Season of burning affects herbage quality and yield on pine-bluestem range. *J. Range Mgmt.* 20:31–33.

Halls, L. K., R. H. Hughes, R. S. Rummell, and B. L. Southwell. 1964. Forage and cattle management in longleaf-slash pine forests. *U.S. Dept. Agr. Farmers Bull.* 2199.

Hanks, R. J., and K. L. Anderson. 1957. Pasture burning and moisture conservation. *J. Soil and Water Cons.* 12:228–229.

Hensel, R. L. 1923. Effects of burning on vegetation in Kansas pastures. *J. Agr. Res.* 23:631–644.

Hervey, D. F. 1949. Reaction of a California annual-plant community to fire. *J. Range Mgmt.* 2:116–121.

Hilmon, J. B., and R. H. Hughes. 1965a. Forest Service research on the use of fire in livestock management in the South. *Tall Timbers Fire Ecol. Conf.* 4:260–275.

———, and ———. 1965b. Fire and forage in the wiregrass type. *J. Range Mgmt.* 18:251–254.

Hopkins, H., F. W. Albertson, and A. Riegel. 1948. Some effects of burning upon a prairie in west-central Kansas. *Trans. Kan. Acad. Sci.* 51:131–141.

Hughes, R. H. 1966. Fire ecology of canebrakes. *Tall Timbers Fire Ecol. Conf.* 5:148–158.

Hulbert, L. C. 1969. Fire and litter effects in undisturbed bluestem prairie in Kansas. *Ecology* 50:874–877.

Jameson, D. A. 1962. Effects of burning on a galleta–black grama range invaded by juniper. *Ecology* 43:760–763.

Leopold, A. S., and F. F. Darling. 1953. Effects of land use on moose and caribou in Alaska. *Trans. N. Am. Wildl. Conf.* 18:553–560.

Lewis, C. E. 1964. Forage response to month of burning. *U.S. Forest Service Research Note* SE-35.

Lightle, P. C. 1960. Brown-spot needle blight of longleaf pine. *U.S. Dept. Agr., Forest Pest Leaflet* 44, rev. 1969.

Lindenmuth, A. W., Jr., and J. R. Davis. 1973. Predicting fire spread in Arizona's oak chaparral. *U.S. Dept. Agr. Forest Service Research Paper* RM—101.

Lotti, T. 1962. The use of prescribed fire in the silviculture of loblolly pine. *Tall Timbers Fire Ecol. Conf.* 1:109–120.

Lynch, J. L. 1941. The place of burning in management of the Gulf Coast wildlife refuges. *J. Wildl. Mgmt.* 5:454–457.

McArthur, A. G., and N. P. Cheney. 1966. The characterization of fires in relation to ecological studies. *Aust. For. Res.* 2:36–45.

McCulloch, C. Y. 1969. Some effects of wildfire on deer habitat in pinyon-juniper woodland. *J. Wildl. Mgmt.* 33:778–784.

McMurphy, W. E., and K. L. Anderson. 1965. Burning Flint Hill range. *J. Range Mgmt.* 18:265–269.

Miller, H. A. 1963. Use of fire in wildlife management. *Tall Timbers Fire Ecol. Conf.* 2:18–30.

Old, Sylvia M. 1969. Microclimates, fire, and plant production in an Illinois prairie. *Ecol. Monog.* 39:355–384.

Owensby, C. E., and K. L. Anderson. 1967. Yield responses to time of burning in the Kansas Flint Hills. *J. Range Mgmt.* 20:12–16.

Peterle, T. J. 1958. Game management in Scotland. *J. Wildl. Mgmt.* 22:221–231.

Phillips, E. P. 1919. A preliminary report on the veld-burning experiments at Groenkloof, Pretoria. *S. Afr. J. Sci.* 16:285–299.

Pompe, A., and R. G. Vines. 1966. The influence of moisture on the combustion of leaves. *Aust. For.* 30:231–241.

Raymond, F. H. 1970. *Brush range improvement—1969.* Sacramento: California Division of Forestry.

Robocker, W. C., and Bonita Miller. 1955. Effects of clipping, burning and competition on establishment and survival of some native grasses in Wisconsin. *J. Range Mgmt.* 8:117–120.

Sampson, A. W., and L. T. Burcham. 1954. Costs and returns of controlled brush burning for range improvement in northern California. *Calif. Div. For., Range Improvement Studies* No. 1.

Schimke, H. E., J. D. Dell, and F. R. Ward. 1969. *Electrical ignition for prescribed burning.* Pacific Southwest Forest and Range Expt. Sta.

Scott, J. D. 1967. Advances in pasture work in South Africa: Pt. 1. *Veld. Herb. Abst.* 37:1–9.

Smith, E. L. 1960. Effects of burning and clipping at various times during the wet season on a tropical tall grass range in northern Australia. *J. Range Mgmt.* 13:197–203.

Southwell, B. L., and R. H. Hughes. 1965. Beef cattle management practices for wiregrass-pine ranges of Georgia. *Ga. Agr. Expt. Sta. Bull.* N.S. 129.

Spencer, D. L., and E. F. Chaletain. 1953. Progress in the management of moose of south central Alaska. *Trans. N. Am. Wildl. Conf.* 18:539–552.

Stoddard, H. L. 1931. *Bobwhite quail, its habits, preservation and increase.* New York: Scribner's.

———. 1963. Bird habitat and fire. *Tall Timbers Fire Ecol. Conf.* 2:163–175.

Thompson, G. A. 1962. Forest Service policy for controlled use of fire. *Tall Timbers Fire Ecol. Conf.* 1:151–154.

U.S. Forest Service. 1956. Glossary of terms used in forest fire control. *U.S. Dept. Agr. Handbook* 104.

Wahlenberg, W. G., S. W. Greene, and H. R. Reed. 1939. Effects of fire and cattle grazing on longleaf pine lands as studied at McNeill, Miss. *U.S. Dept. Agr. Tech. Bull.* 683.

Weaver, H. 1964. Fire and management problems in ponderosa pine. *Tall Timbers Fire Ecol. Conf.* 3:60–79.

———. 1967. Fire and its relationship to ponderosa pine. *Tall Timbers Fire Ecol. Conf.* 7:127–149.

West, O. 1965. *Fire in vegetation and its use in pasture management.* Commonwealth Bur. Pasture and Field Crops. Mimeo.

Wheeler, R. J., Jr. 1948. *The wild turkey in Alabama.* Ala. Dept. Cons.

Williams, R. E. 1955. Development and improvement of Coastal marsh ranges. *U.S. Dept. Agr. Yearbook,* pp. 444–450.

Wright, H. A., and J. O. Klemmedson. 1965. Effect of fire on bunchgrasses of the sagebrush-grass region in southern Idaho. *Ecology* 46:680–688.

Chapter 17

Biological Control of Range Weeds

The processes of natural biological control maintain the so-called balance of nature. Left unchecked, any species has the reproductive capacity to cover much of the earth, but all species are subject to checks on population numbers. The manipulation of grazing animals for the purpose of attaining certain types of vegetation or densities of interacting species is a form of biological control. However, the professional field of biological control concentrates on the use of parasites, predators, or pathogens to reduce population densities of unwanted organisms to levels below economic significance (DeBach, 1964). *Biological control* is further defined as *control of numbers by natural enemies,* according to van den Bosch and Messenger (1973), who list 75 insect species and 21 plant species that have been subjected to substantial or complete control.

The deliberate use of large grazing animals to control vegetation has been treated in Parts One and Two. This chapter examines biological control in the traditional sense. Work on biological control began in the early 1800s, but not until the late 1880s was there a successfully planned project. It was the control of cottony cushion scale on citrus in southern California.

Biological control concentrates on the use of insects to control pests, which may be noxious plants or noxious insects on desirable plants. The word *predator* is used here to include insects that prey on both kinds of pests. Suppression of pests may stem from direct kill, weakening and replacement by competitors, reduced reproductive capacity, and infection by pathogens. Reduction of European rabbits in Australia by the *Myxomatosis* virus is a type of biological control.

PRINCIPLES

Biological control has had its greatest successes when both the species to be controlled and the predator have been introduced. Weeds usually arrive without their natural population controls, hence they thrive and often become more aggressive pests than they were in their original habitats. An objective in biological control is to introduce a natural predator that becomes aggressive because its enemies have been left behind. In the new situations, the total environment may be more favorable to an insect predator than the original environment was, or it may favor a combination of control organisms. For example, secondary invasion of parasitized *Opuntia* by fungi and bacteria speeds the destruction of the weed. Abundant weed populations appear more susceptible to predator destruction than scattered stands.

No sound basis exists for selection of insects to introduce for biological control. The predator and host can be matched closely in terms of climate, competitors, etc., but success or failure must be determined by actual introduction. There is no shortcut in finding the ideal enemy for a rangeland pest — one that keeps a weed at low densities and is relatively free of resident predators and diseases. Huffaker et al. (1971) listed the characteristics of an effective natural enemy as follows: (1) high searching ability, (2) high degree of host specificity, (3) great reproductive capacity relative to the host, and (4) wide adaptability to environment.

Another aspect of biological control, and one similar to management with other means of vegetational manipulation, is that the manager must foster increases in desirable plants to replace those eliminated. Otherwise biological control has little lasting value.

Of practical necessity, biological control should aim for low population numbers rather than eradication. The usual sequences of events after release of a predator are alternating cycles of weed and insect. As the weed population declines, so does the predator, but in most examples the food builds up again faster than the predator. Each crash of both weed and predator occurs with fewer numbers or less density of the host. In the successful examples, such as biological control of *Opuntia* in Australia, the abundance of plant and insect reached an equilibrium at low population densities of both.

Most successful examples of biological control center around one best enemy, but other enemies may improve control. The effective combination of predators may differ over the range of the pest. Importation of diverse natural enemies and studies of their effects on native pests as well as on introduced pests will increase the practical significance of biological control on rangelands.

RISKS

Biological control with introduced species of insects carries considerable potential that the predator may change host plants and attack species of economic importance. Arguments against introductions emphasize this point and the point that chances of success are slight, at best. Huffaker (1957) reviewed papers that showed that host specificity was related to the amounts and kinds of essential oils and alkaloids, which served in different plants as either attractors or detractors. However, an insect's dietary preferences may change, but these changes are difficult to determine because the full food spectrum of an insect seldom is known. Apparently, changes in plant abundance and insect abundance often are mutually related. The risks of the predator becoming a secondary pest increases in direct proportion to its abundance. Extensive testing under quarantine remains the most effective assurance against excessive risk of an introduced insect becoming a pest. The risk of an insect attacking economically valuable plants appears to be reduced when weed and crop are greatly different in morphology, chemistry, and taxonomic relationship. Highly specialized insect feeders present less risk than general leaf and flower feeders (Wilson, 1943), although excellent control of *Hypericum perforatum* by *Chrysolina quadrigemina* is an exception to that rule. *Chrysolina* does not attack ornamental *Hypericum* spp. because of phenological incompatabilities. *Rubus fruticosus* in New Zealand, closely related to many valuable members of the *Rosaceae,* has defied safe biological control.

SOME SUCCESSFUL EXAMPLES

Several highly successful examples of biological control have occurred on rangeland. Three of the four examples described herein concern plant pests, but biological control has been more successful with insect pests, probably because more work has been done with biological control of these pests than with other species.

Opuntia spp.

Several species of *Opuntia* that are native to North and South America were transported to other continents for livestock feed, hedge fences, erosion control, and fruit for human consumption. *Opuntia* escaped cultivation and covered many millions of hectares in Hawaii, Australia, India, Ceylon, Celebes, Mauritius, and South Africa. Australia alone reported 25 million hectares in 1925, of which half were so dense that men and animals could not penetrate the stands (Dodd, 1940).

Australia pioneered in the highly successful biological control of seven *Opuntia* species. *O. stricta* and *O. inermis* were the worst invaders. *O. stricta* did not succumb until the moth, *Cactoblastis cactorum,* was introduced in 1925. *Cactoblastis* did so well that breeding programs of all insect predators on *Opuntia* were omitted in the third year, and the problem was one of distribution of field colonies of *C. cactorum. Opuntia* was greatly and quickly reduced in Australia. The plant species and the moth proceeded through diminishing cycles of regrowth and have remained at low population levels for many years. This is the finest example of plant control by introduced insects.

Hawaii had a problem with the large Mexican cactus, *Opuntia megacantha,* which was used as an emergency livestock feed. A number of slowly spreading insects failed to control it. Not until 1951 were objections to *Cactoblastis cactorum* and the cochineal insect, *Dactylopius tomentosus,* overruled and successful control obtained (Fig. 17-1). The moth became dominant at upper elevations and the cochineal in the lower parts of the cactus stands. However, a few *Opuntia* plants survive at elevations above and below major insect attack zones. These two insects, singly or together, have been successful on other *Opuntia* species in Asia.

Opuntia control illustrates ideal use of biological procedures. This highly specialized plant type had no close relatives of economic value in the invaded countries. Feeders on *Opuntia* in their native home could be imported without their enemies with little fear that they, in turn, would become pests. A favorable

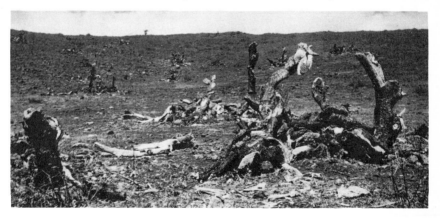

Figure 17-1 *Opuntia* on Hawaii killed by the feeding of *Cactoblastis* and *Dactylopius.*

climate, unlimited food, and a lack of enemies permitted extremely rapid population explosions of the moth and the cochineal in Australia.

In Mauritius, control of the pineapple mealybug with an introduced parasite resulted in loss of the cactus cochineal. Attention to all aspects of predator-prey relations is important in biological control. These aspects include reduction of enemies of the controlling insect so that it can be effective. Considerations in biological control go beyond a single predator-prey relationship.

Hypericum perforatum

This species, called *St. John's wort, Kalamath weed,* or *goatweed,* is known throughout the temperate world. White-skinned animals are photosensitized by it, and the plant crowds out valuable forage species. Before control, *Hypericum* occurred in extensive patches on rangeland, in abandoned fields, and along roads throughout the northwestern United States from western Montana to central California. It first appeared in California about 1900 and covered 1 million hectares in the state by 1952 (Huffaker and Kennett, 1959). In Australia, it spread from a single introduction in 1880 to 200,000 or more hectares by 1930 (Crafts and Robbins, 1962).

Between 1927 and the early 1940s, a large number of insect feeders on *Hypericum* were tested on economically valuable plants in different European districts. Several species passed the tests and were released in Australia, where local control of *Hypericum* was attained. The first introductions into the United States arrived in 1944, and they soon passed starvation tests by not feeding on sugar beets, flax, cotton, and several other crop plants (Holloway, 1948). Four colonies of *Chrysolina hyperici* were released in late 1945. *Chrysolina quadrigemina* took longer to test, and release of it began in 1946. Distribution of colonies to the northwestern states and spread of the insects through the stands of *Hypericum* proceded rapidly.

The adult beetles aestivate in the soil during the summer dry period beginning in late June. Both *Hypericum* and *Chrysolina* become active after the fall rains, and the eggs are laid in October. Hatching and feeding by young larvae follow quickly. In the spring, third- and fourth-stage larvae feed near the ground and pupate in the soil (Holloway and Huffaker, 1951). Destruction of procumbent growth during fall and spring prevents flowering and seed production and reduces the ability of *Hypericum* to compete with other herbaceous plants. *Chrysolina quadrigemina* became the dominant species among the introductions because the life history of the beetle and the phenology of the plant were well synchronized.

Hypericum was reduced to less than 1 percent of its former abundance in California within a decade after the beetle was released (Huffaker and Kennett, 1959). These authors measured the percentage species composition on several sites and found that forage grasses increased in response to decrease in *Hypericum*

(Table 17-1). Plant succession proceeded toward perennial grasses with only a nucleus of *Hypericum* persistent; but in pastures where heavy grazing occurred, undesirable annual species remained (Murphy, 1955). Suppression of *Hypericum* by insects has been less successful in Canada and Australia than in California (Clark, 1953; Holloway, 1964).

Lantana camara and Others

This plant, introduced onto the Hawaiian islands from Central America in about 1805 as an ornamental, escaped and covered thousands of hectares of rangeland by 1900. Insect feeders on leaves, flowers, and seed were introduced in 1902 and again after World War II. Both the early and later introductions partially controlled the *Lantana* on dry areas, but it remains abundant on wet sites (Andres and Goeden, 1971). Where it has been controlled, other woody plants that are more difficult to control have taken its place. Biological control of *Lantana* in Fiji, Australia, and India followed imports of insects from Hawaii (Huffaker, 1964).

A seed feeder, *Apion ulicis,* on *Ulex europaeus* in New Zealand, Hawaii, California, and Oregon destroys as much as 98 percent of the seed crop. This is not sufficient for effective control of most established stands. However, reductions occur over time, and the major advantage with seed and flower feeders may be reduction in the rate of spread of an invading weed. Biological control of annual species such as *Halogeton glomeratus* may be most effective with seed-destroying insects. The review by van den Bosch and Messenger (1973) describes and refers to the current situation in the biological control of other species.

Antonina graminis

The scale, *Antonina graminis*, first found in southern Texas in 1942, severely reduced stands of *Chloris gayana*. Since that time, *Antonina* has been found on 94

Table 17-1 Change in percentage composition of vegetation at one site in northwestern California after release of *Chrysolina quadrigemina* in 1947 *(Selected from Huffaker and Kennett, 1959)*

	Percentage composition					
Species	1947	1949	1951	1953	1955	1957
Hypericum perforatum	57.6	0.0	0.0	0.0	0.1	0.0
Total other forbs, mostly annual	17.8	22.3	49.2	30.1	15.1	27.6
Danthonia californica	9.2	22.7	28.9	30.3	52.6	45.0
Annual grasses	10.8	42.8	19.7	37.9	30.1	25.0
Miscellaneous species	4.6	12.2	2.2	1.7	2.1	2.4

grass species in North America, and it occurs widely in all subtropical regions. Ranchers in Texas have reported a 30 percent loss in grazing capacity due to the scale (Schuster et al., 1971). The losses of *Chloris* were so great that the value of seeding the species was questioned.

A scale parasite, *Neodusmetia sangwani,* was introduced from India in 1959 (Dean et al., 1961). The parasite reduced reproductions of the scale and showed outstanding results within three years of release in any location. However, it has little capacity to find the host and to disperse. Distribution was attained by spreading the parasite on infected grass from an airplane (Schuster et al., 1971).

BIOLOGICAL CONTROL AMONG NATIVES

Much has been written about regulation in population numbers within naturally occurring ecosystems. Wild species tend to be consistently abundant, each species fluctuating in abundance within its own particular pattern. Relative and absolute numbers change in response to environmental changes; then numbers tend to return to a certain magnitude of variation about a stable mean. This concept has been characterized as "contained variation" (Huffaker et al., 1971). It is accomplished through natural controls, often called "the balance of nature."

Every rangeland biome supports countless plant-eating insects. Occasionally one insect species explodes in population numbers. Defoliation of large areas may occur, and at times, patches of plants are killed. It seems reasonable to suggest that natural enemies of insect herbivores prevent many from attaining outbreak proportion. The more subtle effects on vegetation of less than outbreak numbers are poorly known. Several examples of insect impacts on range vegetation illustrate varied plant responses.

The California oak moth, *Phryganidia californica,* cyclically defoliates *Quercus agrifolia,* but few trees are killed (Harville, 1955). Oak woodlands support many and varied insect populations. At least one species of scarab and one weevil occur on each species of chaparral shrub, and Hagen et al. (1971) believed that natural control keeps them below densities damaging to the shrubs. Perhaps a hundred or more species of grasshoppers occur in each of the Western states, but only a few ever reach epidemic numbers. The Mormon cricket, *Anabrus simplex,* suffers considerable mortality from an egg parasite, *Sparasion pilosum,* and predation by the black cricket wasp (LaRivers, 1945). The sagebrush moth, *Aroga websteri,* occasionally defoliates stands of *Artemisia tridentata.* Ritcher (1966) suggested that a kill of the moth's parasites would reduce *Artemisia* in relation to the increased populations of *Aroga* that could be attained. Massey and Pierce (1960) reported insect defoliation of *Chrysothamnus nauseosus* in New Mexico and speculated on the possibility of fostering biological control of the shrub. *Prosopis* stands have been thinned by a twig girdler,

Oncideres rhodosticta (Ueckert et al., 1971), and viable seed of *Prosopis* has been reduced by the leaf-footed bug, *Mozena obtusa* (Ueckert, 1972). *Halogeton glomeratus* was host to numerous insect species in southern Idaho (Tisdale and Zappetini, 1953). *Eremophila gilesii* in southwestern Queensland, Australia, recently was defoliated and ring-barked by a wingless grasshopper (Fig. 17-2). Many more local examples of changes in range vegetation due to large populations of insects could be cited, but neither desirable nor undesirable effects of insect controls in these native situations are well known.

THE FUTURE OF BIOLOGICAL CONTROL

Although only two or three major rangeland weeds have been controlled over wide areas, the future of biological control has much to offer. Possibilities for the biological control of *Halogeton, Centaurea, Cirsium, Carduus, Onopordum, Ulex, Cytisus,* and many other weeds become increasingly attractive as the popularity of chemical controls decreases and as more experience is gained with introduced insects. Each problem needs to be viewed separately and each food-host-consumer relationship examined specifically, whether either or both weed and predator were introduced. The time is ending when range managers deal only with rodents and larger herbivores. The roles of the smaller grazers, especially the insects, will command increasing attention.

Conflicts of interest over rangeland weeds are likely to increase. *Centaurea solstitialis* is an important honey plant; *Opuntia* spp. furnish dairy feed in part of Mexico and emergency feed for range animals during droughts; *Cytisus* is an excellent plant for control of soil erosion; and all plants are in the habitat of

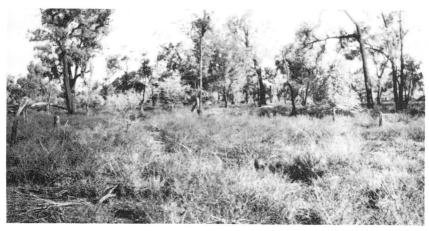

Figure 17-2 *Eremophila gilesii* in Australia killed by an outbreak of wingless grasshoppers.

animals. Arbitration of real or imagined conflicts should precede plant control by any means. The control of any given pest must be considered in an ecosystem context in which other potential pest populations exist, in which various control actions take place, and in which costs and benefits are generated. Every action needs to be preceded with positive answers to questions of ecological effectiveness, necessity, and economic justification (Huffaker, 1971). The time has passed for successive pesticide syndromes and other single-practice crusades on rangeland. The expanded and integrated concept of pest management (Annecke, 1973) embraces the ecosytem framework with consideration of plant pests, food chains, pathogens, insects, lower organisms, and the economics of alternative actions. Biological control has a bright future as a component of pest management (van der Bosch and Messenger, 1973).

LITERATURE CITED

Andres, L. A., and R. D. Goeden. 1971. The biological control of weeds by introduced natural enemies. In *Biological control,* pp. 143–164. New York: Plenum Press.

Annecke, D. P. 1973. Progress towards and ecological approach to pest control. *S. Afr. J. Sci.* 69:82–83.

Clark, L. R. 1953. The ecology of *Chrysomela gemellata* Rossi and *C. hyperici* Forst., and their effect on St. John's wort in the Bright District, Victoria. *Aust. J. Zoo.* 1:1–69.

Crafts, A. S., and W. W. Robbins, 1962. *Weed control.* New York: McGraw-Hill.

Dean, H. A., M. F. Schuster, and J. C. Bailey. 1961. The introduction and establishment of *Dusmetia sangwani* on *Antoninae graminis* in south Texas. *J. Econ. Entomol.* 54:925–954.

DeBach, P. (ed.). 1964. *Biological control of insect pests and weeds.* New York: Reinhold.

Dodd, A. P. 1940. *The biological campaign against prickly pear.* Commonwealth Prickly Pear Board, Brisbane, Aust.

Hagen, K. S., R. van der Bosch, and D. L. Dahlsten. 1971. The importance of naturally-occurring biological control in the western United States. In *Biological control,* pp. 253–293. New York: Plenum Press.

Harville, J. B. 1955. Ecology and population dynamics of the California oak moth, *Phryganidia californica* Packard (Lep: Dioptidae). *Micro-entomology* 20:83–166.

Holloway, J. K. 1948. Biological control of Klamath weed. *Prog. Rept. 10th Annual Western Weed Control Conf.* 19.

———. 1964. Project in biological control of weeds. In *Biological control of insect pests and weeds,* pp. 650–670. New York: Reinhold.

———, and C. B. Huffaker. 1951. The role of *Chrysolina gemellata* in the biological control of Klamath weed. *Econ. Ento.* 44:244–247.

Huffaker, C. B., 1957. Fundamentals of biological control of weeds. *Hilgardia* 27:101–157.

———. 1964. Fundamentals of biological weed control. In *Biological control of insect pests and weeds,* pp. 631–639. New York: Reinhold.

————. 1971. *Biological control.* New York: Plenum Press.

————, and C. E. Kennett. 1959. A ten-year study of vegetational changes associated with biological control of Klamath weed. *J. Range Mgmt.* 12:69–82.

————, P. S. Messenger, and P. DeBach. 1971. The natural enemy component in natural control and the theory of biological control. In *Biological control,* pp. 16–65. New York: Plenum Press.

LaRivers, I. 1945. The wasp *Chlorion laeviventris* as a natural control of the Mormon cricket. *Am. Midland Nat.* 33:743–763.

Massey, C. L., and D. A. Pierce. 1960. *Trirhabda nitidicollis,* a pest of rabbitbrush in New Mexico. *J. Range Mgmt.* 13:216–217.

Murphy, A. H. 1955. Vegetational changes during biological control of Klamath weed. *J. Range Mgmt.* 8:76–79.

Ritcher, P. O. 1966. Biological control of insects and weeds in Oregon. *Ore. Agr. Expt. Sta. Tech. Bull.* 90.

Schuster, M. F., J. C. Boling, and J. J. Marony, Jr. 1971. Biological control of rhodesgrass scale by airplane releases of an introduced parasite of limited dispersing ability. In *Biological control,* pp. 227–250. New York: Plenum Press.

Tisdale, E. W., and G. Zappetini. 1953. Halogeton studies on Idaho ranges. *J. Range Mgmt.* 6:225–236.

Ueckert, D. N. 1972. Natural control of mesquite on Texas rangeland by insects. *Southern Weed Science Society Proceedings,* pp. 453–457.

————, K. L. Polk, and C. R. Ward. 1971. Mesquite twig girdler: A possible means of mesquite control. *J. Range Mgmt.* 24:116–118.

van den Bosch, R., and P. S. Messenger. 1973. *Biological control.* New York: Intext.

Wilson, F. 1943. The entomological control of St. John's wort (*Hypericum perforatum* L.). *Commonwealth of Aust. CSIR Bull.* 169.

Chapter 18

Seeding of Rangelands

Rehabilitation of rangelands by seeding began in the western United States in the late 1800s and has now become an effective and valuable tool. More literature exists on range seeding than any other practice in range management. Practical trials and experiments have failed and succeeded in numbers sufficient to permit analyses of cause and effect relationships and to serve as a foundation for a set of principles. Specific recommendations can be made with assurance of success in the seeding of many range sites.

Before the actual seeding can begin, several questions concerning the need for seeding, changes in management, the seeding site, cost, and expected returns must be asked (Stewart, 1950). The purposes of this chapter are to discuss these questions and then to describe seeding operations. The last part of the chapter surveys techniques and species that are recommended for various regions of the United States.

DECIDING TO SEED

Considerable preparation precedes work in the field. "Is seeding necessary?" and if the answer is "Yes," "Where shall it be done?" are two of the questions that the manager must answer. Other decisions of the manager entail planning for the seeding operation.

The discussion below is organized as an analysis of a series of questions that apply in principle to all the range-improvement practices. Seeding is used as the vehicle for presenting the questions, but grazing management, chemical brush control, fertilization, and other range-improvement practices could be substituted for seeding in the question, "Is seeding necessary?"

Is Seeding Necessary?

Seeding does not substitute for management. If 5 to 10 percent of the present vegetation is desirable, stand improvement should come through changes in management which foster increases of the desirable species (Fig. 18-1). Even where overgrazing has badly depleted the native vegetation, good management permits excellent range to develop on much of the land with little cost. The actual percentages in this rule of thumb depend upon several factors, including the time for plant succession to occur and the income lost while it does so. On areas where heavy animal use, former cultivation, or fire has completely eliminated the important forage plants, seeding may be the only practical reclamation means. The areas where native species will not return and where seeding is necessary will become evident under proper management.

Short (1943) observed in eastern Montana that competition prevented establishment of sown grasses when bunchgrasses covered 15 percent or sodgrasses 7 percent of the land. A few plants of *Agropyron spicatum* growing in the protection

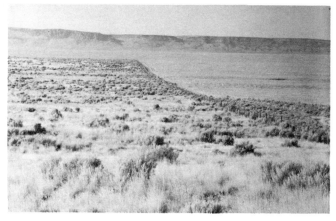

Figure 18-1 The foreground shows a stand of *Agropyron spicatum* in southeastern Oregon which has increased due to reduced grazing in a stand of *Artemisia tridentata*. The background is *Agropyron desertorum* that was seeded after the removal of *Artemisia*.

of *Artemisia tridentata* quickly expand to dominate the vegetation when the brush is sprayed, making seeding unncessary. The degree of competition from native plants which can be tolerated by seeded species varies with soil, exposure, and type of vegetation. Seeding has its greatest potential for profitable returns where desirable native vegetation does not exist, even as a scattered seed source, and where vegetation of inferior quality is destroyed in the rehabilitation process.

Is the Climate Favorable?

Successful seedings are less frequent in areas receiving less than 20 centimeters of precipitation, a third of which should occur during the growing season (Tadmor et al., 1968; Bleak et al., 1965; Robocker et al., 1965). In areas with more than 60 centimeters of precipitation, seeding failures due to lack of moisture are scarce. Precipitation on many rangeland areas throughout the world amounts to 20 to 60 centimeters in most years but not in every year, leading to irregular seeding results. The likelihood of rainfall near the lower limit indicates poor chances of seeding success.

The western Great Plains region from Montana to southern New Mexico experiences average rainfalls of between 28 and 60 centimeters per year (Austin, 1965). One third of 416 seedings during the years 1960–1962 in that region produced less than ten seedlings per square meter, roughly indicating failure. Annual precipitation fluctuates widely in the region. Seedling establishment during the period was higher in northern than in southern parts of the Great Plains (Launchbaugh, 1966).

Is the Habitat Favorable?

Soil characteristics, slope, and exposure limit the production of forage, the use of seeding equipment, and the use of the planted species. Attempts to establish plants on sites that will not support them waste time, effort, and money. Soils of heavy clay or sands are difficult range sites on which to obtain satisfactory seeded stands (Khan, 1968). Alkaline soils, intermittently flooded soils, sterile soils, areas where industrial wastes have accumulated, road cuts and fills, mine spoils, and steep slopes are other difficult habitats. Seeding on these sites and on slopes where machinery tends to increase erosion requires special techniques and frequently is done for objectives other than forage production. Special methods such as terracing, contour furrowing, hand seeding, fertilization, and mulching may be needed to protect site and seedlings and to justify rehabilitation of unfavorable sites (Wein and West, 1971a; 1971b). The challenge in seeding is to revegetate difficult habitats, such as mining-spoil banks (Jacoby, 1969).

Sites that have thin soils, especially southern exposures, are not likely to justify seeding for forage production. However, abandoned croplands are potentially productive rangelands, where successful seedings have been attained, since these lands once were considered suitable for production of crops that require more favorable climate and soil than is needed for many range species.

Habitats with medium-textured soils 30 centimeters deep and high organic-matter content have adequate infiltration capacity and soil moisture for seeding. In mountainous or hill country, these areas are likely to be the lowlands where runoff is slight and run-in water supplements the rainfall. Vigorous growth of *Artemisia, Purshia, Quercus,* and other chaparral species generally indicates favorable sites for seeding. However, in areas where only unpalatable herbs and weedy annual grasses occur and where advanced erosion has destroyed the soil, stands of the introduced and better native species will be obtained with difficulty, if at all. Low herbage growth and undesirable species composition usually indicate that seeding is not the proper solution.

A rule of thumb in selecting sites for seeding is to start with the best habitats and proceed to the less productive ones. The better sites give greater chances for establishment of new stands, high yields of forage, and profits on the investment. Managers should apply intensive methods to small areas before using extensive techniques on large areas.

What Species Should Be Seeded?

The need for additional forage on a ranch and the necessity to match species with habitat determine the species to be seeded. Climatic and habitat restrictions were discussed above. Yearlong ranch operations have a period when forage is scarce, and perhaps that limits the sizes of the operations. Times occur on many ranches when feeding of supplements and hays could be replaced with less costly grazed forages. In selecting species for seeding, the manager needs to provide forage to meet seasonal deficiencies. If an early-growing species or a late-growing species will lengthen the grazing period on green feed and shorten the period of feeding supplements, more is likely to be gained by making the seasonal adjustments in feed than by simply adding more forage into the whole operation. Therefore, the selection of species for seeding rangeland requires analysis of the restraints on production and careful planning of inputs and outputs. Decisions of what to seed and where to seed it are determined, to a large degree, by the deficiencies and sequential feeding requirements in the whole operation.

Of almost equal importance with the climate, site, and need for special feeds is the ability of the species selected to continue producing under grazing pressure. Species and varieties of plants have a great deal of inherent variability in resistance to grazing. Sodgrasses withstand grazing, but most of them produce little seed and are difficult to include in a seeding operation. The manager can vegetatively establish some sodgrasses by planting live pieces of rhizomes, stolons, or plugs of sod. *Buchloe dactyloides* of the western Great Plains and *Trifolium repens* are common cultivated forage plants with stolons. Grasses that spread by rhizomes are illustrated by *Poa pratensis* and *Agropyron smithii*. In the tropics and subtropics around the world, *Cynodon* spp. are widely known for having stolons, rhizomes, or both, depending upon cultivar or variety.

Those range grasses that depend upon seed for regeneration must be grown and grazed under conditions that will permit the production of seed. Many are less resistant to grazing than are sodgrasses, but *Agropyron cristatum* and *Bouteloua gracilis* can withstand occasional heavy use. Species resistant to grazing should be favored in the selection of species to seed rangelands.

One should consider the relative palatability of the plants in a seeding mixture when one selects species to seed. The inclusion of one or two extremely palatable plants with others of lower palatability could result in overutilization and eventual elimination of the favorites. Results from cafeteria grazing studies show that some species and varieties become overused before others are grazed. A range that has been seeded to a mixture must be managed correctly so that the preferred species are perpetrated, just as any mixed forage type needs special management (Fig. 18-2).

Thousands of grasses, legumes, and other forage plants have been introduced from foreign countries and collected from North American rangelands. About 50 grass species have survived rigorous selection by climate, vegetational competition, livestock use, and economic screening to become valued parts of the range seeding resources (Table 18-1). Introduction, adaptation trials, selection, and

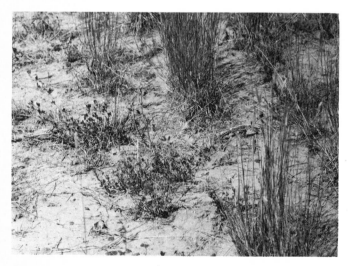

Figure 18-2 Nomad cultivar of alfalfa has been seeded with *Agropyron desertorum*. Livestock graze the *Agropyron* early, before growth of the alfalfa, which furnishes summer feed for antelope.

Table 18-1 Common grasses seeded on rangeland in the United States (*U.S. Department of Agriculture, 1948; Hanson, 1965*)

Species	Common name	Well-known cultivars and date of release	Origin	Average germination percentage	Number pure live seed per kg	Soils*
Agropyron cristatum	Fairway crested wheatgrass	Parkway	Siberia	85	440,000	L,C
Agropyron desertorum	Standard crested wheatgrass	Nordan– 1953	Siberia	85	440,000	L,C
Agropyron elongatum	Tall wheatgrass	Largo–1937 Alkar–1951	Turkey	85	175,000	L,C,A,W
Agropyron inerme	Beardless wheatgrass	Whitmar– 1946	U.S.	75	280,000	L,C
Agropyron intermedium	Intermediate wheatgrass	Greenar– 1945 Nebraska 50–1950	U.S.S.R.	85	220,000	L
Agropyron riparium	Streambank wheatgrass	Sodar–1954	U.S.	92	375,000	S,L,C,A
Agropyron sibiricum	Siberian wheatgrass	P-27–1953	U.S.S.R.	85	550,000	L,C
Agropyron smithii	Western wheatgrass	Arriba	U.S.	60	243,000	S,L,C,W
Agropyron trachycaulum	Slender wheatgrass	Primar– 1946	U.S.	85	350,000	S,L
Agropyron trichophorum	Pubescent wheatgrass	Topar–1953	U.S.S.R.	85	200,000	L,C,A
Andropogon annulatus	Diaz bluestem	Kleberg– 1944	S. Afr.	79	515,000	L,C
Andropogon caucasicus	Caucasian bluestem	. . .	U.S.S.R.	27	1,896,000	L,C
Andropogon gerardi	Big bluestem	Kaw–1950 Champ– 1963 Pawnee– 1963	U.S.	82	420,000	S,L,W S,L,C L,C
Andropogon hallii	Sand bluestem	Woodward– 1955	U.S.	69	275,000	S
Andropogon ischaemum	Yellow bluestem	King Ranch (KR)– 1941	U.S.S.R.	. . .	1,830,000	L

*Indicates adaptation to soils: S = sandy, L = loamy, C = clay, A = alkali, W = wet.

Table 18-1 Common grasses seeded on rangeland in the United States *(U.S. Department of Agriculture, 1948; Hanson, 1965)* (Continued)

Species	Common name	Well-known cultivars and date of release	Origin	Average germination percentage	Number pure live seed per kg	Soils*
Andropogon nodosus	Angleton– 1924	Gordo– 1957	India	...	...	L,C,W
Andropogon scoparius	Little bluestem	Aldous	U.S.	80	835,000	S,L
Arrhenatherum elatius	Tall oatgrass	Tualatin– 1960	U.S.	79	330,000	L,W
Bouteloua curtipendula	Sideoats grama	El Reno– 1944 Uvalde– 1950 Coronado– 1955 Butte–1958 Trailway– 1958 Premier– 1960	U.S.	50	315,000	S,L
Bouteloua gracilis	Blue grama	Lovington	U.S.	60	1,570,000	S,L,A
Bromus carinatus	California brome	Cucamonga– 1949	U.S.	90	88,000	L,C
Bromus catharticus	Rescue grass	Prairie– 1946	S. Am.	85	198,000	S,L
Bromus inermis	Smooth brome	Lincoln– 1942 Manchar– 1943 Achenbach– 1944 Lancaster– 1950 Lyon–1950	Eur.	85	275,000	S,L,W
Bromus marginatus	Mountain brome	Bromar– 1946	U.S.	85	198,000	L,C
Bromus mollis	Soft chess	Blando– 1940	Eur.	...		S,L,C
Buchloe dactyloides	Buffalograss	Mesa–1945	U.S.	45	93,000	C,W

*Indicates adaptation to soils: S = sandy, L = loamy, C = clay, A = alkali, W = wet.

Table 18-1 Common grasses seeded on rangeland in the United States *(U.S. Department of Agriculture, 1948; Hanson, 1965)* (Continued)

Species	Common name	Well-known cultivars and date of release	Origin	Average germination percentage	Number pure live seed per kg	Soils*
Cynodon dactylon	Bermudagrass	Coastal— 1943 Midland— 1953 Suwannee— 1953	Afr.	86	3,480,000	L,C,A,W S
Dactylis glomerata	Orchard grass	Okaroa— 1953 Latar— 1957	Eur.	80	1,190,000	S,L,W
Elymus junceus	Russian wildrye	Mandan— 1940 Vinall—1960	U.S.S.R.	8	375,000	L,C
Eragrostis curvula	Weeping lovegrass	Catalina	Afr.	70	6,443,000	S,L
Eragrostis lehmanniana	Lehmann lovegrass		S. Afr.	60	9,360,000	S,L,C
Eragrostis trichodes	Sand lovegrass	Nebraska 27	U.S.	75	3,418,000	S
Festuca arundinaceae	Tall fescue	Kentucky 31 Alta—1940 Goar—1946 Fawn—1964	Eur.	86	534,000	L,C,A,W
Festuca elatior	Meadow fescue	Ensign— 1944	Eur.	90	507,000	L,C,W
Lolium multiflorum	Italian ryegrass	Wimmera— 1962	Eur.	90	531,000	L
Lolium perenne	Perennial ryegrass	. . .	Eur.	90	545,000	S,L,W
Oryzopsis miliacea	Smilograss	. . .	Eur.	80	1,950,000	L
Panicum antidotale	Blue panicgrass	. . .	Aust.	60	1,500,000	S,L,W
Panicum coloratum	Kleingrass	. . .	Afr.	72	1,095,000	S,L
Panicum maximum	Guineagrass	. . .	Afr.	35	950,000	L,C,W

*Indicates adaptation to soils: S = sandy, L = loamy, C = clay, A = alkali, W = wet.

Table 18-1 Common grasses seeded on rangeland in the United States *(U.S. Department of Agriculture, 1948; Hanson, 1965)* (Continued)

Species	Common name	Well-known cultivars and date of release	Origin	Average germination percentage	Number pure live seed per kg	Soils*
Panicum virgatum	Switchgrass	Blackwell– 1944 Cadda–1955 Nebraska 28–1963	U.S.	62	613,000	S,L,W
Paspalum dilatatum	Dallisgrass	...	S. Am.	70	485,000	L,C,W
Paspalum notatum	Bahiagrass	Pensacola	S. Am.	70	366,000	S,L,C,A,W
Pennisetum ciliare	Buffelgrass	...	S. Afr.	...	970,000	L
Pennisetum purpureum	Napiergrass	...	Afr.	54	3,090,000	L,C
Phalaris arundinacea	Reed canarygrass	...	U.S.	64	1,213,000	S,L,W
Phalaris tuberosa var. *hirtiglumis*	Koleagrass	Perla	N. Afr.	33	805,000	
var. *stenoptera*	Hardinggrass	Wintergreen	S. Afr.	80	1,206,000	L,C
Phleum pratense	Timothy	...	Eur.	80	2,865,000	L,W
Poa ampla	Big bluegrass	Sherman	U.S.	70	2,022,000	L
Poa pratensis	Kentucky bluegrass	...	Eur.	75	4,754,000	S,L,W
Sorghastrum nutans	Indiangrass	Cheyenne– 1945 Nebraska- 54–1957 Holt–1960	U.S.	53	385,000	S,L,W
Stipa viridula	Green needlegrass	Green stipa- grass– 1946	U.S.	24	400,000	S,L

*Indicates adaptation to soils: *S* = sandy, *L* = loamy, *C* = clay, *A* = alkali, *W* = wet.

breeding continue to produce new cultivars, and many not listed in Table 18-1 are available locally. Fortunately, native forage plants are responding to the selection and breeding programs as well as the introduced species. Local strains and varieties often do better in their own habitats than plants from other regions. About 20 native range species have yielded notable strains, such as Primar Slender Wheatgrass, Kaw Big Bluestem, and El Reno Sideoats Grama.

Seeded mixtures of species appear to have several advantages over stands of a single species (Cox and Cole, 1960); the advantages include the following points:

1 A mixed diet is more desirable and often will produce greater livestock gains than a diet composed largely of one species. However, livestock have gained well when forced to eat a single species of relatively low palatability.

2 Periods of growth vary for different species, thus a mixture increases the length of the grazing season on green forage and the uniformity of forage production throughout the season.

3 Differences in depth of root systems may result in greater use of soil moisture and nutrients in some cases, but in other cases, the increased competition may decrease the total forage produced.

4 All pastures have variable habitats. Seeding mixtures increase the chances of sowing plants that will dominate each localized set of habitat factors (Hull, 1971).

5 Some plants benefit others, as, for example, nitrogen fixed by legume rhizobia has a fertilizing effect on grasses. Grasses in legume stands help to prevent bloat in animals.

6 Diseases and insect pests may not attack the grass species equally and are less likely to damage mixtures as much as they do pure stands of one species.

Difficulties with seed mixtures include the following points:

1 More time and labor are necessary to get the seed ready for planting, and the total seed cost may be higher than with a single species. However, economical seed may reduce the need for an expensive species.

2 Differences in seed characteristics make drilling at proper rates and depths difficult.

3 If seed production is an objective, pure stands give best results because harvesting can be uniform and properly timed. The product from a pure stand is easier to clean and to sell at a profitable price.

4 A single species may be the only one adapted to an extreme soil condition or a special seasonal forage need.

Thus, a species is selected to do well on the site where it will be planted and to fulfill a certain purpose. Among other things, the plant should be easy to establish, high in production of palatable forage, resistant to grazing pressure, and able to maintain itself; the seed must be available at a reasonable price. Fortunately, the plants that meet these specifications are also effective in holding the soil and aiding infiltration of water into the soil. Hull (1973a) reported that 4 of the original 37 species seeded on the Davis County, Utah, watersheds in 1936–1939 were still effective soil stabilizers.

Is Proper Management Possible?

Too heavy utilization, poor distribution of animals, improper seasonal control of animals, and other poor managerial practices contribute to the need for most range seedings. Little is gained if the newly seeded stand succumbs to the same faulty grazing practices (Frischknecht and Plummer, 1955). Perennial grasses, for example, require certain management practices in order to become established. Seedlings of the perennial seeded grasses in temperate, semiarid climates develop slowly the first year. They contribute a small portion of the cover, send up few tillers, grow little herbage, and may not flower until the second year. Perennial grasses seeded in tropical and humid climates make rapid growth the first year. During the time of germination and establishment, seedlings in both humid and semiarid regions have open space in the plant cover. Low successional plants, mostly annuals, rapidly occupy the available space. They shade the perennial seedlings and use available moisture, perhaps to a degree that prevents seedling establishment of the planted species. The situation is posed as a problem in control of competition by weeds. In addition, newly seeded stands do not have great capacity to withstand defoliation and trampling.

The manager has several techniques by which he can improve the chances of stand establishment. The most common management recommendation is not to graze the stand until near the end of the second growth period. Young plants may be fatally injured by trampling, by pulling or loosening when they are grazed during wet weather or in muddy soil conditions, and by defoliation, which reduces food reserves. Animal control is essential to the success of range seeding (Johnson, 1959).

Since the beginning of range seeding, instances have been observed in which grazing did not reduce the number of plants that became established. Short (1943) found that complete protection from grazing may not be essential in all cases. Frequently, these instances have been placed in the category of exceptions; for instance, Hull (1944) stated that it would be dangerous to assume that similar favorable results would follow grazing of all seeded areas. Grazing of seeded stands during the first year will do harm more often than not, but the beneficial aspects of grazing should be recognized and used. Where the weeds are dense, a short period of grazing, even heavy grazing, will take the top off the weed crop, reduce shading, increase available space, and make more water available for the seeded plants. Care must be taken to remove the grazing animals before damage is done to the seeded plants. Not all weed growth needs to be removed because mulch or litter controls erosion and ameliorates the microclimate near the soil surface. If properly handled, most seedlings can withstand and may benefit from careful grazings during the establishment period. Unrestricted and careless management during that period is to be avoided. Range seedings on abandoned cropland where debris is minimal may be mowed during the first growing season to reduce competition from weeds. Mowing at a height no lower than 7 centimeters above the soil should be done before the weeds produce seed. The objectives are not to clip the desirable grass seedlings, or to clip them as high as possible, and to cut the weeds as low as possible (Bernardon et al., 1967). The difficult compromise between clipping at a low stubble height for weeds and a high one for desirable grasses often leads to a decision to use herbicides or to graze the weed crop. On steep slopes, grazing and herbicides applied by air may be the only ways to reduce weed competition.

If a legume or other broad-leaved plant is included in the seeded mixture, herbicides should be avoided and grazing encouraged. *Trifoliums* and other legumes belong to the early successional stages. Taller plants must be kept low and sufficient bare ground maintained for legume seedlings each year. Some of the twining subtropical legumes do well in thick grass stands, but these, too, need regular grazing during the first year after seeding.

Pesticides may be needed to assure a seeded stand. Seed-eating birds, rodents, ants, and termites may gather and consume the seed, or an epidemic of grasshoppers may destroy the seedlings. Elimination or reduction of most pest problems starts in the planning stage for seeding rather than after the planting is finished.

In many instances, an apparently poor grass stand the first year after seeding has become an acceptable stand in the second and third years. Seedlings of most perennial grasses on rangelands in temperate regions are inconspicuous and the stands do not thicken sufficiently to reduce the annual weeds for two or three years (Fig. 18-3). A seeded area that has been considered a failure through cursory examination should not be plowed for reseeding until after the second growing season.

Seedings often require shifts in seasonal grazing plans. Rotation schemes and deferred grazing treatments may be sufficient to give new seedlings all the relief from grazing that they need. Fencing to protect a new seeding should be finished and grazing schedules fully planned into the ranch operations before the planting operation. Seedings and fencing of them fit into existing seasonal grazing plans and supplement forage supplies on native pastures (Currie, 1969; Frandsen, 1950; Miller et al., 1957).

Management of grasses for seed production necessitates a management program different from that for forage production. The stand for seed production may be grazed only until tillers begin to elongate early in the year and not again

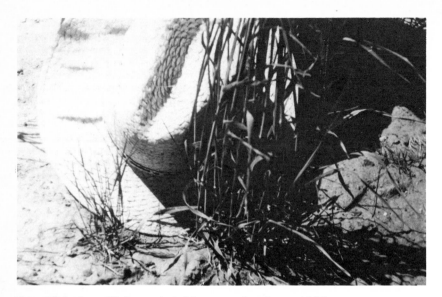

Figure 18-3 A small first-year plant of *Agropyron desertorum* which has not flowered, alongside a fully mature cereal rye plant.

until after the crop is harvested. Thin stands of plants of one species planted in rows 0.5 to 1.0 meter apart and clean tilled produce the largest seed crops (Smika and Newell, 1968). Grazing only partly substitutes for the tillage. Forage-producing stands would be seeded in rows much closer together. Three grasses that give reasonably high yields of seed are *Agropyron cristatum,* 900 kilograms per hectare; *Bromus inermis,* 350 kilograms per hectare; and *Agropyron trachycaulum,* 225 kilograms per hectares.

Predicting Seeding Costs and Returns

The purchase of seed, hiring of equipment, control of brush, and other range-improvement operations require immediate payment of money that, more often than not, must be borrowed. Costs of seed vary widely from year to year. Seeding of burned watersheds and forests in bad fire years takes all available seed within a short time, often causing the market to go from one that is oversupplied to one that is undersupplied. Seed of widely used species may vary from 50 cents to $2 or more per kilogram. Seed of new and promising species may cost five times that amount. Costs of labor, equipment, and application vary according to site and methods. These costs fluctuate widely with changes in economic climate. The total costs for seeding ranges differ from a low of approximately $30 per hectare where seed is purchased and planted to a high of $250 per hectare where brush control and other practices are needed to prepare the seedbed.

Three guidelines commonly are used in analyzing costs and returns of seeding operations. Before the seeding is undertaken, all concerned with financing the scheme will want to be reasonably sure that the returns in increased forage, livestock, game, or some other product will show a profit. One guideline is that costs should not exceed those that can be covered by increased net income within a seven- to ten-year period. A second guideline stipulates that the costs should not exceed the sales value of the land with its new crop. Still a third guideline amortizes the change in rental value on a basis of values in the open market. These three approximations of seeding values give similar answers. In short, the total expenses of the seeding operation should not exceed the costs of buying other land that would give equivalent production (Plath, 1954).

Both the allowable costs and the expected returns depend to a considerable extent upon biological success in the seeding project and upon the way it is managed (Simpson, 1971). Although grazing values may be increased several-fold, the actual increases may be low or high per unit of land. Real values must be favorable in terms of alternate uses of the money; or nonmarket-determined values, such as conserved soil, game products, and esthetic opportunities, must be used to justify expenditures that cannot be reasonably expected to return a profit.

THE SEEDING OPERATION

No attempt will be made in this section to present prescriptions for individual seeding operations. The principles that apply broadly will receive major consideration. The infinite combinations of soil texture, soil fertility, soil moisture-holding capacity, slope, temperature, precipitation, competition among plants, impacts of animals, and other factors require local modification of the principles. Success in seeding depends upon these factors, especially rainfall. But the chances of failure are reduced by following approved and tested recommendations. This section assumes that the decision to seed has been made.

Assembly of Seed, Equipment, and Labor

The seed and necessary tools are assumed to be available in the community. Sources of information about them include local seed stores and offices of the County Agriculture Extension Service, Soil Conservation Service, Bureau of Land Management, and U.S. Forest Service. People in these organizations have and will give the latest information on approved techniques, on the one hand, and on planning for the availability of equipment on the other. For example, there may be only one rangeland drill in the community, which is rented on a tight first-come-first-served schedule. Planning so that seed, the right equipment, and skilled operators are on hand at the right time and place fosters success in the range-improvement operation.

The Seed

The seed source influences seeding success. Plants of the same species from seed grown at widely separated places develop their flowers and herbage at different rates. Seed produced locally gives more satisfactory stands, on the average, than does seed of the same species from other regions. Strains moved southward generally have lower yields and earlier maturity than locally grown seeds. Northern strains may be vulnerable to high temperatures and drought. Strains of southern origin, when moved too far north, may fail to develop mature seed before frost (Riegel, 1940). In general, northern strains are lower in yield and earlier in maturity, while southern strains vary in yield and are later in maturity, than local plants. The rule is not to move seed more than 500 kilometers north or south and certainly not out of the natural range of the species. While these comments do not apply to the seed of introduced species, they, too, have a range of habitats on which they do well, and moving them beyond these restrictions will lead to practical failures.

High-quality seed enhances the chances of obtaining a stand. Good seed is bright in color; moldy, dark, or discolored seed suggests poor quality (Ferguson, 1967). A few seeds should be sectioned with a knife or broken so that it can be determined whether or not the endosperm fills the seed coat and is of healthy appearance. Seed should never be purchased without a visual test of quality. Seed that goes through regular markets must be labeled according to percentages of purity, germination, and adulteration with seed of noxious species. The noxious plants usually listed are those of cultivated crops. Seldom do the weeds of cultivation make a great deal of difference in forage production on rangeland. However, they may spread from rangeland to cropland and therefore are to be avoided.

Seed purity is *the percentage by weight of apparently sound seed of the species.* The impurities include foreign matter that the harvester takes along with the seed and which processing does not remove. Small pieces of straw, chaff, broken seed, small rocks, and parts of insects are common seed impurities. The percentage of impurity can be evaluated in a general way by ocular examination. Most impurities are different in weight, size, and shape from the seed. A manager can estimate the amount of this material by noting the amount that separates from the seed in a float test in water. Accurate measurement of purity requires separation and weighing. Impurities cause drilling problems. They feed through the drill at rates different from that of the seed, separate from the seed due to the shaking of the drill, and clog the seed openings.

The germination percentage is another factor of seed quality. *The proportion of apparently live seed which germinates under standard laboratory test* is *the germination percentage.* Satisfactory germination tests can be accomplished easily at home (Robocker and Zamora, 1971). Two to four samples of each 100 apparently pure live seeds should be placed without crowding on several thicknesses of moist paper towels in a glass-covered dish. The glass cover reduces danger of the seed drying and permits light to enter the chamber. The dish should be placed in indirect light at ordinary room temperature. The seeds should not be allowed to stand in water. The germinated plants should be counted periodically as they are removed over a period of ten days to two weeks or until germination ceases. The final germination percentage is determined by an average of the sample results.

Pure live seed (PLS) content is the most important aspect of seed quality. One obtains this amount by multiplying germination and purity. Thus, a 50-kilogram bag labeled *germination 90 percent and purity 90 percent* contains 81 percent or 40.5 kilograms of pure live seed. A bag of seed with lower quality, say germination 50 percent and purity 75 percent, contains only 37.5 percent pure live seed. The second lot would be worth half as much and would need to be seeded at twice the rate of the first. Notations of purity, germination, and PLS on the seed label are guides for comparing prices and for determining seeding rates.

The listing of pure live seed on the label stipulates that it was determined on a certain date because viability changes with time. Seeds of many grasses retain viability for several years. Certain strains maintain life better than others. Seeds of six grasses remained viable for 20 years even though they were stored without humidity and temperature control (Tiedemann and Pond, 1967). Seeds that remain alive for four or five years under storage give considerable flexibility in time of their use.

Most grass seeds require an after-harvest ripening period during which germination percentages gradually increase from a few months to as long as three years (Table 18-2). In one study, stored grass seeds lost all their viability within 27 years, legumes lived somewhat longer, and 37-year-old seed of *Erodium cicutarium* was the oldest to germinate (Hull, 1973b). Seed of *Stipa* spp. should not be planted until at least a year after harvest. *Oryzopsis hymenoides* may be scarified by acid or mechanical means so that germination can be increased. *Buchloe dactyloides* should be treated with 24 to 48 hours of soaking in a solution of 0.5 percent potassium nitrate, stored wet at 0° to 5°C for six weeks, and dried

Table 18-2 Average percentage germination of different aged seed of three species *(Wilson, 1931)*

| Species | Germination percentage at end of | | |
	1st year	2nd year	3rd year
Bromis inermis	70	74	55
Boutelova gracilis	23	18	4
Agropyron cristatum	47	65	85

immediately. This process increases germination from approximately 10 to 75 percent. *Poa arachnifera* is noted for its short-lived seed, lasting about six months. Seeds of *Andropogon scoparius* and *A. gerardi* seem to drop in viability suddenly at about the fifth or sixth year, and germination often is the highest the second year.

Seed Growing, Harvesting, and Processing

Promising species have been eliminated from widespread use because the seed could not be made available (Canode and Patterson, 1961). Successful seeding on rangeland often begins with the harvesting of a handful of seed, the purchase of a small quantity of seed, or perhaps the receipt of a gift of a few seeds. These seeds are nurtured with care, grown alone in the home garden or nursery, and the quantity of seed gradually increased. A stand of a few square meters to a hectare can be the homegrown, economical source of seed for range improvement or for a venture into the seed-production business. The care and handling learned in the small-scale operation teaches the special techniques needed for success on a larger scale.

Grass seed has been harvested with many types of equipment, most of it homemade. Grain combines will collect small seed of little weight after proper adjustments to the fan, concave distances, and cylinder speed. The various kinds of hand-harvesting equipment include a knife or sickle, a comb and scoop to catch the seed, a pair of paddles, and sweeping or vacuum mechanism to suck up fallen seed and burrs (Nord et al., 1967). A revolving drum with protruding nails strips seed from the standing grass.

The seeds of many grasses need processing before they can be stored or successfully planted (Klebesadel et al., 1962). First, grass seed should be dried. A common harvesting problem is that not all seed ripens at the same time. For example, individual culms of *Panicum antidotale* can have seeds from the milk stage to the completely mature stage. Harvesting should occur when 50 percent or more of the seed is ripe, but harvesting at this time results in gathering moist seeds that have to be dried so that molding in storage is prevented. Second, the bulk seed needs processing. Awns, hairs, empty florets, pieces of stems, and other debris hinder passage of seed through the drills. The *Andropogons* have paired florets, one fertile and one sterile, which constitute a fluffy unit. The sterile floret and long hairs need to be broken from the fertile floret before they can be removed. *Stipa* awns twist together, making the separation of seeds extremely difficult. Seeds of many species planted on rangelands are bulky, fluffy, and light in weight. A modified hammer mill, commonly used to grind grain for feeding, works with many species. Adjustments are made in screen size, clearance of the hammers, and speed depending upon the characteristics of the seed being processed (Schwendiman et al., 1940). After processing, the impurities are removed with a fanning mill.

The Season to Plant

The season of the year in which best seeding results can be expected varies from place to place, from year to year, and among species. All plantings require ample soil moisture and favorable temperature from germination time until the plants have become well established. The seedlings of many species are tender for several weeks after germination and are easily destroyed by drought, soil blowing, flooding, soil crusting, too deep seeding, competition from weeds, frost, hail, disease, and insects. Extreme weather conditions often cause failure regardless of the planting season, and favorable weather may allow an acceptable stand to become established when the rules are not followed completely. In a choice of the time of year in which to seed, the most important considerations are seasonal distribution of rainfall and amount of soil moisture.

Fall seedings are favored in the northern and western parts of the United States and Canada, where the majority of the precipitation occurs in winter and the major growth occurs in a short early-spring period (Klomp and Hull, 1972; Houston, 1957; Kilcher, 1961). Seedlings need the benefit of the full spring growing period. Spring seeding misses that part of the growth period which occurs before machinery can be put onto the land. Fall seeding places the seed into the soil, where it can take advantage of the first warm spring days.

In the Mediterranean-type climate in California, plantings are made in late fall before the first rains. The seeds germinate and the seedlings have a month or two to grow before low winter temperatures slow their progress.

Fall seedings in grain stubble take advantage of the firm seedbed, and the stubble prevents blowing of soil and snow, thus protecting the seedlings from drying and frost damage. Meadows and forested ranges in the western United States are fall seeded. In general, the cool-season grasses do best with fall seeding.

Spring seedings are advisable where the major rainfall occurs in summer and where warm-season grasses are planted (Lavin et al., 1973). These areas include the central Great Plains and the prairies to the east, and the southwestern mountains. Bement et al., (1965) reported successful late-summer establishment of *Agropyron cristatum* in central Colorado. Sandy and well-drained soils can be worked early in the spring, and, hence, spring seedings of both warm- and cool-season grasses on them generally are satisfactory. Heavy or clay soils cannot be worked early in the spring; therefore they are fall seeded.

Site Preparation for Seeding

A well-prepared seedbed that is free of weeds, brush, and other plants enhances the chances for successful seeding (Bryan and McMurphy, 1968; McGinnies, 1968). If the site is worth seeding at all, the extra effort required to remove competing vegetation will be justified in the results. The ideal seedbed for grass has a firm soil (Hyder et al., 1955). If one's heel sinks more than 1 centimeter into the soil with normal walking, the soil is too loose and should be packed (Hyder et al., 1961; McGinnies, 1962).

Methods of seedbed preparation include tilling fully and growing a crop of grain or other annual plant; removing brush, which frequently amounts to tilling the soil; partial tilling in contour or strip applications; constructing microridge relief (Hyder and Bement, 1969); pitting (Anderson and Swanson, 1949); treating road cuts, fills, and steep lands specially; and tilling chemically with Atrazine (Eckert and Evans, 1967; McMurphy, 1969; Eckert et al., 1972).

The preparatory-crop method uses wheat, sorghum, or another annual crop to prepare the land for a seeding of perennial grasses (Stroh and Sundberg, 1971). The aim is to produce a crop that pays part or all of the expenses, reduces weeds, and provides a firm seedbed. The grass is planted into the grain stubble in the fall, after a crop is harvested (Owensby and Anderson, 1965). If needed, disking will reduce excessive fall weeds and part of the litter and loosen baked soil. However, stubble and litter are not to be reduced completely because they provide moisture holding capacity, reduce erosion, and serve as protection to newly established grass seedlings. *Agropyron cristatum* has done well when planted after grain crops in eastern Montana (Friedrich, 1945). Nurse crops, grain, and perennial grass seeded together are to be avoided. The protection from sun and wind afforded by the nurse crop does not balance the competition for soil moisture on most rangeland sites (Stoddard, 1941).

Studies of artificial seeding into closed communities of *Bromus tectorum* and *Artemisia tridentata* in Utah and Nevada found that the early, thick growth of *Bromus* used the available moisture and thereby prevented the establishment of perennial seeded species (Robertson and Pearse, 1945). *Artemisia* stands reduced insolation, wind movement, and evaporation from the soil surface. They also retained snow, hastened infiltration, and retarded surface runoff, but snow disappeared from them as much as two weeks earlier than from the grasslands. Dissipation of the limited supply of stored soil moisture commenced earlier under *Artemisia* than in brush clearings. Successful seedings into closed communities of *Bromus* and *Artemisia* were the exception rather than the rule.

The presence or absence of heavy stands of *Bromus tectorum* in the northern intermountain area usually is a prime factor determining the method of site preparation. Areas without dense stands of *Bromus* usually can be drilled without cultivation, cropping, or chemical tillage. Ranges heavily infested with *Bromus* need treatment before seeding to eliminate the competition. The *Bromus* may be eliminated with a lister or double-moldboard-type drill head that scrapes or turns back a five- to ten-centimeter-wide strip of soil including the *Bromus,* other plants, and surface seed. The new seed is planted in the middle of this narrow cleared strip.

Other, cheaper, methods such as burning, harrowing, spring toothing, etc., have not been successful. Cultivation should be done in the late fall after most of the *Bromus* has germinated or in the early spring before new seed is formed. Freshly plowed land must first be packed with a cultipacker before seeding so that rapid drying is prevented. Drilling is the favored method of seeding on plowed ground, although broadcasting ahead of the cultipacker has given many excellent stands of perennial grass.

Mechanical-brush-control operations leave the soil stirred, often with few competing plants. Seed broadcast onto the rough and loose soil lodges in the cracks and depressions and soon is covered as wind and rain smooth the surface. Burning, either accidental or planned, provides reasonable seedbeds for grasses and legumes in spots of white ash.

Seeding on problem sites, such as ridges, road cuts, road fills, dam faces, and other places of disturbed soil which may be near the angle of repose, requires special techniques. They may be stabilized with burlap sacks filled with soil that has seed mixed with the soil, or the slopes may be covered with sacking, cut brush, or tar from the road-building operation. Special materials, mostly a slurry of wood pulp, seed, and fertilizer sprayed on the slopes with considerable pressure, are used in landscaping new highways. A mulch of wood chips may be used (Klomp, 1968). In other situations, the site preparation may involve only leaving a depression after a tree has been removed or tossing a handful of seed into a pile of brush. Broad pits or basins to hold runoff increase seeding success in dry areas (Slayback and Renney, 1972).

Large amounts of litter and mulch on the ground, for example, where stands of timber have been cleared, need to be removed or incorporated into the soil before grasses are planted. Grass seeds must be in close contact with the mineral soil. However, moderate amounts of litter, as from the aftermath of most harvested grain crops on land to be converted to range, are beneficial to seedling establishment and reduction of wind erosion (Stubbendieck et al., 1973). On problem soils such as moving sands, artificial means may be needed to reduce erosion.

Seeding Rate

Rates of seeding rangeland are low in comparison with rates of seeding cultivated crops and must be modified to suit many variables, including number of seeds per kilogram, purity, germination, conditions of seedbed, growth habits of the grasses, objective of the seeding, and cost of seed. Five to ten kilograms of seed per hectare of large seeded plants are sufficient (Hull, 1972; Launchbaugh, 1970; Mueggler and Blaisdell, 1955). As little as 30 grams to 3 kilograms of seed of the small seeded species—*Eragrostis, Panicum, Poa,* and most legumes—will suffice (Kilcher and Heinrichs, 1968).

A commonly used guide to seeding rates is enough seed for ten established plants per square meter of land. A safety factor of 10 necessitates planting 100 pure live seeds of each species per square meter. With 10,000 square meters per hectare and seed numbering 500,000 per kilogram, the amount of PLS to plant is 2 kilograms per hectare. If the lot of seed has 80 percent purity and 57 percent germination, there is 0.456 kilogram of PLS per kilogram of material. For seeding 2 kilograms of pure live seed per hectare, 4.4 kilograms (2/0.456) of material as it comes from the bag would be seeded. These procedures must be modified to meet local conditions where thick stands are required, where the site will not support ten plants per square meter, or for other purposes. The average number of pure live seed per kilogram is given in Table 18-1.

The relative values or costs of seed lots can be assessed by this procedure. In the above example, material that cost 50 cents per kilogram would cost $2.20 per hectare. Another lot of the same species with 95 percent purity and 95 percent germination would require 2.2 kilograms of material per hectare. If it were selling at a higher price, say 75 cents per kilogram, due to higher quality, it would still cost only $1.65 per hectare and would be the more economical of the two lots of seed.

Seeding Methods

Many techniques have been used to distribute the seed in such a manner that the stand will be even and the seedlings will develop into a closed community of valuable forage plants. A modified grain drill and a specifically made rangeland seeder are the commonly used machines for sowing (Kay and Street, 1961). Drilling ensures uniform distribution and covering of seed. Where the drill must cut through perennial sod, kill annual vegetation to reduce competition, or remove Atrazine from the top soil, the furrow drill with disk openers has a decided advantage (Eckert, 1974). The furrow may be shallow, with 2.5- to 5-centimeter strips scraped bare on either side of the seed row (Hull, 1970), as has been used in stands of *Bromus tectorum* (Nelson et al., 1970). The scraped or scalped strip may be turned back for 10 to 15 centimeters on each side of the seeding furrow, in which case half or more of the land surface is cleaned of vegetation (Fig. 18-4). Examples of the use of the wider strip are the seeding and rejuvenation of *Agropyron smithii* sod in western North Dakota (Houston and Adams, 1971) and in western Nebraska (Schumacher, 1964). The furrow may be a full lister cultivation with rows 1 meter apart and furrows 15 to 25 centimeters deep. The procedure is used in dry climates to reduce competition and to concentrate the water where the new grasses are planted. *Agropyron* is seeded in this fashion into the saltbush-ephedra type along the west side of the San Joaquin Valley in California. A disk in front of the drill spout prevents clogging of the scalper with litter.

Special attachments for the drill, including bands on the disks to control planting depth, agitators in the seedbox to prevent tunneling as the seed feeds into

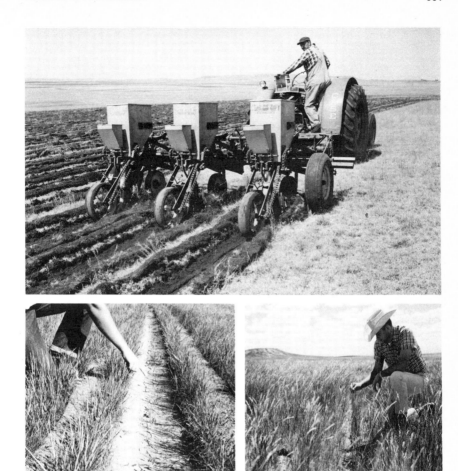

Figure 18-4 Upper photo: A range-interseeding operation in North Dakota. Lower left photo: Young grasses are becoming established in the furrows, and within two or three years, furnish abundant forage, lower right photo. The native stand between the furrows also grows to a greater height after renovation. *(Photos by Soil Conservation Service.)*

the drill spouts, and plugs on every other drill to space the rows approximately 30 centimeters apart, are necessary. This spacing produces a closed stand on favorable sites (McGinnies, 1971). Wide spacing permits planting of small amounts of seed per hectare. Short (1943), at Miles City, Montana, found that 15-, 30-, and 75-centimeter spacings between drill rows resulted in the same total herbage yields in the long run.

A cyclone broadcast seeder continues to be a favorite hand-operated machine for seeding small areas of disturbed soil, such as those on road shoulders, contour furrows, dams, and brush burns. Cyclone spreading of seed may be done by a person on foot, horseback, or in a vehicle. An extension tube and spreader attached to the cyclone seeds narrow strips such as contour furrows. Robertson (1944) successfully broadcast seed with power spreaders that were designed to scatter bait for poisoning insects. Fertilizer broadcasters also have been used. Spreading the seed from aircraft is highly practicable for seeding large areas of land that have been burned over, cut over, and brush controlled. Pelletizing the seed into small clay balls and broadcasting them by air has shown little success (Hull, 1959). Broadcasting results in high losses of seed due to theft of seed by animals and desiccation of the radicle tip before it can enter the soil (Campbell and Swain, 1973; Julander et al., 1969).

Nearly all range grasses are planted less than 2.5 centimeters deep. Small seeded species require a planting depth of 1 or less centimeter. The *Eragrostis* spp., with several million seeds per kilogram, probably should be broadcast onto a rough surface and the seed not covered. Planting and covering of seed of grasses and shrubs is a requirement for successful seeding, but the depth must be shallow enough to permit establishment (Springfield and Bell, 1967; Hull, 1964). Seedlings from planted seed are not as susceptible to pulling by livestock and to environmental extremes at the soil surface as are seedlings from broadcast seed. Planting may be somewhat deeper on coarse-textured soils than on heavy soils (Kinsinger, 1962). A brush drag, trampling by animals, or a light harrowing may be used to cover broadcast seed. The advantages of drilling over broadcasting for the years 1939–1941 near Brookings, South Dakota, are shown in Table 18-3, and the effect of planting depth on the final stand is shown in Table 18-4. Drilled stands of *Agropyron cristatum* in southern Idaho produced ten times more seedlings than did broadcasting (Hull and Klomp. 1967).

Small quantities of seed weighing between a few grams and a kilogram, which are enough to seed a hectare, are difficult to handle in seeding equipment. Tiny, hard seeds tend to settle out of the seed mixture, calibration of amounts through the drill is inaccurate, and many grass seeds do not flow easily. A common procedure is to increase the bulk of the seeding mixture with rice hulls, sawdust, or other inert material that will feed through the drill and maintain the mixture (Lavin and Gomm, 1968). In the tall-grass area, the native species have been cut as a hay crop at the time of seed maturity, and about 500 kilograms per hectare of this material have been spread over the land to be seeded. Disking, cultipacking, or otherwise incorporating this organic material into the soil plants the seed and adds mulch to the seedbed. The hard dough stage or the time when the earliest seeds are ripe are two guides to proper cutting of seed hay. All the seeds will mature in a week or ten days. Although weight and molding can be a problem in the handling of green straw, the hay should be spread onto new land soon after the material is cut so that loss of shattered seed is reduced.

Table 18-3 Percentage emergence and survival of three grass species drilled and broadcast in eastern South Dakota *(Franzke and Hume, 1942)*

Species	Emerged, %		Survived, %	
	Drilled	Broadcast	Drilled	Broadcast
Agropyron cristatum	54	22	23	12
Bromus inermis	31	10	30	9
Agropyron smithii	43	15	67	23
Average	43	15	40	15

Table 18-4 Percentage survival of five species in relation to planting depth on clay soils in eastern South Dakota *(Franzke and Hume, 1942)*

Species	Percentage survival at planting depth		
	Broadcast	5–12 mm	18–25 mm
Agropyron cristatum	None	78	34
Agropyron smithii	None	82	43
Bouteloua gracilis	60	74	None
Bromus inermis	12	86	30
Panicum virgatum	None	65	20

The extensive use of stoloniferous grasses or sodgrasses in revegetation operations requires special methods of planting. *Buchloe dactyloides, Panicum obtusum,* and *Cynodon* spp. have been successfully established at a commercial scale by planting of pieces of stolons and rhizomes or by mashing of small pieces of sod or plugs into moist soil.

REGIONAL SEEDING PRACTICES

Land Resource Regions (Austin, 1965) adequately serve as the basis for brief descriptions of seeding practices on various types of rangeland. The objective of this discussion is to indicate the type of range improvement and the seeding practices for the areas.

The Pacific slope located west of the Cascades and extending into Northern California is wet and has yearlong rainfall. The area is forested but has many cleared hectares planted in fruits, crops, hays, and improved dairy pastures.

Perhaps 10 to 20 percent of the land is used for range sheep and cattle, and deer, elk, and many other wild animals. Seedings may follow logging or cultivation, and they emphasize *Festuca, Bromus, Dactylis, Phleum, Lolium,* and *Trifolium,* all ᵥol-season and moisture-loving species.

The northwestern sagebrush and grass area between the Cascades and the northern Rocky Mountains is about 75 percent rangeland. Irrigated crops, timber, and dry-land grain are the principal crops. Seedings of the *Agropyron* spp. and *Elymus* are the most common on these rangelands. They follow brush control, abandonment from farming, or wildfire. A number of seedings have been established to reduce sugar beet leafhoppers and *Halogeton glomeratus.*

The California region is Mediterranean in its climatic type and supports thick stands of annual grasses, woodland, and chaparral. After brush control in the chaparral type and in forested areas on the Sierra Nevada foothills, seedings to *Phalaris, Lolium, Bromus, Oryzopsis,* and *Trifolium* are common. The annual grassland seldom is seeded.

The Great Basin and Southwestern states constitute the cold and hot deserts in North America. The region is estimated to have greater than 95 percent of the area in shrubs and grasses. *Agropyrons* are seeded in the cold areas. *Eragrostis* and *Bouteloua* species are used in the south, although range seeding is not highly successful in areas with less than 20 to 25 centimeters of rainfall.

Seeding in the Rocky Mountains usually aims to rehabilitate wet and dry meadows, to obtain a forage crop after brush control or timber harvesting, and to protect the soil after wildfire. Seeding mixtures usually contain *Agropyrons, Bromus, Poa,* and *Dactylis.*

The Great Plains region from the base of the Rocky Mountains eastward to the Corn Belt has much in common throughout its length from Canada to Mexico. On the drier western side, the favorite species for range revegetation are *Agropyrons, Boutelouas,* and *Buchloe dactyloides. Elymus junceus* is included in the north. To the eastward, these species are replaced by *Andropogons, Panicums,* and *Sorghastrum nutans.* In central and western North Dakota, *Bromus inermis* covers many hectares of land between the *Agropyrons* to the west and the *Andropogons* to the east. Much seeding is done through the region to rehabilitate short-grass sod into mixed prairie and to convert cropland into grassland. Perhaps 50 percent of the area is cropland, but this percentage varies from near zero on the western side to nearly 100 percent in the true prairie region.

Most seeding in southern and eastern Texas follows mechanical brush control. Various species of *Andropogons, Panicums, Loliums* and others are planted. To the east and into the Southeastern states, the plantings include *Cynodons, Paspalums, Panicums,* and *Pennisetums.* These species may be used in conjunction with short-rotation timber crops or in rotation with cultivated crops.

Seedings on rangeland in other parts of the world are mainly in tropical and subtropical climates where species of *Panicum, Paspalum, Pennisetum, Di-*

gitaria, and *Brachiaria* are mixed with legumes such as *Phaseolus* and *Desmodium.* Legumes of the genera *Trifolium* and *Medicago* dominate plantings in Mediterranean climates. Varieties of *Cenchrus ciliaris* and *Stylosanthes humilis* cover many hectares of rangelands in Australia and Africa. Shrub species that show value for browse have received increasing attention throughout the world, especially in arid climates (Cable, 1972; Statler, 1967; Nord et al., 1971).

LITERATURE CITED

Anderson, D., and A. R. Swanson. 1949. Machinery for seedbed preparation and seeding on southwestern ranges. *J. Range Mgmt.* 2:64–66.

Austin, M. E. 1965. Land resource regions and major land resource areas of the United States. *U.S. Dept. Agr. Handbook* 296.

Bement, R. E., R. D. Barmington, A. C. Everson, L. O. Hylton, Jr. and E. E. Remmenga. 1965. Seeding of abandoned croplands in the central great plains. *J. Range Mgmt.* 18:53–59.

Bernardon, A. E., D. L. Huss, and W. G. McCully. 1967. Effects of herbage removal on seedling development in cane bluestem. *J. Range Mgmt.* 20:69–72.

Bleak, A. T., N. C. Frischknecht, A. P. Plummer, and R. E. Eckert, Jr. 1965. Problems in artificial and natural revegetation of the arid and shadscale vegetation zone of Utah and Nevada. *J. Range Mgmt.* 18:59–65.

Bryan, G. G., and W. E. McMurphy. 1968. Competition and fertilization as influences on grass seedlings. *J. Range Mgmt.* 21:98–101.

Cable, D. R. 1972. Fourwing saltbush revegetation trials in southern Arizona. *J. Range Mgmt.* 25:150–153.

Campbell, M. H., and F. G. Swain. 1973. Factors causing losses during the establishment of surface-sown pastures. *J. Range Mgmt.* 26:355–359.

Canode, C. L., and J. K. Patterson. 1961. Grass seed production from seeded rangelands. *J. Range Mgmt.* 14:88–92.

Cox, M. P., and R. S. Cole. 1960. The South Dakota method of specifying mixtures for range seeding. *J. Range Mgmt.* 13:294–296.

Currie, P. O. 1969. Use seeded ranges in your management. *J. Range Mgmt.* 22:432–434.

Eckert, R. E., Jr. 1974. Atrazine residue and seedling establishment in furrows. *J. Range Mgmt.* 27:55–56.

————, and R. A. Evans. 1967. A chemical-fallow technique for control of downy brome and establishment of perennial grasses on rangeland. *J. Range Mgmt.* 20:35–41.

————, G. J. Klomp, R. A. Evans, and J. A. Young. 1972. Establishment of perennial wheatgrasses in relation to Atrazine residue in the seedbed. *J. Range Mgmt.* 25:219–224.

Ferguson, R. B. 1967. Relative germination of spotted and nonspotted bitterbrush seed. *J. Range Mgmt.* 20:330–331.

Frandsen, W. R. 1950. Management of reseeded ranges. *J. Range Mgmt.* 3:125–129.

Franzke, C. J., and A. N. Hume. 1942. Regrassing areas in South Dakota. *S. Dak. Agr. Expt. Sta. Bull.* 361.

Friedrich, C. A. 1945. Seeding crested wheatgrass on cheatgrass land. *N. Rocky Mtn. Forest and Range Expt. Sta. Research Note* 38.

Frischknecht, N. C., and A. P. Plummer. 1955. A comparison of seeded grasses under grazing and protection on a mountain brush burn. *J. Range Mgmt.* 8:170–175.

Hanson, A. A. 1965. Grass varieties in the United States. *U.S. Dept. Agr. Handbook* 170.

Houston, W. R. 1957. Seeding crested wheatgrass on drought depleted range. *J. Range Mgmt.* 19:131–134.

————, and R. E. Adams. 1971. Interseeding for range improvement in the northern Great Plains. *J. Range Mgmt.* 24:457–461.

Hull, A. C., Jr. 1944. The relation of grazing to establishment and vigor of crested wheatgrass. *J. Am. Soc. Agron.* 36:358–360.

————. 1959. Pellet seeding of wheatgrasses on southern Idaho rangelands. *J. Range Mgmt.* 12:155–163.

————. 1964. Emergence of cheatgrass and three wheatgrasses from four seeding depths. *J. Range Mgmt.* 17:32–35.

————. 1970. Grass seedling emergence and survival from furrows. *J. Range Mgmt.* 23:421–424.

————. 1971. Grass mixtures for seeding sagebrush lands. *J. Range Mgmt.* 24:150–152.

————. 1972. Seeding rates and row spacings for rangelands in southeastern Idaho and northern Utah. *J. Range Mgmt.* 25:50–53.

————. 1973a. Duration of seeded stands on terraced mountain lands, Davis County, Utah. *J. Range Mgmt.* 26:133–136.

————. 1973b. Germination of range plant seeds after long periods of uncontrolled storage. *J. Range Mgmt.* 26:198–199.

————, and G. J. Klomp. 1967. Thickening and spread of crested wheatgrass stands in southern Idaho ranges. *J. Range Mgmt.* 20:222–227.

Hyder, D. N., and R. E. Bement. 1969. A micro-ridge roller for seedbed modification. *J. Range Mgmt.* 22:54–56.

————, D. E. Booster, F. A. Sneva, W. A. Sawyer, and J. B. Rodgers. 1961. Wheel-track planting on sagebrush-bunchgrass range. *J. Range Mgmt.* 14:220–224.

————, F. A. Sneva, and W. A. Sawyer. 1955. Soil firming may improve range seeding operations. *J. Range Mgmt.* 8:159–163.

Jacoby, P. W., Jr. 1969. Revegetation treatments for stand establishment on coal spoil banks. *J. Range Mgmt.* 22:94–97.

Johnson, W. M. 1959. Grazing intensity trials on seeded ranges in the ponderosa pine zone of Colorado. *J. Range Mgmt.* 12:1–7.

Julander, O., J. B. Low, and O. W. Morris. 1969. Pocket gophers on seeded Utah mountain range. *J. Range Mgmt.* 22:325–329.

Kay, B. L., and J. E. Street. 1961. Drilling wheatgrass into sprayed sagebrush in northeastern California. *J. Range Mgmt.* 14:271–273.

Khan, C. M. A. 1968. Sand dune rehabilitation in Thal, Pakistan. *J. Range Mgmt.* 21:316–321.

Kilcher, M. R. 1961. Fall seeding versus spring seeding in the establishment of five grasses and one alfalfa in southern Saskatchewan. *J. Range Mgmt.* 14:320–322.

————, and D. H. Heinrichs. 1968. Rates of seeding Rambler alfalfa with dryland pasture grasses. *J. Range Mgmt.* 21:248–249.

Kinsinger, F. E. 1962. The relationship between depth of planting and maximum foliage height of seedlings of Indian ricegrass. *J. Range Mgmt.* 15:10–13.

Klebesadel, L. J., C. I. Branton, and J. J. Koranda. 1962. Seed characteristics of bluejoint and techniques for threshing. *J. Range Mgmt.* 15:227–229.

Klomp, G. J. 1968. The use of woodchips and nitrogen fertilizer in seeding scab ridges. *J. Range Mgmt.* 21:31–36.

————, and A. C. Hull, Jr. 1972. Methods of seeding three perennial wheatgrasses on cheatgrass range in southern Idaho. *J. Range Mgmt.* 25:266–268.

Launchbaugh, J. L. , ed. 1966. A stand establishment survey of grass plantings in the Great Plains. *Nebr. Agr. Expt. Sta. Great Plains Council Report* 23.

————. 1970. Seeding rate and first-year stand relationships for six native grasses. *J. Range Mgmt,* 23:414–417.

Lavin, F., and F. B. Gomm. 1968. Stabilizing small seed dilution mixtures. *J. Range Mgmt.* 21:328–330.

————, ————, and T. N. Johnsen, Jr. 1973. Cultural, seasonal, and site effects on pinyon-juniper rangeland plantings. *J. Range Mgmt.* 26:279–285.

McGinnies, W. J. 1962. Effect of seedbed firming on the establishment of crested wheatgrass seedings. *J. Range Mgmt.* 15:230–234.

————. 1968. Effect of post-emergence weed control on grass establishment in north-central Colorado. *J. Range Mgmt.* 21:126–128.

————. 1971. Influence of row spacing on crested wheatgrass seed production. *J. Range Mgmt.* 24:387–389.

McMurphy, W. E. 1969. Pre-emergence herbicides for seeding range grasses. *J. Range Mgmt.* 22:427–429.

Miller, H. W., A. L. Hafenrichter, and O. K. Hoglund. 1957. The influence of management methods on seedings of perennials in the annual range area. *J. Range Mgmt.* 10:62–66.

Mueggler, W. F., and J. P. Blaisdell, 1955. Effect of seeding rate upon establishment and yield of crested wheatgrass. *J. Range Mgmt.* 8:74–76.

Nelson, J. R., A. M. Wilson, and C. J. Goebel. 1970. Factors influencing broadcast seeding in bunchgrass range. *J. Range Mgmt.* 23:163–170.

Nord, E. C., P. F. Hartless, and W. D. Nettleton. 1971. Effects of several factors on saltbush establishment in California. *J. Range Mgmt.* 24:216–223.

————, E. R. Schneegas, and H. Graham. 1967. Bitterbrush seed collecting—By machine or by hand. *J. Range Mgmt.* 20:99–103.

Owensby, C. E., and K. L. Anderson. 1965. Reseeding "Go-back" land in the Flint Hills of Kansas. *J. Range Mgmt.* 18:224–225.

Plath, C. V. 1954. Reseed now? *J. Range Mgmt.* 7:215–217.

Riegel, A. 1940. A study of the variations in the growth of blue grama grass from seed produced in various sections of the Great Plains Region. *Kan. Acad. Sci. Trans.* 43:155–171.

Robertson, J. H. 1944. An efficient method of broadcasting range grass seeds. *Intermountain Forest and Range Expt. Sta. Research Paper 8.*

——, and C. K. Pearse. 1945. Artificial reseeding and the closed community. *Northwest Sci.* 19:58–66.

Robocker, W. C., D. H. Gates, and H. D. Kerr. 1965. Effects of herbicides, burning, and seeding date in reseeding an arid range. *J. Range Mgmt.* 18:114–118.

——, and B. A. Zamora. 1971. Small alternating temperature germinator. *J. Range Mgmt.* 24:465–466.

Schumacher, C. M. 1964. Range interseeding in Nebraska. *J. Range Mgmt.* 17:132–137.

Schwendiman, J. L., R. F. Sackman, and A. L. Hafenrichter. 1940. Processing seed of grasses and other plants to remove awns and appendages. *U.S. Dept. Agr. Cir.* 558.

Short, L. R. 1943. Reseeding to increase the yield of Montana rangelands. *U.S. Dept. Agr. Farmers' Bull.* 1924.

Simpson, J. R. 1971. Costs and returns in a study of common property range improvements. *J. Range Mgmt.* 24:248–251.

Slayback, R. D., and C. W. Renney. 1972. Intermediate pits reduce gamble in range seeding in the Southwest. *J. Range Mgmt.* 25:224–227.

Smika, D. E., and L. C. Newell. 1968. Seed yield and caryopsis weight of side-oats grama as influenced by cultural practices. *J. Range Mgmt.* 21:402–404.

Springfield, H. W., and D. G. Bell. 1967. Depth to seed fourwing saltbush. *J. Range Mgmt.* 20:180–182.

Statler, G. D. 1967. *Eurotia lanata* establishment trials. *J. Range Mgmt.* 20:253–255.

Stewart, G. 1950. Reseeding research in the intermountain region. *J. Range Mgmt.* 3:52–59.

Stoddart, L. A. 1941. Nurse crops not advisable in range reseeding. *Farm and Home Sci.* 2(2):6, 11.

Stroh, J. R., and V. P. Sundberg. 1971. Emergence of grass seedlings under crop residue culture. *J. Range Mgmt.* 21:226–230.

Stubbendieck, J., P. T. Koshi, and W. G. McCully. 1973. Establishment and growth of selected grasses. *J. Range Mgmt.* 26:39–43.

Tadmor, N. H., M. Evenari, and J. Katznelson. 1968. Seeding annuals and perennials in natural desert range. *J. Range Mgmt.* 21:330–331.

Tiedemann, A. R., and F. W. Pond. 1967. Viability of grass seed after long periods of uncontrolled storage. *J. Range Mgmt.* 20:261–262.

U. S. Department of Agriculture. 1948. *Grass. Yearbook of Agriculture.*

Wein, R. W., and N. E. West. 1971a. Phenology of salt desert plants near contour furrows. *J. Range Mgmt.* 24:299–304.

——, and ——. 1971b. Seedling survival on erosion control treatments in a salt desert area. *J. Range Mgmt.* 24:352–357.

Wilson, C. P. 1931. The artificial reseeding of New Mexico ranges. *N. Mex. Agr. Expt. Sta. Bull.* 189.

Chapter 19

Rangeland Fertilization

Fertilization of rangelands aims to increase forage production totally and season-ally, to improve nutritive qualities of forage, to enhance seedling establishment, and to alter palatability in order to aid animal control. Few trials of range fertilization existed before the 1950s, and these yielded varied but generally unspectacular results. Yields of hay from mixed prairie were increased by applica-tions of barnyard manure at Havre, Montana, beginning in 1925 (Heady, 1952) and at Manyberries, Alberta, Canada, in 1928 (Clarke and Tisdale, 1936, 1945). The results appeared unprofitable. Bentley (1946) reported an increase in legumes from fertilized plots in the California annual grassland and later de-scribed a range-fertilization program that started in 1941 (Bentley and Green, 1954). Dickey et al. (1948) obtained a profitable first-year return from 225 kilograms per hectare of ammonium phosphate sulfate (16-20-0) on annual grass-land at Pleasanton, California. Results from many other early exploratory trials went unreported, but they generated widespread testing of rangeland fertiliza-tion.

Nearly all papers on range fertilization report favorable biological results but wide and often unpredictable variations. Duncan and Hylton (1970), based on an extensive review, described results of range fertilization which varied because of yearly climatic variations, soil series, growth habits of the plant species, stage of plant maturity at the time of sampling, plant parts sampled, fertilizer rates and types, sampling methods and reporting units, season of fertilizer application, and means by which the fertilizer was applied. An almost infinite number of permutations of these causes of variation, many of which remain unmeasured, complicates summarization of results from rangeland fertilization. Instead of presenting recipes for fertilizing small areas of rangeland, the objective in this chapter is to analyze the widespread biological problems with range fertilization, the major responses to fertilization, and the management of fertilized rangeland within the firm or ranch context.

WIDESPREAD FERTILIZER PROBLEMS

The major causes of uncertainty about responses to range fertilization appear to be the variation of soil deficiencies from place to place and the fluctuation of responses with changes in rainfall and temperatures.

Nutrient Deficiencies in Range Soil

The growth of the range forage crop within its own particular environmental conditions best indicates the available plant nutrients in the soil. Addition of nutrients to the soil and measurement of plant responses determine the deficiencies that existed in the untreated soil. While these deficiencies may be indicated by soil test, greenhouse trial, and tissue analysis, a field test gives results directly usable in specifying fertilizer practice. The bulk of information obtained from experience and testing on North American rangelands shows that the major soil-nutrient deficiencies are too little available nitrogen, phosphorus, and sulfur. As management of rangeland becomes more intense, range soil-fertility problems will become more complex, as soil-nutrient problems have deepened in crop agriculture.

Nitrogen deficiency seems universal. A review of perhaps 150 papers showed that, in most instances, herbage growth increased as a result of nitrogen fertilization. Phosphorus deficiency clearly came second and sulfur deficiency third in importance. Both nitrogen and phosphorus were deficient in many areas, and supplying one without the other was of little value. Potassium, calcium, and magnesium amendments to soils under crops and pastures commonly increase production, but these elements appear unimportant in rangeland fertilization. The trace elements—zinc, iron, boron, manganese, copper, and molybdenum—have had an even smaller response than potassium and calcium in rangeland fertilization, although they are included in the mix of soil amendments for a few crops, orchards, and vineyards on a local basis. Widespread deficiencies of the trace elements occur in many rangeland soils in Australia.

The fertility of rangeland soils probably varies more than the fertility of agricultural soils. This is particularly true when the definition of soil fertility embraces soil physical characteristics, moisture content, organic matter, and the living inhabitants as well as the amount and availability of chemical elements. While a narrow definition emphasizes the delivery of chemical salts to plant tissues, management of soil fertility must include the factors controlling that delivery. In this respect, rangelands include widely variant conditions. Many are too extreme in dryness, wetness, texture, acidity, salinity, or alkalinity for agricultural crops. Fertilizer use is just one factor in successful rangeland management. Its effectiveness depends upon the degree to which fertilizer practices correlate with other limits in production. Every range pasture presents a different combination of these soil-fertility factors.

Relationships with Weather

Precipitation, soil moisture, and temperature change daily, monthly, and yearly, needing special attention in rangeland fertilization programs. Perhaps the best indication of the importance of these factors was given by Martin and Berry (1970) for the California annual grassland. In summarizing 54 field experiments during 15 years of work in 20 counties, they placed the limits of profitable fertilization within the 330- to 760-millimeter average rainfall belt. Less rainfall gave insufficient water for efficient fertilizer use, and more rainfall leached the applied fertilizers before they could be used. Smika et al. (1965) suggested that 380 millimeters of rainfall in western North Dakota produced maximum herbage without added nitrogen but 500 millimeters were required with 90 kilograms per hectare of nitrogen. Patterson and Youngman (1960) gave the limit of profitable fertilizer use on *Agropyron desertorum* in eastern Washington at 330 millimeters of precipitation. In a year with rainfall outside the limits, 330 to 760 millimeters, rangeland fertilization would be expected to give poor results, although the average yearly rainfall for the area might be within those limits.

Other writers have implied or found similar results but made no attempt to quantify the precipitation limits beyond the statement that results were disappointing in drought years in semidesert grassland (Herbel, 1963; Arizona Interagency Range Technical Sub-committee, 1969), in the mixed prairie of southern Texas (Reynolds et al., 1953), and in the *Bromus tectorum* type of northeastern California (Kay, 1966). Although few workers have suggested specific limits to rangeland fertilization based on rainfall, there appears to be a possibility of using rainfall as a guide to fertilization.

The carryover of fertilizer in the soil beyond the first year is another aspect of response to fertilizer which closely relates to rainfall. Low rainfall in areas and years allows the added minerals to remain in the soil more than one year. The carryover may last several years (Table 19-1). Numerous reports of carryover effects in the northern Great Plains of the United States and Canada indicate that accumulated increased herbage yields over a number of years are more important than initial increases. Responses persisted as much as six years in mixed prairie (Smoliak, 1965; Read, 1969) and three to four years in seeded ranges in the same region (Houston, 1957; Thomas, 1961). Yields of *Agropyron inerme* and other species took four to eight years to return to normal after a single fertilizer application in southern British Columbia (Mason and Miltimore, 1969, 1972; Hubbard and Mason, 1967). Other studies reporting carryover include work on meadows in northeastern Oregon (Hedrick et al., 1965), high meadows in Utah (Bowns, 1972), in Arizona (Lavin, 1967), and slash pine plantations in Florida (Hughes et al., 1971). Significant nitrogen carryover effects seldom occur in the California annual grassland, although McKell et al. (1970) obtained increased herbage yields three years after application of chicken manure and Jones (1963) obtained carryover effects with high rates of nitrogen. Apparently, the presence of ammoniacal forms of nitrogen and elemental sulfur decreases the possibilities of leaching losses.

Carryover of sulfur and phosphorus occurs more commonly than retention of nitrogen, as shown by increased herbage yields, the depth to which nitrogen and phosphorus were leached (Black and Wight, 1972), and the amount of nitrogen needed to balance immobilization and losses each year (Power, 1972). Sulfur leached gradually over a three-year period (Conrad et al., 1966). Flood irrigation of native meadows reduced carryover of nitrogen to near zero and phosphorus to one-fifth in a year's time in eastern Oregon. Carryover effects of fertilizers on

Table 19-1 Annual herbage production of *Agropyron intermedium* in the pine zone near Flagstaff, Arizona, after one fertilization with 74 kg/ha of nitrogen *(Lavin, 1967)*

| Year | Annual herbage production, kg/ha | | |
	Control	Nitrogen-fertilized	Difference
1957	994	2,270	1,276
1958	1,632	2,573	941
1959	548	775	227
1960	708	833	125
1961	256	285	29
Total	4,138	6,736	2,598

Calamagrostis rubescens disappeared in two years in southern British Columbia (Freyman and van Ryswyk 1969).

Yearly variations in response to fertilizers have been referred to above. Cosper et al. (1967) reported about 130 percent yearly difference in herbage yield from both fertilized and unfertilized mixed prairie in Wyoming; the yearly variation amounted to 2,051 and 953 kilograms per hectare, respectively. Similarly wide fluctuations in production characterize annual grassland (Hoglund et al., 1962) and, in fact, all native forage-producing areas (Table 19-2).

A different sort of variation was reported by Lorenz and Rogler (1972, 1973) for mixed prairie in western North Dakota. A significant response to phosphorus did not occur until the fourth year of treatment and thereafter continued throughout the experiment. Probably the capacity of the soil to immobilize phosphorous became saturated after four applications, and additional amounts then were more readily available to plants than in the early treatments.

Application of fertilizer on different dates has not given large differences in results. Cooper (1956) found no difference between fall and winter applications on flood-meadows in eastern Oregon. Early fall gave the greatest amount of winter feed in the California annual type (Jones, 1960). Sneva (1973b) reported no difference between fall, winter, and spring applications on *Agropyron desertorum* and *A. sibiricum*. Apparently fertilizers need to be applied when rainfall will take the minerals into the soil and near the beginning of growth so that the plants can take advantage of the added minerals. The seed yield of *Elymus junceus* increased when the species was fertilized after harvest each year (Lawrence and Kilcher, 1964).

RESPONSES TO FERTILIZATION

The major benefits from rangeland fertilization center on increased amounts of seed and herbage that have higher nutritive qualities than the same feeds grown without fertilization. Feed may be produced earlier with fertilizers than without them. Secondarily, or more locally, fertilization is used to promote seedling establishment and distributional control of animals.

Increases in Herbage

Nearly all reports of fertilizer trials describe increases in herbage production (Table 19-3). Mediterranean annual grassland responds to fertilization throughout its range (Hoglund et al., 1952; Woolfolk and Duncan, 1962; Jones, 1963; Martin and Berry, 1970; Luebs et al., 1971; Ofer and Seligman, 1969). However, certain treatments in many experiments produced no increases in herbage, and a few treatments depressed yields.

Table 19-2 Yearly fluctuations in increased herbage production from fertilizer treatments of the same amounts

Vegetational type	Location	Fertilizer type and amount, kg/ha	Increase in herbage production, kg/ha	Year	Source
Coastal prairie	Texas	Nitrogen—336	280 252	1964 1965	Powell and Box (1967)
True prairie	Kansas	Nitrogen—90	1,570 2,190	1957 1959	Launchbaugh (1962)
Palouse prairie	Washington	Nitrogen—90	113 3,537[*]	1956 1957	Patterson and Youngman (1960)
California annual	California	Nitrogen—135; phosphorus—29	404[†] 3,677	1960–1961 1961–1962	Luebs et al. (1971)
Alpine meadow	Utah	Nitrogen—67	289 1,214 242	1966 1967 1968	Bowns (1972)
Mixed prairie seeded to *Agropyron desertorum*	North Dakota	Nitrogen—67	618 1,489 1,605 434 2,876 2,077 2,541 3,527 2,048 1,688 985 2,443 1,860	1949 1950 1951 1952 1953 1954 1955 1956 1957 1958 1959 1960 Average	Lorenz and Rogler (1962)

[*]*Bromus tectorum* amounted to 3,189 kg/ha.
[†]Rainfall approximated 200 mm in 1960–1961 and 580 mm in 1961–1962.

The northern mixed prairie in the United States and Canada constitutes another region where much range fertilization occurs. A sample of the many papers from that region illustrates the herbage increases and variations in results which prevail (Lodge, 1959; Smoliak, 1965; Cosper et al., 1967; Burzlaff et al., 1968; Goetz, 1969, 1970; Lorenz and Rogler, 1972; Power, 1972). Fertilization of the true prairie increases herbage production by stimulating cool-season species, undersirable forbs, or both at the expense of warm-season species (Huffine and

Table 19-3 The apparently optimal fertilizer treatment reported by the cited author(s)

Vegetational type	Location	Fertilizer type and amount, kg/ha	Increase in herbage production, kg/ha	Source
True prairie	Nebraska	Nitrogen—27; phosphorus—9	560	Warnes and Newell (1969)
	Oklahoma	Nitrogen—112	122	Gay and Dwyer (1965)
Mixed prairie	Nebraska	Nitrogen—67	603	Burzlaff et al. (1968)
	North Dakota	Nitrogen—75	954	Goetz (1969)
	Alberta	Nitrogen—138	840	Lutwick et al. (1965)
Palouse prairie	British Columbia	Nitrogen—269	418	Mason and Miltimore (1969)
Mountain meadow	Oregon	Nitrogen—224	4,094	Nelson and Castle (1958)
Sagebrush-grass	Utah	Nitrogen—67	650	Hooper et al. (1969)
Desert grassland	Arizona	Nitrogen—90; phosphorus—72	614	Freeman and Humphrey (1956)
Pinon-juniper seeded to *Agropyron intermedium*	Flagstaff, Arizona	Nitrogen—111	1,337	Lavin (1967)

Elder, 1960; Gay and Dwyer, 1965; Powell and Box, 1967; Dee and Box, 1967; Drawe and Box, 1969; Graves and McMurphy, 1969; Warnes and Newell, 1969; Owensby et al., 1970). Cool-season species and weeds were not encouraged in a Nebraska test (Rehm et al., 1972).

Although herbage increases resulting from nitrogen applications have been reported for Palouse prairie and other variants of the western mountain bunchgrass type, recommendations for rangeland fertilization generally are less than enthusiastic (Smith and Lang, 1962; Thomas et al., 1964; Cook, 1965; Wilson et al., 1966; Hubbard and Mason, 1967). Wet meadows respond to fertilization, especially if water level and irrigation do not leach the minerals from the soil, as shown by Leamer (1963) in New Mexico; Cooper and Sawyer (1955) and Rumburg

(1963) in eastern Oregon; Russell et al. (1965) and Moore et al. (1968) in Nebraska; Martin et al. (1965) in California; and Bowns (1972) in southwestern Utah.

Fertilization stimulated annual *Bromus tectorum* but not perennial *Agropyron spicatum* in eastern Washington. Increased yield of *B. tectorum* varied unpredictably over 11 years (Kay, 1966). Annual species responded more than did *Phalaris tuberosa* to low fertilization rates in California. At high rates, *Phalaris* rapidly increased in yield (Martin et al., 1964). Trials of rangeland fertilization gave discouraging results in the semi-desert grassland (Freeman and Humphrey, 1956; Holt and Wilson, 1961; Herbel, 1963; Bahe et al., 1973). Forest sites usually give favorable herbage-yield responses to fertilization, as illustrated on *Calamagrostis rubescens* in British Columbia (Freyman and van Ryswyk, 1969), on pine woodland in northeastern Oregon (Hedrick et al., 1965), and on pine woodland in the southern United States (Hughes et al., 1971).

Fertilization of seeded introduced *Agropyron* spp., *Elymus junceus, Bromus inermis,* and a few other species appears to be a practical means of increasing herbage production in the northern Great Plains (Kilcher, 1958; Smika et al., 1960; Rogler and Lorenz, 1969; Power and Alessi, 1970), in the sagebrushgrass type in Oregon (Sneva et al., 1958; Cooper and Hyder, 1958; Sneva 1973a, 1973b, 1973c), and in Utah (Cook, 1965), but had no practical results in Nevada (Eckert et al., 1961). *Agropyrons* in the pine zone responded with increased yields in Arizona (Lavin, 1967) and with no significant increases in northeastern Utah (Hull, 1963). *Dactylis glomerata* responded to nitrogen in western Oregon (Hedrick, 1964) and to nitrogen, phosphorus, and sulfur in the Blue Mountains of eastern Oregon (Geist, 1971). Increased yields of *Cynodon* and other introduced species commonly occur after fertilization in the southern United States (Adams and Stelly, 1962).

Increases in Forage Quality

Some 50 papers on effects of range fertilization report that improved forage quality results from additions of nitrogen to the soil. In a few locations, phosphorus and sulfur, in addition to nitrogen, enhance quality. Duncan and Hylton (1970) reviewed the subject, showing that increases in yield and quality relate directly to each other. *Quality* in this context refers to *percentage crude protein as determined by plant nitrogen quantities*. Vegetational types from which these results have been reported include the California annual grassland, planted species throughout the range region, mixed prairie, mountain meadows, herbaceous vegetation under tree canopies, true prairie, coastal prairie, and Palouse prairie. The citations for these statements essentially duplicate those in the previous section on yield increases.

Increased crude protein levels due to fertilization may not be particularly beneficial since the increase occurs when crude protein levels of unfertilized forages are adequate for efficient animal growth. As the growth cycle advances, the protein level in fertilized herbage normally drops faster than the level in unfertilized herbage. Improved curing of feed on the ground comes more readily from improved botanical composition—more legumes—than from fertilization per se.

Uses of fertilizers include correction of deficiencies for animal nutrition, such as phosphorus fertilization to relieve phosphorus deficiencies in range cattle (Reynolds et al., 1953) and to reduce the ratio of potassium to calcium and magnesium where grass tetany occurs (Azevedo and Rendig, 1972). Nitrate poisoning may result from massive nitrogen fertilizations. Houston et al. (1973) found that *Chenopodium leptophyllum* reached a dangerous level (2,000 ppm) of nitrate-nitrogen when 224 kilograms of nitrogen per hectare were applied. *Lepidium densiflorum,* another annual forb, required a fertilizer application of 672 kilograms of nitrogen per hectare to be dangerous. The perennial grasses always remained below the toxic level.

The effects of fertilization on digestibility vary. Poulton et al. (1957) found little difference in digestibility of either *Dactylis glomerata* or *Medicago sativa* with nitrogen fertilizations that ranged from zero to 450 kilograms of nitrogen per hectare. Conversely, hay from fertilized *Bouteloua gracilis* rangeland in New Mexico showed increased digestibility of dry matter, protein, and energy by wether lambs (Kelsey et al., 1973). After an extensive review of nutritive values resulting from pasture fertilization, Blaser (1964) suggested that TDN, or digestible energy, changed little with nitrogen fertilization because increases in crude-protein digestibility balanced decreases in soluble carbohydrates. Other pasture workers have reported increases in soluble carbohydrates from nitrogen fertilization (Jones, D. I. H. et al., 1961). Improved quality of feed after fertilization may be related to characteristics, such as succulence, increased green period, narrow leaf-stem ratio, and botanical composition of the feed, other than chemical contents.

Changes in Botanical Composition

Additions of phosphorus, sulfur, and potassium on rangeland usually favor legumes and other forbs, sometimes with little effect on grass yield (Fig. 19-1). Nitrogen fosters the grasses and reduces the legumes (Table 19-4). These results occur with *Cynodon-Trifolium* pastures in the southern United States (Adams and Stelly, 1962; Adams et al., 1966), in *Dactylis glomerata–Trifolium* pastures in western Oregon (Hedrick, 1964), in meadows in eastern Oregon (Cooper, 1957; Cooper and Hunter, 1959), in the California annual grassland (Jones, M. B. et al., 1961), and in annual range in Israel (Ofer and Seligman, 1969).

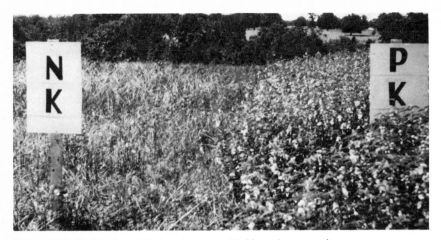

Figure 19-1 Fertilization with phosphorus resulted in an increase of a native unpalatable legume and a decrease in grass on the right, while nitrogen fertilization caused little change in the composition.

At the present stage of range-fertilization practice, few managers use varying combinations of elements to manipulate balances among legumes, other forbs, and grasses. One exception is in the foothill grasslands in California, where fertilization programs aim to change the botanical composition toward more legumes and thereby attain greater yield and higher feed quality. One procedure adds phosphorus to favor clovers, which furnish nitrogen to the grasses (Jones and Evans, 1960; Jones and Winans, 1967). A second procedure, on granitic soils, is the application of 67 kilograms of sulfur per hectare at three-year intervals (Bentley and Green, 1954; Bentley et al., 1958; Conrad et al., 1966).

Fertilization alters the proportion of cool-season species in the true and mixed prairies. In the true prairie, increases in undesirable weeds usually accompany increases in cool-season grasses (Huffine and Elder, 1960; Powell and Box, 1967; Drawe and Box, 1969; Owensby et al., 1970). Rehm et al. (1972) found no increases in cool-season species in Nebraska during four years of fertilizing a seeded mixture of native warm-season species. Nitrogen fertilization of northern Great Plains grassland results in a desirable spring response of the cool-season grasses, especially *Agropyron smithii,* (Rogler and Lorenz, 1957; Cosper et al., 1967). Increased forbs may improve the habitat for seed-eating birds, as sulfur fertilization and increased legumes have favored quail in California (Shields and Duncan, 1966).

Rumberg and Cooper (1961) found meadow hay in eastern Oregon to be mostly *Hordeum brachyantherum* and *Elymus triticoides* where fertilization was 448 to 672 kilograms of nitrogen per hectare. The clovers disappeared and the sedges started decreasing at 224 kilograms of nitrogen per hectare .

Table 19-4   Influence of rangeland fertilization upon botanical composition

Vegetational type and location	Fertilizer type and amount, kg/ha	Species	Percentage composition without treatment	Percentage composition with treatment	Source
California annual type, San Joaquin range, 1959	Sulfur−67; nitrogen−90	Grasses	58.2	71.1	Woolfolk and Duncan (1962)
		Legumes	1.2	0.5	
		Erodium	39.3	27.1	
		Other forbs	1.2	1.3	
1960	Sulfur−67; nitrogen−90	Grasses	27.0	40.5	
		Legumes	1.6	0.1	
		Erodium	60.9	52.1	
		Other forbs	10.5	7.2	
Annual grassland, Israel	Nitrogen−79	Grasses	33	65	Ofer and Seligman (1969)
		Legumes	50	15	
		Other forbs	17	20	
	Phosphorus−59	Grasses	33	20	
		Legumes	50	74	
		Other forbs	17	6	
	Nitrogen−79; phosphorus−59	Grasses	33	70	
		Legumes	50	15	
		Other forbs	17	15	
Palouse prairie, Washington	Nitrogen−45	*Agropyron inerme*	66	14	Patterson and Youngman (1960)
		Festuca idahoensis	4	4	
		Poa secunda	17	25	
		Bromus tectorum	13	58	
Mixed prairie, Wyoming	Nitrogen−37	*Bouteloua gracilis*	76	60	Rauzi et al. (1968)
		Poa secunda	19	37	
Mixed prairie, Alberta	Nitrogen−336; phosphorus−168; potassium−336	Grasses	48.0	57.4	Smoliak (1965)

Rehabilitation of Depleted Areas

The use of fertilizers to rehabilitate rangeland, that is, to increase seedling establishment, increase cover, change the botanical composition, and reduce erosion, seems to be a questionable practice. Cook (1965) found no benefits to seedling emergence and survival of introduced *Agropyron* spp. and *Elymus jun-*

ceus on foothill ranges in Utah. Hull (1963) reported similar results from work at higher elevations in the same region. Ayeke and McKell (1969) suggested that high nitrogen and phosphorus content did not increase the first growth of *Lolium multiflorum* and *Oryzopsis miliacea*. Although Thompson and Schaller (1960) recommended banding phosphorus for seedling establishment in the southern Great Plains, most authors of studies of the central North American grasslands have found fertilization at the time of seeding to have no effect or a detrimental effect because weed growth was stimulated (Welch et al., 1962; Lorenz and Rogler, 1962; Cosper et al., 1967; Johnston et al., 1967; Warnes and Newell, 1969; Bryan and McMurphy, 1968). Tiedemann and Kock (1973) questioned the use of fertilizer to aid in restoration of cover in pine-fir forests after fires.

Palatability

Animals commonly prefer fertilized areas, and many plot results have been lost because the fertilized plots were selected and overused by animals. Deer in the Black Hills of South Dakota grazed earlier and more frequently in nitrogen-fertilized areas than in unfertilized places (Thomas et al., 1964). *Calamagrostis rubescens* showed high palatability when fertilized in southern British Columbia (Freyman and van Ryswyk, 1969), and fertilization reduced differences between palatable and unpalatable species on the Santa Rita Experimental Range (Holt and Wilson, 1961). Cattle walked less, took bigger bites, picked fewer acorns, and spent less time grazing on fertilized than on unfertilized pastures (Green et al., 1958). Fertilization on mountain rangeland can attain better distribution of grazing (Smith and Lang, 1958, 1962; Hooper et al., 1969).

Seasonal Growth

Fertilization changes plant growth rate during certain seasons. The most striking and consistent result from many fertilizer trials on the California annual grassland has been increased fall, winter, and early-spring growth from supplemental nitrogen. Phosphorus and sulfur must be adequate. The result is feed composed mostly of grasses during the seasons when little grass is expected (Martin and Berry, 1970). The length of the green feed season is extended by earlier range readiness (Hoglund et al., 1952; Jones, 1960, 1963). Rapid early growth prevents the extension of green feed into the dry season and the growth of summer weeds because the soil moisture is depleted rapidly (McKell et al. 1959). Wilson et al. (1966) speculated that the annual *Bromus tectorum* could be made to produce abundant early growth in southeastern Washington, thereby shortening the winter feeding period. The beginning of growth in the semidesert grassland follows summer rains, and fertilization cannot advance that time. However, fertilization extends the green period into the fall (Honnas et al., 1959; Lavin, 1967). In areas with severe winters, applications of fertilizer in fall, winter, and spring are equally effective (Cooper, 1956).

Manipulating the times of range readiness, leaf drying, and plant maturity obviously has an important relationship to the beginning, ending, and rotation of grazing (Goetz, 1970). However, Sneva (1973a) gives a word of caution and recommends that fertilization not be used to facilitate early grazing of *Agropyron desertorum* or high early-spring stocking rates. Stimulated early growth depletes stored carbohydrates. If fertilized *Agropyron desertorum* is grazed earlier than unfertilized stands, grazing also should be terminated earlier.

MANAGEMENT OF FERTILIZED AREAS

Whether fertilization of rangeland produces sufficient forage increases to be profitable remains an unanswered question under most conditions. Papers describe unprofitable results for *Bromus tectorum* and *Agropyron desertorum* (Kay and Evans, 1965; Kay, 1966; Eckert et al., 1961), for semidesert grassland (Freeman and Humphrey, 1956), for mixed prairie (Clarke and Tisdale, 1936; Smike et al., 1963; Nichols and McMurphy, 1969; Rauzi et al., 1968), for seeded *Bromus inermis* and *Agropyron desertorum* (Thomas, 1961), for Palouse prairie (Patterson and Youngman, 1960), for seeded mountain grasslands (Hull, 1963, and for *Andropogon*-dominated prairies (Bryan and McMurphy, 1968; Powell and Box, 1967). These 13 papers make little attempt at a budgetary analysis, but they do express the authors' evaluations of their own results.

Another group of papers express confidence that fertilization yields a profit, but all caution that certain restrictions must be met. For the California annual grassland, Martin and Berry (1970) claimed that precipitation should be within the limits of 330 to 760 millimeters during the year of application. Dickey et al. (1948) did their work within those limits. Sulfur fertilization of annual range at the San Joaquin Experimental Range turned a profit because it doubled the grazing capacity at a low cost per hectare. Addition of sulfur and nitrogen produced more grazing days than did addition of sulfur alone, but the practice was unprofitable because it cost more than did adding only sulfur (Conrad et al. 1966).

Fertilization of western North Dakota mixed prairie appears to yield a profit (Rogler and Lorenz, 1969). Kilcher (1958) reported profits from fertilized *Agropyron desertorum* in all four years of his study in southern Saskatchewan but in only some years for two other species. In southern British Columbia, adequate returns occurred on one of four sites (Hubbard and Mason, 1967). Herbel (1963) suggested fertilization on only the best sites and in wet years for the semidesert grassland. Fertilization of wet meadows appeared consistently profitable in eastern Oregon (Cooper and Sawyer, 1955), but was profitable in only half the years in northeastern California (Martin et al., 1965).

Most attempts to analyze fertilization inputs for profitability have given costs for additional feed produced during the years of the study or costs and returns at a selected time. For example, Kay (1966) found that the cost of obtaining 900 kilograms of increased forage from fertilizing *Bromus tectorum* varied from $8.07 to $50.52 for the years 1956 to 1965. Fertilization of *Agropyron inerme* on nine sites for four years in southern British Columbia yielded forage costing between $6.40 and $98 per ton (Mason and Miltimore, 1969). The production of increased forage on 11 seeded grasses in eastern Oregon cost $6.70 to $17.60 per 900 kilograms in the 1950s (Cooper and Hyder, 1958). Hooper et al. (1969) found that fertilizing blocks of 4 to 6 hectares on mountain rangelands in Utah gave a profit when values were attached to increased use of the fertilized blocks and the surrounding unfertilized areas. Reynolds et al. (1953) found that supplementing cattle with phosphorus by adding disodium phosphate to the drinking water was more practical than fertilizing the range.

FINAL COMMENTS

The few papers that definitely show that range fertilization produces a profit in the livestock operation are in great contrast with most of the 150 or more papers on range fertilization. Very likely, the problems lie in the management of this practice. No doubt exists that sites make a difference (Herbel, 1963); that production fluctuates as much on fertilized as on unfertilized range (Bentley et al., 1958); that rainfall limits responses (Martin and Berry, 1970); that range forage that must be grazed has costs and values different from those of hay (Nelson and Castle, 1958); that fertilization, grazing, and weather interact (Jones and Evans, 1960); and that grazing, even close grazing, of fertilized areas is essential (Hedrick, 1964). Definition of these causes of variation serves to reduce risks of losses from range fertilization. Further research and experience should sharpen knowledge of the limits of fertilizer applications.

The increased forage produced by range fertilization must be used by additional animals and not by animals that substitute the fertilized pasture for unfertilized green forage, which then grows to maturity without being grazed. Forage from fertilized pastures abounds at nearly the same time that unfertilized range reaches its peak in quantity and quality. Therefore, the manager must increase the numbers of animals on a whole-ranch basis in order to take full advantage of the increased forage. Significant weight-gain differences of animals on properly managed fertilized and unfertilized ranges are difficult to attain. More likely, increased numbers of animals and kilograms of product per hectare, rather than increased animal weights, generate the profit. The manager must integrate fertilization into his whole-ranch program and invest where inputs will do the most good. The biological basis for range fertilization lacks many details, and the managerial aspects have hardly been touched. The land manager should start with plots or small pastures and gradually gather the specific information that he needs.

Range fertilization seeks an ideal: the ability to furnish each plant with the nutrients it needs on each particular soil as required within the vagaries of weather; the ability to control species composition of the forage; and the delivery of that forage to animals in ways that produce profit for the ranch enterprise. These are the problems, the objectives, and the challenges of range fertilization.

LITERATURE CITED

Adams, W. E., and M. Stelly. 1962. Fertility requirements of coastal Bermudagrass and crimson clover grown on Cecil sandy loam. I. Yield response to fertilization. *J. Range Mgmt.* 15:84–87.

———, ———, R. A. McCreery, H. D. Morris, and C. B. Elkins, Jr. 1966. Protein, P, and K composition of coastal Bermudagrass and crimson clover. *J. Range Mgmt.* 19:301–305.

Arizona Interagency Range Technical Sub-committee. 1969. Guide to improvement of Arizona rangeland. *Ariz. Agric. Ext. Serv. Bull.* A-58.

Ayeke, C. A., and C. M. McKell. 1969. Early seedling growth of Italian ryegrass and smilo as affected by nutrition. *J. Range Mgmt.* 22:29–32.

Azevedo, J., and V. V. Rendig. 1972. Chemical composition and fertilizer response of two range plants in relation to grass tetany. *J. Range Mgmt.* 25:24–27.

Bahe, Billy, J. L. Strochlein, and P. R. Ogden. 1973. Response of lehman lovegrass to time of fertilizer application. *J. Range Mgmt.* 26:222–224.

Bentley, J. R. 1946. Range fertilization—One means of improving range forage. *California Cattleman,* Sept. p. 6, 24.

———, and L. R. Green. 1954. Stimulation of native annual clovers through application of sulfur on California foothill range. *J. Range Mgmt.* 7:25–30.

———, ———, and K. A. Wagnon. 1958. Herbage production and grazing capacity on annual-plant range pastures fertilized with sulfur. *J. Range Mgmt.* 11:133–140.

Black, A. L., and J. R. Wight. 1972. Nitrogen and phosphorus availability in a fertilized rangeland ecosystem of the northern Great Plains. *J. Range Mgmt.* 25:456–460.

Blaser, R. E. 1964. Symposium on forage utilization: Effects of fertility levels and stage of maturity on forage nutritive value. *J. An. Sci.* 23:246–253.

Bowns, J. E. 1972. Low level nitrogen and phosphorus fertilization on high elevation ranges. *J. Range Mgmt.* 25:273–276.

Bryan, G. G., and W. E. McMurphy. 1968. Competition and fertilization as influences on grass seedlings. *J. Range Mgmt.* 21:98–101.

Burzlaff, D. F., G. W. Fick, and L. R. Rittenhouse. 1968. Effect of nitrogen fertilization on certain factors of a western Nebraska range ecosystem. *J. Range Mgmt.* 21:21–24.

Clarke, S. E., and E. W. Tisdale. 1936. Range pasture studies in southern Alberta and Saskatchewan. *Herbage Reviews* 4:51–64.

————, and ————. 1945. The chemical composition of native forage plants of southern Alberta and Saskatchewan in relation to grazing practices. *Can. Dept. Agr. Pub.* 769.

Conrad, C. E., E. J. Woolfolk, and D. A. Duncan. 1966. Fertilization and management implications on California annual-plant range. *J. Range Mgmt.* 19:20–26.

Cook, C. W. 1965. Plant and livestock responses to fertilized rangelands. *Utah Agric. Expt. Sta. Bull.* 455.

Cooper, C. S. 1956. The effect of source, rate and time of nitrogen application upon the yields, vegetative composition and crude protein content of native flood-meadow hay in eastern Oregon. *Agron. J.* 48:543–545.

————. 1957. A legume for native flood meadows: I. Establishment and maintenance of stands of white-tip clover (*T. variegatum*) in native flood meadows and its effect upon yields, vegetative and chemical composition of hay. *Agron. J.* 49:473–477.

————, and A. S. Hunter, 1959. A legume for native flood meadows: II. Phosphorus fertilizer requirements for maintaining stand of white-tip clover (*Trifolium variegatum*). *Agron. J.* 51:350–352.

————, and D. N. Hyder. 1958. Adaptability and yield of eleven grasses grown on the Oregon high desert. *J. Range Mgmt.* 11:235–237.

————, and W. A. Sawyer. 1955. Fertilization of mountain meadows in eastern Oregon. *J. Range Mgmt.* 8:20–22.

Cosper, H. R., J. R. Thomas, and A. Y. Alsayegh. 1967. Fertilization and its effect on range improvement in the northern Great Plains. *J. Range Mgmt.* 21:216–222.

Dee, R. F., and T. W. Box. 1967. Commercial fertilizers influence crude protein content of four mixed prairie grasses. *J. Range Mgmt.* 20:96–99.

Dickey, P. B., O. K. Hoglund, and B. A. Madison. 1948. Effect of fertilizers on the production and season of use of annual grass range in California. *J. Am. Soc. Agron.* 41:186–188.

Drawe, D. L., and T. W. Box. 1969. High rates of nitrogen fertilization influence coastal prairie range. *J. Range Mgmt.* 22:32–36.

Duncan, D. A., and L. O. Hylton, Jr. 1970. Effects of fertilization on quality of range forage. *U.S. Dept. Agr. Misc. Pub.* 1147:57–62.

Eckert, R. E., Jr., A. T. Bleak, and J. H. Robertson. 1961. Effects of macro- and micronutrients on the yield of crested wheatgrass. *J. Range Mgmt.* 14:149–155.

Freeman, B. N., and R. R. Humphrey. 1956. The effects of nitrates and phosphates upon forage production of a southern Arizona desert grassland range. *J. Range Mgmt.* 9:176–180.

Freyman, S. and A. L. van Ryswyk. 1969. Effect of fertilizer on pinegrass in southern British Columbia. *J. Range Mgmt.* 22:390–395.

Gay, C. W., and D. D. Dwyer, 1965. Effects of one year's nitrogen fertilization on native vegetation under clipping and burning. *J. Range Mgmt.* 18-273–277.

Geist, Jon M. 1971. Orchardgrass responses to fertilization of seven surface soils from the central Blue Mountains of Oregon. *U.S. Dept. Agr. Forest Service Research Paper.* PNW-122.

Goetz, H. 1969. Composition and yields of native grassland sites fertilized at different rates of nitrogen. *J. Range Mgmt.* 22:384–390.

————. 1970. Growth and development of northern Great Plains species in relation to nitrogen fertilization. *J. Range Mgmt.* 23:112–117.

Graves, J. E., and W. E. McMurphy. 1969. Burning and fertilization for range improvement in central Oklahoma. *J. Range Mgmt.* 22:165–168.

Green, L. R., K. A. Wagnon, and J. R. Bentley. 1958. Diet and grazing habits of steers on foothill range fertilized with sulfur. *J. Range Mgmt.* 11:221–227.

Heady, H. F. 1952. Reseeding, fertilizing, and renovating in an ungrazed mixed prairie. *J. Range Mgmt.* 5:144–149.

Hedrick, D. W. 1964. Response of an orchardgrass-subclover mixture in western Oregon to different clipping and fertilizing practices. *J. Range Mgmt.* 17:147–152.

————, J. A. B. McArthur, J. E. Oldfield, and J. A. Young. 1965. Seasonal yield and chemical content of forage mixtures on a pine woodland meadow site in northeastern Oregon. *Ore. Agr. Expt. Sta. Tech. Bull.* 84.

Herbel, C. H. 1963. Fertilizing tobosa on flood plains in semidesert grassland. *J. Range Mgmt.* 16:133–138.

Hoglund. O. K., H. W. Miller, and A. L. Hafenrichter. 1952. Application of fertilizers to aid conservation on annual forage range. *J. Range Mgmt.* 5:55–61.

Holt, G. A., and D. G. Wilson. 1961. The effect of commercial fertilizers on forage production and utilization on a desert grassland site. *J. Range Mgmt.* 4:252–256.

Honnas, R. C., B. L. Branscomb, and R. R. Humphrey. 1959. Effect of range fertilization on growth of three southern Arizona grasses. *J. Range Mgmt.* 12:88–91.

Hooper, J. F., J. P. Workman, J. B. Grumbles, and C. W. Cook. 1969. Improved livestock distribution with fertilizer—a preliminary economic evaluation. *J. Range Mgmt.* 22:108–110.

Houston, W. R. 1957. Renovation and fertilization of crested wheatgrass stands in the northern Great Plains. *J. Range Mgmt.* 10:9–11.

————, L. D. Sabatka, and D. N. Hyder. 1973. Nitrate-nitrogen accumulation in range plants after massive N fertilization on shortgrass plains. *J. Range Mgmt.* 26:54–57.

Hubbard, W. A., · d J. L. Mason. 1967. Residual effects of ammonium nitrate and ammonium phosphate on some native ranges of British Columbia. *J. Range Mgmt.* 20:1–5.

Huffine, W. W., and W. C. Elder. 1960. Effect of fertilization on native grass pastures in Oklahoma. *J. Range Mgmt.* 13:34–36.

Hughes, R. H., G. W. Bengtson, and T. A. Harrington. 1971. Forage response to nitrogen and phosphorus fertilization in a 25-year-old plantation of slash pine. *U.S. Dept. Agr. Forest Service Research Paper.* SE-82.

Hull, A. C., Jr. 1963. Fertilization of seeded grasses on mountainous rangelands in northeastern Utah and southeastern Idaho. *J. Range Mgmt.* 16:306–310.

Johnston, A., S. Smoliak, A. D. Smith, and L. E. Lutwick. 1967. Improvement of southeastern Alberta range with fertilizers. *Canadian J. Plant. Sci.* 47:671–678.

Jones, D. I. H., G. Griffith, and R. J. K. Walters. 1961. The effects of nitrogen fertilizer on the water soluble carbohydrate content of perennial ryegrass and cocksfoot. *J. Br. Grassland Soc.* 16:272–275.

Jones, M. B. 1960. Responses of annual range to urea applied at various dates. *J. Range Mgmt.* 13:188–192.

————. 1963. Yield, per cent nitrogen, and nitrogen uptake of various California annual grassland species fertilized with increasing rates of nitrogen. *Agron. J.* 55:254–257.

————, and R. A. Evans, 1960. Botanical composition changes in annual grassland as affected by fertilization and grazing. *Agron. J.* 52:459–461.

————, W. E. Martin, L. J. Berry, and V. Osterli. 1961. Ground cover and plants present on grazed annual range as affected by nitrogen fertilization. *J. Range Mgmt.* 14:146–148.

————, and S. S. Winans, 1967. Subterranean clover versus nitrogen fertilized annual grasslands: Botanical composition and protein content. *J. Range Mgmt.* 20:8–12.

Kay, B. L. 1966. Fertilization of cheatgrass ranges in California. *J. Range Mgmt.* 19:217–220.

————, and R. A. Evans. 1965. Effects of fertilization on a mixed stand of cheatgrass and intermediate wheatgrass. *J. Range Mgmt.* 18:7–11.

Kelsey, R. J., A. B. Nelson, G. S. Smith, and R. D. Pieper. 1973. Nutritive value of hay from nitrogen-fertilized blue grama rangeland. *J. Range Mgmt.* 26:292–294.

Kilcher, M. R. 1958. Fertilizer effects on hay production of three cultivated grasses in southern Saskatchewan. *J. Range Mgmt.* 11:231–234.

Launchbaugh, J. L. 1962. Soil fertility investigations and effects of commercial fertilizers on reseeded vegetation in west-central Kansas. *J. Range Mgmt.* 15:27–34.

Lavin, F. 1967. Fall fertilization of intermediate wheatgrass in the southwestern ponderosa pine zone. *J. Range Mgmt.* 20:16–21.

Lawrence, T., and M. R. Kilcher. 1964. Effect of time of fertilizer application on the seed and forage yield of Russian wild ryegrass. *J. Range Mgmt.* 17:272–273.

Leamer, R. W. 1963. Effect of fertilization on yield on an irrigated mountain meadow. *J. Range Mgmt.* 16:204–208.

Lodge, R. W. 1959. Fertilization of native range in the northern Great Plains. *J. Range Mgmt.* 12:277–279.

Lorenz, R. J., and G. A. Rogler. 1962. A comparison of methods of renovating old stands of crested wheatgrass. *J. Range Mgmt.* 15:215–219.

————, and ————. 1972. Forage production and botanical composition of mixed prairie as influenced by nitrogen and phosphorus fertilization. *Agron. J.* 64:244–249.

————, and ————. 1973. Interaction of fertility level with harvest date and frequency on productiveness of mixed prairie. *J. Range Mgmt.* 26:50–54.

Luebs, R. E., A. E. Laag, and M. J. Brown. 1971. Effect of site class and rainfall on annual range response to nitrogen and phosphorus. *J. Range Mgmt.* 24:366–370.

Lutwick, L. E., A. D. Smith, and A. Johnston. 1965. Fertilizer experiments on native rangelands using increasing-rate spreader. *J. Range Mgmt.* 18:136–139.

Martin, W. E., and L. J. Berry. 1970. Effects of nitrogenous fertilizers on California range as measured by weight gains of grazing cattle. *Calif. Agric. Expt. Sta. Bull.* 846.

————, C. Pierce, and V. P. Osterli. 1964. Differential nitrogen response of annual and perennial grasses. *J. Range Mgmt.* 17:67–68.

————, V. V. Rendig, A. D. Haig, and L. J. Berry. 1965. Fertilization of irrigated pasture and forage crops in California. *Calif. Agr. Expt. Sta. Bull.* 815.

Mason, J. L., and J. E. Miltimore. 1969. Yield increases from nitrogen on native range in southern British Columbia. *J. Range Mgmt.* 22:128–131.

————, and ————. 1972. Ten year yield response of beardless wheatgrass from a single nitrogen application. *J. Range Mgmt.* 25:269–272.

McKell, C. M., V. W. Brown, R. H. Adolph, and C. Duncan. 1970. Fertilization of annual rangeland with chicken manure. *J. Range Mgmt.* 23:336–340.

————, J. Major, and E. R. Perrier. 1959. Annual-range fertilization in relation to soil moisture depletion. *J. Range Mgmt.* 12:189–193.

Moore, A. W., E. M. Brouse, and H. F. Rhoades. 1968. Influence of phosphorus fertilizer placement on two Nebraska sub-irrigated meadows. *J. Range Mgmt.* 21:112–114.

Nelson, J., and E. N. Castle. 1958. Profitable use of fertilizer on native meadows. *J. Range Mgmt.* 11:80–83.

Nichols, J. T., and W. E. McMurphy. 1969. Range recovery and production as influenced by nitrogen and 2,4-D treatments. *J. Range Mgmt.* 22:116–119.

Ofer, Y., and N. G. Seligman. 1969. Fertilization of annual range in northern Israel. *J. Range Mgmt.* 22:337–341.

Owensby, C. E., R. M. Hyde, and K. L. Anderson. 1970. Effects of clipping and supplemental nitrogen and water on loamy upland bluestem range. *J. Range Mgmt.* 23:341–346.

Patterson, J. K., and V. E. Youngman. 1960. Can fertilizers effectively increase our range land production? *J. Range Mgmt.* 13:255–257.

Poulton, B. R., G. J. MacDonald, and G. W. VanderNoot. 1957. The effect of nitrogen fertilization on the nutritive value of orchardgrass hay. *J. An. Sci.* 16:462–466.

Powell, J., and T. W. Box. 1967. Mechanical control and fertilization as brush management practices affect forage production in south Texas. *J. Range Mgmt.* 20:227–236.

Power, J. F. 1972. Fate of fertilizer nitrogen applied to a northern Great Plains rangeland ecosystem. *J. Range Mgmt.* 25:367–371.

————, and J. Alessi. 1970. Effects of nitrogen source and phosphorus on crested wheatgrass growth and water use. *J. Range Mgmt.* 23:175–178.

Rauzi. F., R. L. Lang, and L. I. Painter. 1968. Effects of nitrogen fertilization on native rangeland. *J. Range Mgmt.* 21:287–291.

Read, D. W. L. 1969. Residual effects from fertilizer on native range in southwestern Saskatchewan. *Can. J. Soil Sci.* 49:225–230.

Rehm, G. W., W. J. Moline, and E. J. Schwartz. 1972. Response of a seeded mixture of warm-season prairie grasses to fertilization. *J. Range Mgmt.* 25:452–456.

Reynolds, E. B., J. M. Jones, J. H. Jones, J. F. Fudge, and R. J. Kleberg, Jr. 1953. Methods of supplying phosphorus to range cattle in south Texas. *Texas Agr. Expt. Sta. Bull.* 773.

Rogler, G. A., and R. J. Lorenz. 1957. Nitrogen fertilization of northern Great Plains rangelands. *J. Range Mgmt.* 10:156–160.

————, and ————. 1969. Pasture productivity of crested wheatgrass as influenced by nitrogen fertilization and alfalfa. *U.S. Dept. Agr. Tech. Bull.* 1402.

Rumburg, C. B. 1963. Production of regrowth forage on native flood meadows. *Agron. J.* 55:245–247.

————, and C. S. Cooper. 1961. Fertilizer-induced changes in botanical composition, yield, and quality of native meadow hay. *Agron. J.* 50:255–258.

Russell, J. S., E. M. Brouse, H. F. Rhoades, and D. F. Burzlaff. 1965. Response of sub-irrigated meadow vegetation to application of nitrogen and phosphorus fertilizer. *J. Range Mgmt.* 18:242–247.

Shields, P. W., and D. A. Duncan. 1966. Fall and winter food of California quail in dry years. *Calif. Fish and Game* 52:275–282.

Smika, D. E., H. J. Haas, and J. F. Power. 1965. Effects of moisture and nitrogen fertilizer on growth and water use by native grass. *Agron. J.* 57:483–485.

———, ———, and G. A. Rogler. 1960. Yield, quality, and fertilizer recovery of crested wheatgrass, bromegrass, and Russian wildrye as influenced by fertilization. *J. Range Mgmt.* 13:243–246.

———, ———, and ———. 1963. Native grass and crested wheatgrass production as influenced by fertilizer placement and weed control. *J. Range Mgmt.* 15:5–8.

Smith, D. R., and R. L. Lang. 1958. The effect of nitrogenous fertilizers on cattle distribution on mountain range. *J. Range Mgmt.* 11:248–249.

———, and ———. 1962. Nitrogen fertilization of upland range in the Bighorn Mountains, Wyoming. *Wyo. Agr. Expt. Sta. Bull.* 388.

Smoliak, S. 1965. Effects of manure, straw and inorganic fertilizers on northern Great Plains ranges. *J. Range Mgmt.* 18:11–15.

Sneva, F. A. 1973a. Crested wheatgrass response to nitrogen and clipping. *J. Range Mgt.* 26:47–50.

———. 1973b. Wheatgrass response to seasonal applications of two nitrogen sources. *J. Range Mgmt. 26:137–*139.

———. 1973c. Nitrogen and paraquat saves range forage for fall grazing. *J. Range Mgmt.* 26:294–295.

———, D. H. Hyder, and C. S. Cooper. 1958. The influence of ammonium nitrate on the growth and yield of crested wheatgrass on the Oregon high desert. *Agron. J.* 50:40–44.

Thomas, J. R. 1961. Fertilizing brome grass–crested wheatgrass in western South Dakota. *So. Dak. Agr. Expt. Sta. Bull.* 504.

———, H. R. Cosper, and W. Bever. 1964. Effects of fertilizers on the growth of grass and its use by deer in the Black Hills of South Dakota. *Agron. J.* 56:223–226.

Thompson, L. F., and C. C. Schaller. 1960. Effect of fertilization and date of planting on establishment of perennial summer grasses in North Central Oklahoma. *J. Range Mgmt.* 13:70–72.

Tiedemann, A. R., and G. O. Klock. 1973. First-year vegetation after fire, reseeding, and fertilization on the Entiat Experiment Forest. *U.S. Dept. Agr. Forest Service Research Note* PNW-195.

Warnes, D. D., and L. C. Newell. 1969. Establishment and yield responses of warm-season grass strains to fertilization. *J. Range Mgmt.* 22:235–240.

Welch. N. H., E. Burnett, and E. B. Hudspeth. 1962. Effect of fertilizer on seedling emergence and growth of several grass species. *J. Range Mgmt.* 15:94–98.

Wilson, A. M., G. A. Harris, and D. H. Gates. 1966. Fertilization of mixed cheatgrass-bluebunch wheatgrass stands. *J. Range Mgmt.* 19:134–137.

Woolfolk, E. J., and D. A. Duncan. 1962. Fertilizers increase range production. *J. Range Mgmt.* 15:42–45.

Chapter 20

Soil and Water Conservation

Rangelands the world over have experienced more extensive damage by wind and water erosion than is normally expected from geological causes. This acceleration of damage is a result of overgrazing, of direct harvesting of fuel wood in deserts and forests, of cultivation, and of other upsets in the natural systems (Fig. 20-1). Soil erosion from uncultivated rangelands during and immediately following severe droughts may be greatly accelerated due to previous mismanagement.

The distinction between erosion as a normal process and as accelerated destruction is difficult to determine. However, normal geologic erosion is severe only in the rare instances when climate changes or when land has risen or subsided rapidly; otherwise it is barely detectable. No soil would exist on sloping land if geological erosion were faster than soil formation.

Much erosion has been attributed to the results of burning. Certainly, increased erosion is likely to occur immediately following destruction of vegetation. Fire or any other factor that reduces foliage also reduces interception, transpiration, and cover, thereby increasing the amount of water available for surface overflow. But fire has been a factor in most vegetational types of the world far

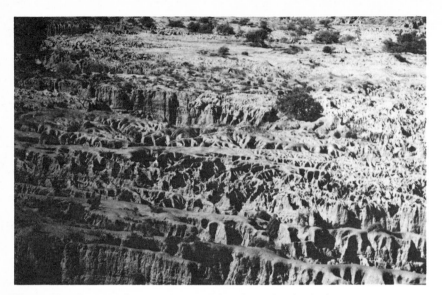

Figure 20-1 Severe soil destruction caused by faulty farming in the valley, and overgrazing in the watershed, Vlekpoort, Republic of South Africa.

longer than man has been exerting his influence. If fire effects were permanent or greater than could be repaired between burns, soil and vegetation would disappear. Some 30 widely scattered experiments indicate that removal of forest cover by any means increases streamflow and modifies the water regime, but these effects continue to diminish after the first year (Raeder-Roitzsch, 1968). A few vegetational types may change from brush to grass with increased fire; thus fire may result in decreased erosion.

Until the last few decades, erosion was promoted by (1) lack of knowledge about its causes and cures, (2) a limited population that either had little overall effect on resources or in which people could move to a new site as an old one was destroyed, and (3) uninformed land regulations or customs. The rock terraces in the Middle East illustrate the fact that soil management and erosion have been problems since cultivation began. These neatly contoured rock walls are mostly abandoned and hold little soil. We do not know if they were used to keep in place soil that was originally formed there, to hold soil hauled from the lowlands by the donkey load, to catch soil eroding from above, or for a combination of these purposes. Much of the terraced land in the Middle East is on limestone that is highly fissured, with deep soil in the cracks. Perhaps early cultivators found that a relatively small effort in terracing these slopes paid handsomely in grapes and olives, both of which depend on deep soil. Nor is it clear whether loss of soil from these terraces caused the downfall of civilizations or came after wars had reduced populations and forced them to leave, abandoning the land for short or extended periods. However, it is certain that abandoned man-made structures are reduced by the forces of nature. Rangeland structures that are made to alter normal flows of water need constant care. Others that restore flows to normal gradients gradually become a part of the natural landscape.

THE EROSION PROCESS

Soil erosion relates to the protection from and resistance of soil to the forces of water and wind. These forces have two actions: dislodgement of soil particles and transport (Bennett et al., 1951). In many respects, water and wind are similar in their actions of dislodgment and transport. Occasionally water and wind interact, as with driven rain, and seldom does a range area show erosion by one force and not the other.

Erosion by Water

The impact of falling raindrops is the most widespread of the dislodgement forces. Five centimeters of rain per hectare deliver enough force to lift eighteen centimeters of soil to a height of 1 meter (Nichols and Gray, 1941). If the raindrops are large, the force is delivered in blows that dislodge soil particles and splash them in all directions. When the raindrops are tiny, little dislodgement of soil particles occurs. On level land with rain falling vertically, splash is equal in all directions and there is little net loss of soil, but the greater the slope, the more downhill the creep of material. On 10 percent slope, the downgrade splash is about three times the upgrade movement. A violent storm could splash as much as 250 tons per hectare (Ellison, 1950). Perhaps accumulation of soil within a healthy bunchgrass plant is due to this action. Splash effects show as muddy walls following a rain and as flattening of a pile of sand.

Splash erosion destroys soil structure, places particles in suspension, and keeps mixing water and soil. This action of mixing water and soil commonly is called *puddling*. As muddy water infiltrates the soil, the suspended particles tend to plug the soil pores, sometimes completely preventing further intake of water. A dry, unstructured soil, such as dust, traps air, which also prevents wetting except on the puddled surface. When the sealed layer dries, it forms a crust. All this tends to waterproof the land and to increase surface runoff. Gross splash can be used as a soil erodability index (Yamamoto and Anderson, 1973).

The overland flow of water transports soil materials and nutrients dislodged by raindrops and further loosens soil particles by abrasion. The first sheet erosion of soil may not be noticed readily, but it results in concentration of water, loss of fertility, and scouring action that soon is evidenced by rills and grooves in the land.

The deeper water-cut channels become gullies, the worst of which often occur toward the bottoms of watersheds. Gullies gradually work headward as soil sloughs from the steep sides and is carried away. Large gullies often are objects of concerted schemes for action, such as the Vlekpoort scheme in South Africa, the program on the damaged land near Kondoa in Tanzania, and the treatment of the gullied areas in the United States in the 1930s.

Erosion-control structures such as sizable dams or gully plugs often are bypassed with new gullies unless steps are taken to reduce peaks of surface flow from the watershed. Terraces and contour structures, which aim at controlling surface water flow, fail all too often. They may fill with silt or be breached by a burrowing animal. They are not effective in preventing downhill splash erosion, which may flatten a contour terrace. Any furrow break concentrates flow, which cuts a new gully in its downhill rush of water.

As a principle, surface water flow, or runoff, should be prevented by soil and vegetational management that promotes as much infiltration as possible where the rain falls. Splash or puddle erosion, fertility erosion, and sheet erosion may be as damaging to productivity as large gullies, but the damage is difficult to assess and seldom determined. Measured soil loss is usually that scoured from gullies and channels. Good vegetational management of the watershed must be the first practice. It will lessen potential erosion in crisis areas and promote healing on most of the watershed. Those few areas that do not respond may be treated with dams, terraces, or other practices.

Since runoff is inevitable and necessary and erosion is a natural process, the reasonable approach is to manage runoff and erosion according to the productivity objectives of an area. These may vary from promoting as much runoff as possible with no erosion to preventing both runoff and erosion completely, even preventing geological erosion. *Runoff* in this chapter refers only to surface or overland flow of water.

Some soils, especially those with a loose sandy layer over dense clay and those with high silt content which also have low absorptive capacity and low organic matter, are highly erodable. Stability of soil structure influences erodability. Aggregated clays tend to be difficult to erode until the structure is broken. The topography makes a great difference in erosion rate, as multiplying the slope by 4 roughly results in twice the velocity of flow, 4 times the eroding power, 32 times the material carried, and 64 times the size of material that can be moved. The force of running water is dependent on volume and rate of flow, which are related to intensity and duration of rainfall.

Soil texture, soil structure, slope, and rainfall are, to a degree, beyond man's control, so he usually resorts first to management of the amount and kind of plant cover on the soil. For example, Ellison (1950) suggested from widespread studies in Texas and Oklahoma that a grass stand with 7 tons of herbage and litter per hectare yielded only 1.2 tons of splashed soil per hectare. Infiltration of water into the soil was 6 centimeters in 15 minutes. Nearby, on bare soil, 170 tons of soil per hectare were splashed and water intake was 2.5 millimeters in 15 minutes. From similar work, Allred (1950) suggested that approximately 2,800 kilograms per hectare of plant material is adequate to keep splash erosion below 15 tons per hectare, which he considered adequate protection. Soil algae and lichens in his study reduced the amount of mulch needed to hold soil in light storms, but they often were broken by heavy rain.

Soils that do not rapidly absorb water may be subject to high runoff and erosion. Nonwettable soils have been reported in several western states, Florida, New Zealand, and Australia (DeBano et al., 1967). Hydrophobic conditions may be associated with microorganisms or chemical substances in live plant materials and mulch. Nonwettability can be intensified by fire, as shown in California chaparral and desert scrub (Adams, Strain, and Adams, 1970). It seems to be associated with a range of 200° to 425°C in the soil temperature gradient during a fire. Preliminary research has shown that application of wetting agents can increase infiltration, decrease runoff and erosion, and increase grass establishment (DeBano et al., 1967). The practicality of large-scale application of wetting agents is yet to be determined.

Erosion by Wind

Wind erosion is similar to water erosion in causes, results, and cures. It occurs where the soil is exposed to the dislodging force of moving air and varies with structure of dry soil; surface roughness; slope; cover on the soil; and velocity, angle of incidence, and duration of air movement. A 40-kilometer-per-hour wind has four times the power to pick up soil as has a 20-kilometer-per-hour wind. Dune sands begin to move with wind velocities of 15 to 25 kilometers per hour. As soil particles are moved by air, they have an abrasive action that dislodges more soil. Control can be attained by decreasing exposure to wind with tillage practices or by planting vegetation that covers the soil and adds organic matter that promotes improved soil structure.

In arid and semiarid regions, where much bare soil exists, maintenance of shrub types of vegetation is the principal way to control soil erosion by wind. Shrubs occupy area, reducing exposure of the soil to wind. The most efficient shrubs for this purpose are the ones that have their greatest width at ground level. Shrubs present a frontal or vertical silhouette from any direction, thus reducing wind velocity. Wind-tunnel experiments suggest that relatively narrow shrubs with a low diameter-height ratio—less than 2—give sufficient roughness to reduce wind erosion and provide an herbaceous grazing resource between the shrubs (Marshall, 1970).

RECOGNITION OF EROSION

Anyone working on rangeland needs to be able to recognize erosion. Perhaps the first obvious signs are pedestal plants with roots showing and movement of soil away from rocks and burned woody stems. The newly exposed rocks and stem bases usually are light in color, thereby indicating the depth of soil that has been removed. Often fine debris will have accumulated in small nearby contour ridges and lodged at the uphill side of any obstruction to water flow. Rills or small grooves of V shape will be present, and pebbles or gravel may be accumulating on the soil surface during early stages of accelerated erosion. More or less level areas are sites of soil accumulation when gentle slopes begin to erode. More serious are subsoil and bedrock exposure, mud flows from slopes, mud bars along streams, gorged channels, floods with higher peaks, undercut stream banks, lowering of the water table, and large gullies that are head cutting. Any of these should be recognized as a warning that erosion is active. Normally, the steeper the land, the more essential it is to recognize erosion when it starts, to appraise its causes, and to take remedial steps (Gleason, 1953).

CONTROL OF EROSION WITH COVER

Because erosion begins at the soil surface, maintenance of soil cover is the most important way to prevent erosion and to heal eroded areas. A cover composed of vegetation and surface organic material breaks the beating action of rain, intercepts some of the rain, keeps the surface soil moist longer than does bare soil, improves soil structure by adding organic matter, and protects the soil from wind. Vegetation reduces the rate of water flow across the surface by damming it and continually breaking larger volumes of flow into smaller volumes. Even unattached organic material that may float and move with runoff water tends to lodge, making tiny debris basins. Thus, more time is taken for flow from hillside to channel, resulting in lower flood peaks, more water infiltrating into soil, more storage of water in soil, and gradual release of water for later channel flow.

Through long experience, most soil conservationists on rangeland have learned to concentrate their efforts on managing vegetation rather than on making downstream structures of concrete and stone. Conservation practices that employed cover, plantings, and farming techniques were subsidized by the federal government on 10 million hectares in 1967. Dams, terraces, waterways, dikes, ditches, shaping of slopes, and drainages were applied to slightly over 1.2 million hectares (Agriculture Stabilization and Conservation Service, 1968). The large area involved in the 1967 government subsidy program supports the notion that major effort is aimed at reducing the effects of eroding forces on each square meter of soil rather than at stopping runoff water and soil somewhere downstream.

Amounts of Cover Needed

Although cover and amounts of mulch or organic residues have been used to suggest proper utilization of ranges, there still is little specific information about the relation of mulch quantity to the condition of the soil surface. Protection requirements for granitic soils in southwestern Idaho appeared to be 70 percent cover of soil with plants and mulch in perennial wheatgrass *(Agropyron inerme)* and 90 percent cover in annual grass *(Bromus tectorum)*. Normally these requirements mean that spots of bare soil should be no larger than 10 centimeters in diameter in the wheatgrass type and 5 centimeters in the annual type. Runoff was most closely related to cover, and erosion to the size of bare soil patches (Packer, 1951). Few studies on mountain ranges have suggested less than 60 percent cover for control of overland water flow and erosion. Plant and mulch cover accounted for 52 to 80 percent of the explained variance in erosion in a number of studies (Packer and Laycock, 1969).

Erosion is prevented mainly in proportion to the amount of soil surface protected from raindrop impact with a cover of mulch, plants, and stone. Of secondary importance in preventing erosion are bulk density and soil pore space, as illustrated below by measurements with artificial rainfall on subalpine range in central Utah (Meeuwig, 1965) and at other summer range sites in Idaho and Montana (Meeuwig, 1970).

	Four summer range sites			
Cover, %	85.0	73.9	70.6	63.1
Bulk density (0–25 cm), %	0.96	1.02	0.99	1.04
Noncapillary porosity (0–25 cm), %	18.8	19.6	15.1	17.7
Sediment, kg/ha	194	508	942	1,106

Effects of Changing Cover Type

Managers of rangeland frequently are concerned with changes in vegetational type and the effects these changes have on runoff and erosion. In the chaparral type of southern California, removal of the shrub cover by fire leaves the steep slopes highly susceptible to erosion (Fig. 20-2). Some slopes, steeper than the angle of repose, immediately begin to show creep as material rolls downhill. Similar soil movement occurs in the mountains of New Zealand's South Island. Even where slopes are not so steep, increases in surface runoff and erosion often occur during the bare-soil period between destruction of one vegetational type and establishment of the next. Significant drops in runoff and sediment production occur as vegetative cover becomes reestablished. Means of cover replacement are discussed in the chapter on seeding.

Where grass replaces woody plants on deep soil and adequate rainfall exists to wet the whole soil profile, increased water yield will occur. Grasses, normally being less deep-rooted than woody plants, remove water from only the upper parts of the soil profile, resulting in less needed to recharge the profile and more runoff. Rowe and Reimann (1961) suggested that the soil must be at least 1 meter deep for significant differences in water yield between grass and chaparral types to exist. Kittredge (1954) stated that on deep soil a grass cover will give about the same erosion loss as pine, but five times the runoff. Where rainfall is light and soils are shallow, the type of plant is of little consequence to the water budget.

Following cover-type change, adjustments in the hydrological regime may take only a year or decades may be needed to achieve complete soil and slope stability. For example, deep woody roots take several years to decompose. When they do and only grass roots remain, land slipping may occur as deep soil support is reduced (Rice and Foggin, 1971). Land slipping may occur several years after the vegetation has been converted to grass. Soil movements from stream channels reduce the support for upper slopes, which begin to erode or to seek new stable gradients, sometimes taking years or decades to do so. Removal of phreatophytes certainly increases water yield, 43 percent in one case (Rowe, 1963), but it also increases channel scouring and watershed instability. Adjustments in stands of water, but these may result in unstable watersheds. Additional means of manipulating water outflow include changing the vegetation from perennials to annuals, which transpire for only a part of the year, changing the vegetation to species that have a different rooting depth, and defoliating transpiring vegetation.

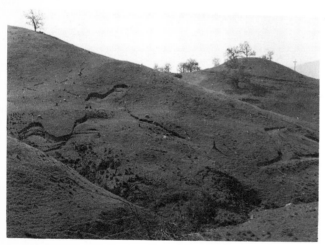

Figure 20-2 Landslips occurred on this site after the woody cover was removed.

MECHANICAL STRUCTURES TO CONTROL WATER EROSION

Gullies may be especially active in different positions along their length. At the head of a gully, grass and other herbaceous cover often hold the top few centimeters of soil with a mass of fibrous roots. Woody plants and tap-rooted species hold a thicker layer of soil than do the grasses, but gullies deeper than approximately ½ meter grow by undercutting the soil slumping along the sides and head. Other gullies may be cutting fastest in their lower elevations. Young gullies that are growing both upstream and downstream need control measures at these critical points. Older gullies that are continuous with the main drainages should be attacked first where they are most active, normally in the lowest segments. Control measures that do not treat all critical points are likely to fail (Heede, 1970).

Mechanical structures are necessary to control gullies or large flows in emergency situations. Examples of such structures would be a series of small dams used to raise the water table in a mountain meadow that had been cut with a gully. Dams of this type may be constructed from materials available at the site or from prefabricated, interlocking metal strips that can be delivered by helicopter or packed by horses to inaccessible places. The U.S. Forest Service has used dams of this type in meadows high in the Sierra Nevada Mountains, and in other places. Their best use is near the headlands in small gullies, but even there the outlets and spillways need protection. These dams are placed so that the water held by each nearly reaches the dam above. Gully-filling projects that exploit nearby topsoil and expose subsoil, without watershed management above the gullies, should be avoided.

Thousands of soil and water conservation structures were built by the Civilian Conservation Corps and other agencies between 1934 and 1942. In 1949 and 1961, about 900 such structures in the Gila and Membres River basins in Arizona and New Mexico were examined for structural soundness, erosion-control effectiveness, and vegetational response (Peterson and Branson, 1962). Treatments included earth-filled dams; gully plugs of various materials; and water spreaders made of rock, soil, brush, concrete, and wire. Over half of the structures had been breached within a few years after construction, and the total quantity of trapped sediment amounted to less material than was used in the original construction of the structures. Failures were due to poor siting, improper design, faulty construction, and lack of maintenance. The success of conservation structures in this and other areas show that they can be effective in controlling erosion and are necessary in certain situations.

The Vlekpoort Reclamation Scheme

Several erosion-control principles are illustrated by the extended program to control deep gullies in the upper reaches of the Vlekpoort River, South Africa

(Labuscagne and de Villiers, 1966). The first step in 1946 was to build dams in the larger gullies. One 4.3-meter dam, as an example, had sedimentation to the dam overflow in one year but did not fill to a stable gradient until 1953. At that time, sediments extended 915 meters upstream from the dam. During 1959 and 1960, extensive plantings with *Phragmites communis* and *Sorghum almum* were made in the sediments furthest from the dam and along the stream banks. Revegetation resulted in renewed sediment deposition both downstream and upstream from the plantings. By 1963, sediments reached 1,617 meters upstream, where they were 7.5 meters above the spillway level.

This example shows that relatively large dams are necessary to initiate deep-gully control and that vegetation planted in the accumulated sediment increases the dams' effectiveness. Shaping of gully sides was not done in this scheme, although frequently it is recommended. Sedimentation builds the V-shaped gullies into U-shaped ones and eventually into flat valleys with ever-increasing width. Coincident with valley filling, depth and velocity of water flow decrease, further promoting sedimentation. Introduced plant species need to be the kinds that will survive flooding and sedimentation. They usually are rhizomatous and nodal rooting. Mature stems from tall-growing and coarse grasses, such as those mentioned above, are excellent local sources of mulch that can spread over bare surfaces to enlarge the erosion-control area. Once a stable gradient is achieved, normal bed-load or eroding material will cross it, so the final solution is to reduce erosion from slopes above the gullies. This suggests that the source of trouble may be faulty management above the gullies, with excess runoff scouring the valley.

In Malawi, an opposite situation occurs. There the spectacular erosion is in the uplands. Broad, often water-logged valleys are holding the sediments and actually increasing in size. The few eroding spots in the valleys are small in size and are healing at the lower edges as rapidly as they are head cutting. Although an initial erosion-control scheme may aim its efforts downstream, the major problems and final solutions usually are on the headwater slopes.

Control of Bank-Cutting

Streams that are cutting their banks on the curves during peak flows may be controlled, but the necessary procedures are expensive. The banks need to be shaped or sloped so they will hold riprap of rocks or heavy materials. Plantings of *Salix* spp., *Alnus* spp., and other riparian woody plants above and in the riprap add stability to banks. Finally, fencing to prevent grazing and to promote a tangle of growth on the stream bank is advisable.

Contour Terraces and Trenches

In 1930, following disastrous summer floods from the western slopes of the Wasatch Mountains in Utah, several watersheds were closed to grazing, and fire control was intensified to prevent further depletion of vegetative cover. On selected highly eroded spots labeled *flood source areas,* about 700 hectares in extent, contour trenches were constructed and seeded to interrupt the gully system and to keep rain where it fell. Specifications for the terraces included zero-grade, spacing and depth sufficiently close to hold 4 centimeters of rain, and check dams at 8-meter intervals across but slightly lower than the terrace dike. Success of the whole rehabilitation program was evident in 1936 and 1945, when storms of greater rainfall rates than the storms of 1930 occurred with no flooding (Bailey and Copeland, 1961).

As the above example showed, increased vegetation on the slopes and terraces reduced the need for special structures in the drainages (Fig. 20-3). Where gradients are less than 15 to 20 percent or 7.5 to 10 degrees, an out-sloped type of terrace is recommended. The in-sloped type may be used on steeper land, to about 35 degrees. However, any manipulation of soil and vegetation on land inclined greater than 20 to 25 degrees should be approached with caution, lest soil disturbance cause even greater erosion.

Contour-basin terraces of the in-sloped type constructed after fire on the San Dimas Experimental Forest in southern California failed when unaided by barley plantings. The barley plantings alone, as contour-row plantings, proved to be the best erosion-control measures tested (Hill, 1963). These examples suggest that terraces on steep land can be effective if they result in improvement of vegetative cover. They should be applied only where quick development of cover is absolutely necessary, normally in small areas to give a measure of relief to larger areas that will recover without expensive treatment.

For terraces to succeed on mountain lands, they need to be on deep soil (75 centimeters) with mass stability or no slumping, be of ample size, and have an

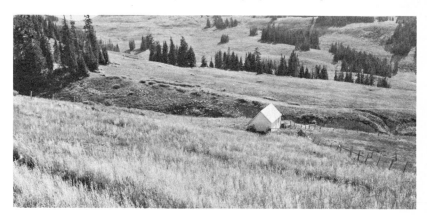

Figure 20-3 This is Watershed B on the Great Basin Experimental Range, Ephraim, Utah. Watershed studies began here in 1912. Two years after contour trenching and seeding in 1952, as shown in the photo, little erosion had occurred. *(Photo by U.S. Forest Service.)*

infiltration capacity that will accommodate the ponded water without overflow. Seeding and terracing are likely to be mutually beneficial to each other and to watershed stability, especially in areas of low rainfall. Success of Trigo pubescent wheatgrass *(Agropyron trichophorum)* in an area of 200 millimeters of rainfall in California was much better with deep, lister-type furrows on the contour than with shallow-drilled rows (Cornelius and Burma, 1970).

Contour Furrows, Plantings, and Ridges

Other mechanical structures or treatments of rangeland for the purposes of eliminating, reducing, or deflecting runoff and controlling erosion include contour furrows, strips that are simply plowed, plantings, and ridges. These structures, although used widely on rangeland in the past, are seldom used today. Ranges in excellent condition usually do not need them, since control of runoff and erosion by the vegetational cover normally is adequate, reliable, and permanent.

Contour-plowed furrows are used on slopes of less than 20 percent in the northern Great Plains to control erosion and to encourage *Agropyron smithii* and other rhizomatous grasses. Seeding may be a part of the operation because the cleared strips are excellent seedbeds. The furrows are 7.5 to 15 centimeters deep, of similar width, and spaced 1.3 or fewer meters apart. Sod turned by furrowing may be rolled or packed to reduce weeds the first year. These furrows should be end blocked and should not cross gullies, trails, or low places where gullies could develop. Somewhat deeper furrows may be used to protect downstream structures.

Runoff and Erosion from Roads

Range roads, especially those in mountainous areas originally constructed for logging purposes, are major sources of runoff and sediment. Many are considered temporary at the time of building, so little care is taken to construct proper roadbeds, drainages, and erosion-control structures. Often new roadbeds are subjected to sudden and severe storms, frost heaving, and snow-melt runoff before vegetation and stable soil conditions are reestablished. In order to lessen damage to the roads themselves and to reduce sediments in the watersheds, several practices are recommended.

First, the road fill should use rocks and soil with as little organic debris as possible. Second, a drainage system should be constructed which removes water from the road in small streams; keeps water away from fill areas; and discharges the runoff onto vegetated slopes, against obstructions such as fallen trees, slash, and brush clumps, and through protective, unlogged strips before it reaches a major drainage. Third, raw surfaces of cuts and fills should be seeded, mulched, staked, terraced, wattled, or even cribbed to stabilize them initially against heavy rains and runoff. These practices are most effective if established before the first rain. Mulching is the most effective during the first season.

Careful selection of road locations can do much to reduce drainage and erosion problems. Building of roads on heavy clay soils should be avoided. Attention to both vertical and horizontal curvature largely determines the amount of cut and fill surface, which is directly related to erosion potential. Fill slopes, especially, should be stabilized with planted species. The nearer the road curves are to the natural landscape profiles, the more the road fits the natural beauty of the landscape, usually with the least damage to landscape stability.

SAND CONTROL

Permanent control of sand movement normally is accomplished with plantings of sand-loving plants, such as *Ammophila* spp. along seacoasts or *Tamarix* spp. as used on the sands in Saudi Arabia. Native species, such as *Calamovilfa longifolia* and *Andropogon hallii,* are used in the Nebraska Sand Hills. Plantings should begin on the windward side of the zone of deposition (McLaughlin and Brown, 1942). *Ammophila arenaria* was most successful on sand dunes along the Pacific Northwest coast, and success was enhanced by planting at a spacing of 12 by 60 centimeters and fertilizing during low winter temperatures (Brown and Hafenrichter, 1948). In the deep-sand areas of the north central United States, matured grass hay is spread as a mulch and anchored by mixing it with the sand. A cover crop of sorghum, sudan grass, or even cereal grain is sometimes raised. Then the sand-loving grasses are seeded directly into the stubble for a more permanent cover.

Other type barriers, such as snow fencing or slatted wooden fences, as well as plantings, tend to hold sand in place or to stop sand from moving. These work well if the sand is in narrow strips or the areas small. Large sand deserts, such as the Great Nafud in Saudi Arabia, can hardly be controlled or stabilized to protect a road or a canal, for example. Justification for sand stabilization projects is difficult where square kilometers of sand are moving toward low-value developments. One approach in such situations is to build structures that tend to channel or intensify the wind into smaller areas (Whitfield, 1938), thereby causing the wind velocity to increase, as through a funnel. Such channeling has been accomplished by placing sealing strips of asphalt or tar parallel with the prevailing wind. The tendency is for the wind to move the sand from between the strips at a velocity that carries the sand beyond the road (Fig. 20-4). Picket fences at a slight angle to the wind also promote scouring of the dunes. The distance between pickets should be about the same as the width of the picket so that nearly the same proportion of air goes through and over the fence. Bags filled with sand and placed on dune crests lower as wind removes the sand from around them. If the dunes are isolated and surrounded by hard land, listing or roughening the hard land to hold the sand is essential to lowering of the dune profile.

The location of fences for both snow and sand control on irregular terrain determines the pattern of deposition. When the fence is placed on the windward

ROAD

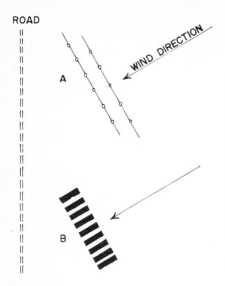

Figure 20-4 Arrangement of barriers to control movement of sand by wind. A: Barriers to stop sand movement by wind before the sand covers the road. If the barriers are irregular in top line, concentrated wind will result in sand blowouts, increasing unevenness of the dune, and difficulty in holding the barrier. A single fence causes a sharp crest, while a double fence properly spaced results in a gently rounded dune crest. B: Barriers or asphalted strips of sand arranged parallel with the prevailing wind will promote increased wind velocity between the barriers and sand crossing the road. Asphalted and bare strips are of the same width.

side of a hill crest, the resulting dune or snow drift will be short and high. Fences on a crest result in long accumulations downhill to leeward. Barriers placed on the lee of the crest are likely to be covered (Schmidt, 1970).

The objectives in sand control are to lower dune crests, to reduce slopes to at least a 3:1 horizontal-vertical ratio, and to spread the sand as evenly as possible. When these objectives are accomplished, vegetational control is most effective and, except in a few situations, fencing or other devices to control sand become temporary. On the other hand, fencing, proper use, and other animal-management practices are continually needed on unstable and vulnerable sandy sites if forage production is to be maintained.

WINDBREAKS AND SHELTERBELTS

Windbreaks and shelterbelts have had a long history in the control of wind erosion. Denmark began planting trees in the 1860s to control sand movement after destruction of heather stands and faulty cultivation practices resulted in large areas of moving sand. Russia used shelterbelts even earlier. Experience and research showed that the most effective windbreaks were filters with 30 to 40 percent holes rather than complete barriers to air movement. Effectiveness was increased with more height rather than with more width, since the wider the windbreak planting, the less permeable it usually was. This relationship has resulted in windbreak effects being measured in terms of changes to leeward according to distance in units of windbreak height. At ten times the height, measurements suggest 20 percent less evaporation from soil, 3 percent higher relative humidity, higher air temperatures, less wind damage, and increased yields of several crops (Zethner-Moller, 1968). Twenty times the height would appear to be a reasonable distance between windbreaks which would give at least a little protection to all areas. A single windbreak should be 30 to 100 meters from the major area to be protected.

Windbreaks are common sights in the plains and prairie portions of the United States. Most farmsteads and feedlots have them on the northern and western sides for protection in the winter from severe storms and in the summer from hot winds. Their contrasting colors and shapes provide beauty, and they furnish areas for recreational sports and wildlife habitat. On the one hand, increased wood supply and protection from cold winds reduce fuel costs. On the other hand, windbreaks may harbor pests of various kinds, they occupy space, and the land on either side is unsuitable for cultivation because of shade and root competition.

The windbreak itself may be a single row of trees, as along the windward side of a field, or a planting of several species in a dozen or more rows. Normally, fewer rows are used in the Western, drier areas than in the Eastern prairies. Rows should be 3 to 6 meters apart—a distance selected to accommodate shallow cultivation between them for weed control. Spacings within the rows are 1 meter for shrubs, 1 to 3 meters for low deciduous trees, 2 to 3 meters for conifers, and 3 to 4 meters for tall trees. Each row may be a different species, but 20 to 50 percent of the planting should be evergreen. Most windbreaks are planted in straight lines. Contour plantings and irregular shapes, accomplished with groups of different species at the ends and along the sides, enhance soil protection and beauty. Except in single-row shelterbelts, alternating species within a row should be avoided. Other don'ts about windbreaks include not placing tall, spreading species adjacent to lower species; grazing; burning; spraying with herbicides; allowing overpopulations of rodents; or planting too close to ditches, terraces, and drains. Local and state laws prohibit plantings that result in blind highway corners, grow into or increase maintenance of utility lines, and cause snow to drift onto roadways.

An example of a good seven-row windbreak in central Kansas is as follows: (1) *Cotoneaster* spp., (2) *Juniperus virginiana,* (3) *Pinus nigra,* (4) *Morus* spp., (5) *Populus* spp., (6) *Ulmus parvifolia,* (7) *Juniperus virginiana.* This planting gives contrasting colors in leaves, flowers, and fruits for beauty, food and shelter for wildlife, and wind control during winter and summer. Windbreaks vary widely in composition and layout because of wide differences in soils and climates. Before a windbreak is established, local practice should be investigated.

WATER-USE PRACTICES

A number of practices closely related to those for mechanical control of erosion are used to make more efficient use of water in semiarid and arid areas. These include cutting contour furrows, pitting, water spreading, and water harvesting. They are based on the principle that one way to manage runoff is to manipulate the depression storage capacity of the land. Interrupted contour terraces, which were described earlier, also serve this purpose.

Pitting or Interrupted Contour Furrows

Range pitting is accomplished by turning fine- and medium-textured soil with a disk for a length of 0.6 to 1 meter, to a depth of 7.5 to 16 centimeters, in rows 0.6 to 1 meter apart (Fig. 20-5). Adjacent disks are on separate eccentrics so that as one enters the soil, another is lifted. Pitting with a one-way eccentric disk and scalping with a sod drill proved effective in the western Great Plains beginning about 1939 (Barnes and Nelson, 1945; Rauzi et al., 1962). Pitting with either a disk or a tined pitter is used to minimize wind effects and to trap moisture in South Australia (Young, 1969). This technique also is known as *constructing interrupted contour furrows*. It normally is restricted to areas with less than 20 percent slope.

Pits 1.5 meters long and 1.5 to 2.5 meters wide were found to increase herbage production of *Cenchrus ciliaris* by two and one-half times over the conventional small pits and five times over untreated range in the 15- to 20-centimeter summer rainfall zone in southern Arizona. The pits were constructed so that all runoff water passed through them (Slayback and Cable, 1970). The resulting short, irregularly-spaced disk furrows or pits have no regular drainage from one to another. They are placed on the contour to hold as much water as possible. On flat ground, they may be placed perpendicular to prevailing winter winds in order to catch snow.

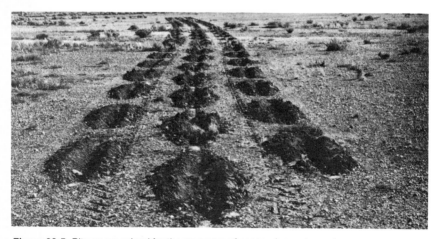

Figure 20-5 Pits on rangeland for the purposes of conserving water and increasing forage production.

The purpose of pitting is to increase forage production by breaking soil crusting, encouraging water infiltration, and decreasing water runoff. This purpose may be accomplished even if the pits fill with sand, which has a high infiltration rate. Pitting is most commonly used in the northern Great Plains area of the United States, but even there, a question of its economic value exists. Productivity increases, but whether it increases enough to compensate for pitting costs has not been determined. Pits normally fill with sand or soil in about five years, but their effect may last longer.

Efforts to rehabilitate bare and badly eroded flat land in the Ord River Catchment of northern West Australia have resulted in several adaptations of implements for the purpose of promoting water penetration into soil. One is an opposed-disk plow with a central deep ripper and attached seeder box. It is similar in action to the Arcadia Model B contour-furrowing machine. The disks are operated as a pitter to make interrupted contour furrows that do not channel water. The deep ripper provides broken ground under the bank of loose soil, making it more stable than a heap of loose soil on compacted ground. This machine is combined with a chisel plow that loosens the soil for one machine width on the upslope side. The "pits" and plowed strips have retained seed and water-collection characteristics for five years and have been effective in rehabilitating large areas of bare soil (Fitzgerald, 1968).

Low contour dikes about 50 centimeters in height, sometimes called *broad-base furrows,* and contour furrows in medium- to heavy-textured soils, at intervals of 1 to 1.6 meters, to depths of 20 to 25 centimeters increased yield of herbage from 560 to 1,600 kilograms per hectare under a wide variety of conditions from Montana to Arizona (Branson et al., 1966). Favorable results were due to reduced runoff, higher soil moisture, and seeding of new species on the disturbed soil. Ripping and pitting with disks and spike-toothed implements were not so effective. The decrease in water catchment in furrows was rapid for about five years, but effects were evident in the vegetation for much longer. Sandy soils gave little response. Sites dominated by *Atriplex nuttallii* showed the most improvement, and those with *Eurotia lanata, Bouteloua eripoda,* and *Stipa comata* did not respond favorably.

Leaching Basins

Level lands in western New South Wales, Australia, which have lost patches of topsoil often form into alternating low ridges and shallow basins with impermeable surfaces devoid of vegetation. The surfaces may be sealed due to high sodium content. Few mechanical techniques except dikes that impound water that gradually leaches some of the salts, thereby permitting vegetation to invade or seedings to be successful, have been successful on these areas. In a Montana area with high salts, forage production increased as leaching in furrowed soil reduced calcium, magnesium, and sodium (Branson et al., 1966).

Water Spreaders

A water spreader is a system for spreading flood waters to irrigate land, to reduce and store sediment, or to obtain deep storage of ground water, as is done in the San Gabriel Valley, California. Native species may be encouraged for hay growth by water spreading in wet or dry meadows in the western United States. Crops of grain, vegetables, fruits, and fiber are planted on land where water is spread in Australia, Israel, Saudi Arabia, and other countries with desert climates. Seldom are water spreaders economically justified for grazing purposes alone; yet the interrelationships between and needs for better water management and range use require that they be described as a part of rangeland management.

Many attempts at water spreading have failed because of inadequate designs. Engineers often have attempted to handle the whole flow of a waterway with structures that have all too often been inadequate in an unusual storm. The results are destroyed dikes, breached check dams, broken terraces, and new gullies. For example, unless the water checks are extremely large and well protected at flow points, the type of system shown in Figure 20-6 will sooner or later be overtopped and destroyed because the tendency is always for the flow to cut back to its original

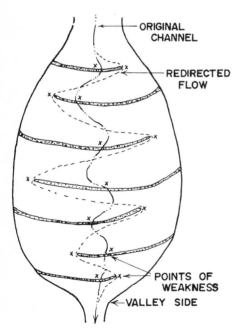

Figure 20-6 Points of weakness are shown in a simple water-spreading system. The greatest pressure of water occurs against the center and at the end of each dike, around which water tends to flow rapidly. No provision, except the height of the dikes, is made to handle large floods. Extremely flat land (1 percent or less slope) is required for the water to spread; otherwise floods will develop a new channel around the dikes. This sketch illustrates a type of water spreading that frequently fails. Ancient systems in the Middle East suggest that the terraces should be tied to both banks and a central, wide, adequate spillway should be used to allow overflow to the next terrace. The basins above each terrace eventually will fill with silt, resulting in a new slope gradient for the whole area. A break then may cause a deep gully where none existed before.

course. When the break comes, a gully larger than the previous one may be formed.

Diverting water from large watersheds, say 1 square kilometer and larger, requires structures that will contain large flash floods or will divert only a part of the flow. The potential damage from large flows, the greater percentage runoff from small areas than from large watersheds, and probably the heavy work of construction and maintenance led the ancient peoples of the Middle East to concentrate on small areas. In one Israeli study, only one diversion canal was found among old systems that had served more than 5 hectares. Larger developed areas were served by several canals.

Ancient development of runoff water for local agriculture seemed to have followed three stages beginning at about 900 B.C. The first stage was the construction of diversions and simple dikes with wide spillways across broad, flat valleys. Apparently, sedimentation soon caused the dikes to be raised so that water would be prevented from overtopping and damaging the structures. Breaching, sometimes not until systems were abandoned, resulted in cutting of deep gullies. The second stage was a water-spreader system for flood water lifted from the gully by a dam placed upstream with water led to the fields through long canals. The third stage was development of ''runoff farms'' from small drainages on adjacent hillsides. The main drainage system was abandoned as a source of water because sediment from the main channel filled the ditches (Shanan et al., 1961).

These sequential developments were due in part to the gradual but complete sedimentation of the systems to a point where slope gradients could no longer be managed with available terraces. As the land surface builds higher with sedimentation, the terraces must be raised in height, and the tendency is for greater gully cutting when a breach occurs. Studies in New Mexico (Hubbell and Gardner, 1950) showed that sedimentary deposits in water-spreading systems can significantly reduce deposition in channels and reservoirs. However, rapid deposition of 2.5 or more centimeters damaged the forage crop, but this damage varied among species, with *Agropyron smithii* being the least susceptible.

Ancient water-spreading systems in the Negev Desert divided large watersheds and flows into smaller ones by means of separate terraces, diversions, and pipes that could be opened or closed as needed. The architects of these systems applied the principle that the easiest way to handle flood waters was to keep quantities small by reducing volume of flow near the source. No doubt they found large reservoirs or other large structures exceedingly difficult to construct and therefore attacked eroding forces at a scale they could handle. Water forces increase exponentially as the volume increases downstream and become correspondingly more difficult to control. Division included employment of terraces or ditches that subdivided the watersheds, diversions that subdivided the water flow into separate fields, or both types of structures in the same system (Fig. 20-7).

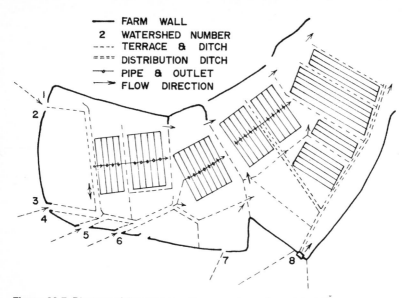

Figure 20-7 Diagram of the ancient water-spreader system at Avdat in Israel as restored for hydrological studies and trials with range grasses, field crops, and fruit trees (Evenari et al., 1968). The farm wall encloses an area approximately 200 by 400 meters. Water from watersheds I–V in part or in total may be used in the first set of plots or bypassed to other fields. After all the fields are irrigated or when the flow is greater than the internal capacity of the system, water may be shunted through or around it without damage. Numbers I–VII in this system divide a single large watershed into seven smaller ones and permit adequate irrigation in any selected field from a small flow. Number VIII shows partial development of another watershed. This is the type of water-spreader system that has been used successfully by various desert civilizations in the Middle East for approximately 3,000 years. Such systems require attention during each water flow, take considerable maintenance, and, on a long-term basis, are destroyed by siltation.

Work in Israel has suggested that a ratio of spreader land (hectares) to watershed should be approximately 1:20–30. This ratio is calculated on the basis of 15 percent runoff from an average of 100 millimeters of annual precipitation and the assumption that the crop needs 400 millimeters of water, therefore

$$100 \text{ mm} \times 0.15 \times 20 \text{ ha} = 30 \text{ mm on 1 ha}$$
$$+ \ 100 \text{ mm of original rainfall} = 400 \text{ mm/ha}$$

This ratio can be adjusted as data or experience become available on rainfall, runoff, and needs. The ratio will be narrower, say 1:10 or 1:15 in areas of 25 to 30 centimeters of rainfall.

Another principle that has emerged from the Israeli work is that the proportion of the precipitation which runs off is greater from smaller watersheds (10 to 20 percent) than from larger ones (1 to 5 percent), due to high percolation into the larger stream beds. In other words, small watersheds give a higher percentage water yield and more frequent flows than do larger watersheds (Tadmor et al., 1960). This was indicated in the comparisons of flows from lysimeters and watersheds varying in size from 32 square meters to 20 or more hectares. Runoff began after 4 to 6 millimeters of rain in small watersheds of less than 25 hectares, while at least 10 to 12 millimeters of rain were required to initiate runoff from large watersheds (Evenari et al., 1961). These are points in favor of keeping the spreader systems as small as possible.

Increased flow from small watersheds over large ones could bring relatively more sediment to dams or other structures in the smaller catchments. Records in the United States show that the larger watersheds produce less sediment per square kilometer than do small watersheds, as follows (Attaullah, 1968):

Watershed size, km^2	Number of measurements	Average annual sediment production, m^3/km^2
<26	650	1,375
26–259	205	570
259–2,590	123	360
>2,590	118	180

Water infiltration into stream beds and sediment entrapment increase as length of drainages increase. Without additional water, flood flows tend to get smaller as they progress downstream. Less volume results in less channel scouring and sediment carrying capacity. What begins as a high proportion of rainwater running off and low water volume in a watercourse at the head of a watershed becomes a lower proportion of runoff but more concentrated volume downstream. The volume, in turn, tends to diminish as the flow proceeds.

Reasons for failure of water-spreading systems appear to be inadequate design, lack of maintenance, poor judgment, or lack of management of water during each flow. The ancient systems were probably manned immediately when enough precipitation occurred to cause runoff. The successful ones today are managed carefully during each flow. Automatic water-spreader operations seem to be beyond economic feasibility. Their principal values are for local irrigation, raising watertables, and diverting water so that gullies will heal.

Water Harvesting

Hand in hand with water spreading (distributing concentrated flow to land outside the stream channel) in regions with less than approximately 200 millimeters of precipitation are watershed practices to minimize infiltration and to increase the runoff. These are commonly known as *water-harvesting practices*. For example, it is known that a rough soil surface, such as a stony surface, retards runoff, promotes infiltration, and slows evaporation. Piling of stones so that their cover of the soil surface was reduced from 10 to 25 percent to 1 to 2 percent increased runoff by 20 to 100 percent in the Negev Desert near Avdat. This is a logical explanation for the piling of stones by ancient peoples in the region. Increased runoff also increased erosion, but this occurred more during the first rains, after rocks were removed, than later, when the disturbed surface had been wetted several times. The same study also showed that the puddled and crusted soil on the areas where stones were removed produced more runoff from gentle slopes than from steep slopes, probably due to differences in horizontal surface area presented to the rain. In these studies, the erosion rate was not high, equivalent to 1 centimeter of soil in 100 years, but even this rate can produce an erosion pavement in a few centuries.

Water harvesting may be used to increase the water available for individual shrubs or a patch of grass. A small area, a microwatershed, say 10 to 1,000 square meters in size, bounded by low dikes, with finely scratched drainage lines oriented toward a corner collecting basin, has furnished enough water for establishment and production of singly planted fruit trees, saltbushes, or grasses in the Negev Desert (Evenari et al., 1968). Small watersheds of this type may be paved or covered with plastic to deliver all precipitation to cisterns for watering plants, livestock, game, and birds.

Evaporator-type solar stills are water-harvesting devices for producing fresh water from salt water in desert areas. They are useful in situations where drinking-water needs for animals and people justify considerable expense. A model of one is shown in Figure 20-8.

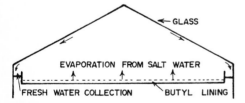

Figure 20-8 Cross section of a greenhouse-type solar distillation unit used to obtain fresh water from salt water in desert areas. Brackish water is led through shallow, Butyl rubber–lined troughs. Heat from the sun vaporizes part of the water, which condenses on the inside of the glass. Fresh-water droplets run down the inside of the glass to the collection troughs. This type of solar still furnishes fresh water for Coober Pedy in the desert center of Australia, at a rate of 90 to 110 liters per year per 0.1 square meter of still, and the fresh water costs $2 to $5 per 1,000 liters.

LITERATURE CITED

Adams, Susan, B. R. Strain, and M. S. Adams. 1970. Water-repellent soils, fire, and annual plant cover in a desert scrub community of southeastern California. *Ecology* 51:696–700.

Agriculture Stabilization and Conservation Service. 1968. *Summary; 1965, 1966, 1967: Agr. Cons. Program.* U.S. Dept. Agr.

Allred, B. W. 1950. What should Texas expect from range conservation? *Texas J. Sci.* 2:7–14.

Attaullah, M. 1968. Watershed management as related to useful life of reservoirs. *Procedures of the 1st West Pakistan Watershed Management Conference,* Pakistan For. Inst., Peshawar, pp. 49–52.

Bailey, R. W., and O. L. Copeland. 1961. *Vegetation and engineering structures in flood and erosion control.* Intermtn. For. and Range Expt. Sta.

Barnes, O. K., and A. L. Nelson. 1945. Mechanical treatments for increasing the grazing capacity of shortgrass range. *Wyo. Agr. Expt. Sta. Bull.* 273.

Bennett, H. H., F. G. Bell, and B. D. Robinson. 1951. Raindrops and erosion. *U.S. Dept. Agr. Cir.* 895.

Branson, F. A., R. F. Miller, and I. S. McQueen. 1966. Contour furrowing, pitting, and ripping on rangelands of the western United States. *J. Range Mgmt.* 19:182–190.

Brown, R. L., and A. L. Hafenrichter. 1948. Factors influencing the production and use of beachgrass and dunegrass clones for erosion control: I. Effect of date of planting. *J. Am. Soc. Agron.* 40:512–521. II. Influence of density of planting. *J. Am. Soc. Agron.* 40:603–609. III. Influence of kinds and amounts of fertilizer on production. *J. Am. Soc. Agron.* 40:677–684.

Cornelius, D. R., and G. D. Burma. 1970. Seeding and seedbed ridging to improve dry grazing land in central California. *Proceedings of the XI International Grassland Congress,* pp. 107–111.

DeBano, L. F., J. F. Osborn, J. S. Krammes, and J. Letey, Jr. 1967. Soil wettability and wetting agents—Our current knowledge of the problem. *U.S. Forest Service Research Paper* PSW-43.

Ellison, W. D. 1950. Soil erosion by rainstorms. *Science* 111:245–249.

Evenari, M., L. Shanan, and N. H. Tadmor. 1968. "Runoff farming" in the desert. I. Experimental layout. *Agron. J.* 60:29–32.

———, ———, ———, and Y. Aharoni. 1961. Ancient desert agriculture in the Negev. *Science* 133:979–996.

Fitzgerald, K. 1968. The Ord River Catchment Regeneration Project. *W. Aust. Dept. Agr. Bull.* 3599.

Gleason, C. H. 1953. Indicators of erosion on watershed land in California. *Trans. Am. Geophys. Union* 34:419–426.

Heede, B. H. 1970. Morphology of gullies in the Colorado Rocky Mountains. *Bull. Internatl. Assoc. Sci. Hydrology XV* 2:79–89.

Hill, L. W. 1963. *The San Dimas Experimental Watershed.* Pacific Southwest Forest and Range Expt. Sta.

Hubbell, D. S., and J. L. Gardner. 1950. Effects of diverting sediment-laden runoff from arroyos to range and crop lands. *U.S. Dept. Agr. Tech. Bull.* 1012.

Kittredge, J. 1954. Influences of pine and grass on surface runoff and erosion. *J. Soil and Water Cons.* 9:179–185.

Labuscagne, P. W., and C. P. M. de Villiers. 1966. The vegetation factor in sediment deposition above a soil reclamation weir. *Proceedings of the 9th International Grassland Congress,* pp. 567–571.

Marshall, J. K. 1970. Assessing the protective role of shrub-dominated rangeland vegetation against soil erosion by wind. *Proceedings of the 11th International Grassland Congress,* pp. 19–23.

McLaughlin, W. T., and R. L. Brown. 1942. Controlling coastal sand dunes in the Pacific Northwest. *U.S. Dept. Agr. Cir.* 660.

Meeuwig, R. O. 1965. Effects of seeding and grazing on infiltration capacity and soil stability of a subalpine range in central Utah. *J. Range Mgmt.* 18:173–180.

———. 1970. Sheet erosion on intermountain summer ranges. *U.S. Dept. Agr. Forest Service Research Paper* INT-85.

Nichols, M. L., and R. B. Gray. 1941. Some important farm machinery and soil conservation relationships. *Agr. Engin.* 22:341–343.

Packer, P. E. 1951. Status of research on watershed protection requirements for granitic mountain soils in southwestern Idaho. *Intermtn. Forest and Range Expt. Sta. Research Paper* 27.

———, and W. A. Laycock. 1969. Watershed management in the United States: Concepts and Principles. *Lincoln Col. Papers in Water Resources* 8:1–22.

Peterson, H. V., and F. A. Branson. 1962. Effects of land treatments on erosion and vegetation on range lands in parts of Arizona and New Mexico. *J. Range Mgmt.* 15:220–226.

Raeder-Roitzsch, J. E. 1968. Watershed research the world over—Results to-date and possible applications in West Pakistan. *Proceedings of the 1st West Pakistan Watershed Management Conference,* Pakistan For. Inst., Peshawar, pp. 299–320.

Rauzi, F., R. L. Lang, and C. F. Becker. 1962. Mechanical treatments on shortgrass rangeland. *Wyo. Agr. Expt. Sta. Bull.* 396.

Rice, R. M., and G. T. Foggin III. 1971. Effect of high intensity storms on soil slippage on mountainous watersheds in southern California. *Water Resources Res.* 7:1485–1496.

Rowe, P. B. 1963. Streamflow increases after removing woodland-riparian vegetation from a southern California watershed. *J. For.* 61:365–370.

———, and L. F. Reimann. 1961. Water use by brush, grass and grass-forb vegetation. *J. For.* 59:175–181.

Schmidt, R. A., Jr. 1970. Locating snow fences in mountainous terrain. *Proceedings of the International Symposium on Snow Removal and Ice Control Research,* Dartmouth College, Hanover, N.H., pp. 222–225.

Shanan, L., N. H. Tadmor, and M. Evenari. 1961. The ancient desert agriculture of the Negev. VII. Exploitation of runoff from large watersheds. *J. Natl. Univ. Inst. Agr., Rehovot, Ktavim* 11:9–31.

Slayback, R. D., and D. R. Cable. 1970. Larger pits aid reseeding of semidesert rangeland. *J. Range Mgmt. 23:333*–335.

Tadmor, N. H., L. Shanan, and M. Evenari. 1960. The ancient desert agriculture of the Negev. VI. The ratio of catchment to cultivated area. *J. Natl. Univ. Inst. Agr., Rehovot, Ktavim* 10:193–221.

Whitfield, C. J. 1938. Sand dunes of recent origin in the southern Great Plains. *J. Agr. Res.* 56:907–917.

Yamamoto, T., and H. W. Anderson. 1973. Splash erosion related to soil erodability indexes and other forest soil properties in Hawaii. *Water Resources Res.* 9:336–345.

Young, G. J. 1969. Pitting aids re-vegetation of pastoral country. *S. Aust. J. Agr.* 73:99–103.

Zethner-Moller, O. 1968. The effects of shelterbelts and windbreaks illustrated by examples from Denmark. *Proceedings of the 1st West Pakistan Watershed Management Conference,* Pakistan For. Inst., Peshawar, pp. 237–243.

Chapter 21

Putting Rangeland Management into Practice

Range scientists concentrate on gaining an understanding of the processes of rangeland ecosystems. Rangeland professionals provide that knowledge to the actual managers and administrators of rangeland. The exchange of information between the providers and the users has been slow. Many scientists have neither the interest nor the time to sell their products. Range managers, as a group, often are more concerned with what can be done biologically than with what the land managers choose or can afford to do. The traditions of rangeland use change slowly for these and many other causes. One might ask the question after reading this far in *Rangeland Management:* ''If these practices (Chapters 8-20) are so good, why haven't they found wider application?'' This chapter briefly introduces a few of the possible answers to that question by discussing the practices as a group within their economic, social, and political contexts. Most rangeland in the United States is better suited to all types of use today than it was 20 years ago. The aim here is to suggest ways of making rangeland management even more effective. However, it is not an analysis of educational and extension techniques.

The Operating Ecosystem

The ranch, federal land allotment for grazing, game reserve, or other social and political rangeland unit operates as an entity. The manager makes decisions allocating land, labor, and capital. Most ranches are also households concerned with consumption of products, profits, and even the principal itself during droughts and economic depressions. The consuming part of the ranch ecosystem requires numerous intangible items, as well as physical products, which constitute a good family living. The rangeland unit or ranch combines the business administration of an operating firm, the social concerns of family living, the politics of a community, with economic tenets throughout.

For obvious reasons, this book examines rangeland practices one at a time and one following another. A few attempts at cost-benefit analysis show differences among techniques, for example, among mechanical-brush-control practices. Further economic comparisons are not made because choices among practices have little meaning when they emphasize a single technique, one pasture among many, or livestock and not all animals. The unity of the whole operating firm, including alternate uses of resources and complementary effects throughout the system, must be the framework for selection of range practices. The selection of a practice cannot be determined by analyses of values within the practice itself.

A common pattern of evaluating range practices proceeds about as follows: A single pasture or, more often, a single range site within a pasture, is selected for improvement, and the technique is applied. Careful records of costs as well as production records of forage and perhaps livestock are maintained. After a few years, a balance sheet is produced showing that the range-improvement practice was profitable. Most published case histories of this type suggest that ranchers can increase net income by using the practice. While the data and analyses are accurate for the single pasture, extension of the conclusions to the whole operating ecosystem may not be justified. The single practice needs to be placed into relative position with other practices and uses of money to produce profit.

SELECTING THE PARTS OF A RANGE-IMPROVEMENT PROGRAM

Each range site, pasture, and ranch will respond to several techniques. Change of animal numbers, fencing and water development to improve distribution of animals, planning of the sequence of grazing, and altering of the mixture of animal species are the major tools for controlling impacts of the animals. Noxious plant control, seeding, and fertilization have many variations and may be combined in numerous sequences to attain range improvement. Obviously, they originate different costs and they generate different returns. Just as obviously, the chosen practice should yield the greatest return per dollar spent. Heady and Jensen (1954) illustrated this point with an example from pastures in Tennessee. Mowing of *Poa* yielded $16 for each $1 spent, mowing plus seeding of other grasses gave $5.70 for each $1 invested, and mowing plus seeding plus fertilization yielded only 49 cents for each $1 spent. Although fertilization increased forage production, the added cost caused the whole set of practices to be unprofitable.

Range improvement generally entails a sequence of techniques in which each adds to the cost and to the returns of the whole group of practices. Analysis of costs and returns from fencing, pond construction, spring development, and trail construction on the Cache National Forest in Utah suggested that some of these practices are profitable and some are not (Workman and Hooper, 1968). Fertilization may be as valuable to gain better distribution of animals as it is to increase herbage production (Hooper et al., 1969). The sequence of events in converting chaparral to grass in California commonly begins with chaining and/or burning, which is followed with seeding to grasses and legumes, spraying with 2,4-D, and improved livestock management (Burma, 1970). A range economics problem— one where the answers help the managers choose among practices—is finding the break-even point with sequential practices. Although the costs of improvements are easier to obtain than the increased returns and accumulated capital values, techniques are available for analyzing benefits and returns from multiple rangeland practices. However, because of lack of data, numerous assumptions must be made in most analyses.

INTENSITY OF THE PRACTICE

Range managers must recommend the intensity at which practices are to be applied. For livestock alone, all *Artemisia tridentata* might be removed from a pasture, but for livestock, antelope, and sage grouse, 15 to 25 percent of the vegetation should be *Artemisia*. Therefore the application level for *Artemisia* control relates to the improvement objective. Other practices follow the same principle. Each range program turns out to be a stream of costs and benefits through time which is influenced by intensity of application (Caton et al., 1960).

If the measurement of value is increased forage and the practice is fertilization, the response curve commonly shows large increases in forage at low rates of fertilizer application, a point where no increase is obtained with an additional bit of fertilizer, and decreases in production with still more fertilizer. This common situation of diminishing returns as intensity of application increases applies to most range practices. Of particular appropriateness to this discussion is the observation that too many experiments in their objectives and range managers in their recommendations aim for intensity of practice that will yield the greatest biological return. However, the point where marginal product equals marginal cost is nearly always at a rate of practice intensity less than the rate for maximum biological response. Recommendations for intensity of practices should be in terms of the margin as the optimum level, not the high point of biological production.

Probabilities of risk or failure and uncertainty where probabilities are unknown seldom can be stated for range practices. Very few papers describing research, practical experiments, and actual range practice analyze the risk and uncertainty of failure. Yet everyone talks privately about the causes of failure, and the land manager must live with failures, much as he does with variations in weather. His usual approach is to average returns over a number of years. However, he must always face the question of the level of application next year. He needs to know the consequence of too little or too much when he builds fence, constructs watering points, fertilizes, seeds, etc. These answers seldom are available.

The economic significance of risks is to lower the rate of practice intensity to a point somewhere below where marginal product equals marginal cost. This constitutes a form of insurance against loss. If the manager demands a certain percentage return on investment in range-improvement practices, as most managers do, the level of application is further reduced below the marginal point.

Sound range recommendations require analyses that give the biological maximum, the point of increase in product value equal to the cost of producing that value, quantified risk and uncertainty, and reasonable returns on investment. When the rancher examines a new practice in all of these terms, the application rate may be zero. Ranchers are conservative in accepting range practices for many reasons, one of which is that full economic analysis often has not been made. They are reluctant to do trial and error testing when profit and loss in their operations are at stake. Systems analyses of various types are being applied to range practices, and they promise to yield improved evaluation procedures.

SELECTING RANGELAND PRODUCTS

Rangeland throughout the world produce forage and habitat for domestic and wild animals, recreational opportunities for people, water for downstream users, and places of abode for people. Some rangelands may be changed to timberland, changed to cultivated land, or covered permanently by houses and highways. Other lands may be switched from timber and agricultural uses to rangeland uses. The public, largely through the marketplace but recently by extensive legislation on environmental impacts, determines the uses of the land and the trends in changing use.

The consequences of these changing demands are increased land values, higher taxes, and statutory regulation of rangeland use. Production costs increase, and the manager often finds that he must choose new or different combinations of products in order to stay in business. For example, ranch operators find that they must alter fence construction to meet the public demand for game protection, leave brush for animal habitat, and provide access to their land to maintain public confidence. In order to make the most of these changes, they may charge for camping, hunting, and other recreational uses of the land.

The flow and the probability of income from livestock over time function in accordance with current and future stocking rates (McConnen, 1965). Any function of timing must consider variations in climate, economic environment, and altered public regulation. Impending changes in public demand for rangeland products cause managers to postpone new practices because they fear uncertainty and undermining of long term stability. A rancher's resources are limited. Expansion toward a new product requires limitations of other products. Opportunity costs of sacrificed products are costs to any new programs. Livestock often give the highest returns from the rancher's scarcest resource, labor, while alternate products may require relatively more labor. The rancher, as he changes products, must choose practices that give the greatest returns per dollar spent. He is inclined to stay with tested practices rather than embark on unknown new products. The dilemma over substituting new for old rangeland products slows acceptance of all management techniques.

SUMMARY

Rangeland managers accept recommended practices slowly. The following points do two things: support this view and offer suggestions or opportunities for more effective management. The major problem is establishing each practice within the framework of the rangeland ecosystem, considered in its largest sense, biological, social, political, and economic.

1 Recommended practices often are considered separately and not in their full managerial and economic contexts.

2 Analysis of costs and returns of a practice on a piece of land fails to place the practice in an operating system.

3 Maximum economic return seldom accrues from maximum bilogical return.

4 Maximum rangeland profit in the long run may be well below the point on the curve where marginal product value equals marginal cost.

5 Risk and uncertainty costs reduce profit and increase conservative attitudes toward change.

6 Data and economic analyses are insufficient to show adequate choices among alternative range practices and among a sequence of practices.

7 Comparisons of costs and returns from alternative products are largely unknown among range practices.

8 Operators hesitate to make any change that might undermine long-term stability.

9 Rapidly changing social, political, and economic structures lead to uncertainty and continued use of established procedures by the manager.

10 Goals of each rangeland manager differ; some managers may aim for large profits, while others may give first preference to a good life with little concern for accumulating wealth, and still others aim for protection of the rangeland ecosystem. Range management accommodates all of these views.

LITERATURE CITED

Burma, G. D. 1970. Controlling brush and converting to grass. *Proceedings of the 11th International Grassland Congress*, pp. 172–175.

Caton, D. D., C. O. McCorkle, and M. L. Upchurch. 1960. Economics of improvement of western grazing land. *J. Range Mgmt.* 13:143–151.

Heady, E. O., and H. R. Jensen. 1954. *Farm management economics*. Englewood Cliffs, N.J.: Prentice-Hall.

Hooper, J. F., J. P. Workman, J. B. Grumbles, and C. W. Cook. 1969. Improved livestock distribution with fertilizer—A preliminary economic evaluation. *J. Range Mgmt.* 22:108–110.

McConnen, R. J. 1965. Relation between the pattern of use and the future output from a flow resource. *J. Farm Econ.* 47:311–323.

Workman, J. P., and J. F. Hooper. 1968. Preliminary economic evaluation of cattle distribution practices on mountain rangelands. *J. Range Mgmt.* 21:301–304.

Appendix I

Scientific and Common Names of Plants

The following alphabetical list includes the genera and species of plants mentioned in the text. See Table 18-1 for common names of well-known cultivars. Common names are based on usage in the following literature.

Beetle, A. A., 1970. Recommended plant names. *Univ. Wyo. Agr. Expt. Sta. Res. J.* 31.
Hanson, A. A. 1965. Grass varieties in the United States. *U.S. Dept. Agr. Handbook 170.*
Munz, P. A. 1959. *A California flora.* Berkeley: Univ. of California Press.

Scientific Name	Common Name
Abies concolor	white fir
Acacia	acacia
Acacia aneura	mulga
Acacia farnesiana	huisache acacia
Acacia gregii	catclaw acacia
Acacia rigidula	blackbrush acacia
Acer saccharum	sugar maple
Achillea lanulosa	yarrow

Scientific Name	Common Name
Adenostoma fasciculatum	chamise
Agropyron	wheatgrass
Agropyron cristatum	crested wheatgrass
Agropyron desertorum	crested wheatgrass
Agropyron elongatum	tall wheatgrass
Agropyron inerme	beardless wheatgrass
Agropyron intermedium	intermediate wheatgrass
Agropyron riparium	streambank wheatgrass
Agropyron sibiricum	Siberian wheatgrass
Agropyron smithii	western wheatgrass
Agropyron spicatum	bluebunch wheatgrass
Agropyron trachycaulum	slender wheatgrass
Agropyron trichophorum	pubescent wheatgrass
Aira caryophyllea	silver hairgrass
Alnus	alder
Aloysia lycioides	aloysia
Ambrosia artemisiifolia	common ragweed
Amelanchier alnifolia	Saskatoon serviceberry
Ammophila	beachgrass
Ammophila arenaria	European beachgrass
Andropogon	bluestem
Andropogon annulatus	Dias bluestem
Andropogon caucasicus	Caucasian bluestem
Andropogn divergens	pinehill bluestem
Andropogon geradi	big bluestem
Andropogon hallii	sand bluestem
Andropogon ischaemum	yellow bluestem
Andropogon nodosus	Angleton bluestem
Andropogon scoparius	little bluestem
Andropogon tener	slender bluestem
Aplopappus tenuisectus	burro goldenweed
Arctostaphylos	manzanita
Aristida glabrata	Santa Rita threeawn
Aristida stricta	pineland threeawn
Arrhenatherum elatius	tall falseoat
Artemisia	sagebrush
Artemisia frigida	fringed sagewort
Artemisia tridentata	basin big sagebrush
Arundinaria tecta	switch cane
Aspergillus	bacteria
Astragalus	milkvetch
Astragalus miser var. *oblongifolius*	weedy milkvetch
Atriplex	saltbush
Atriplex confertifolia	shadscale saltbush
Atriplex nuttallii	nuttall saltbush

Scientific Name	Common Name
Atriplex polycarpa	allscale saltbush
Artiplex vesicaria	Australian saltbush
Avena barbata	slender wildoat
Axonopus affinis	common carpetgrass
Balsamorrhiza sagittata	arrowleaf balsamroot
Berberis trifoliata	agarito barberry
Berberis vulgaris	European barberry
Beta maritima	sugar beet
Betula	birch
Bouteloua	grama
Bouteloua barbata	sixweeks grama
Bouteloua curtipendula	sideoats grama
Bouteloua eriopoda	black grama
Bouteloua gracilis	blue grama
Bouteloua rothrockii	rothrock grama
Brachiaria	signalgrass
Brassica	mustard
Bromus	brome
Bromus carinatus	California brome
Bromus catharticus	rescuegrass
Bromus inermis	smooth brome
Bromus marginatus	mountain brome
Bromus mollis	soft chess
Bromus rigidus	ripgut brome
Bromus rubens	red brome
Bromus tectorum	cheatgrass
Buchloe	buffalograss
Buchloe dactyloides	common buffalograss
Calamagrostis rubescens	pine reedgrass
Calamovilfa longifolia	prairie sandreed
Carduus	thistle
Carduus nutans	musk thistle
Carex filifolia	threadleaf sedge
Carex geyeri	elk sedge
Cassia	senna
Cassia armata	desert senna
Casuarina	beefwood
Ceanothus	ceanothus
Ceanothus sanguineus	redstem ceanothus
Ceanothus velutinus	showbrush ceanothus
Cenchrus ciliaris	buffelgrass
Centaurea	starthistle
Centaurea solstitialis	yellow starthistle
Cercocarpus	mountain mahogany
Cercocarpus betuloides	birchleaf mountain mahogany

Scientific Name	Common Name
Cercocarpus breviflorus	Wright mountain mahogany
Cercocarpus ledifolius	curlleaf mountain mahogany
Chenopodium leptophyllum	narrowleaf goosefoot
Chloris gayana	rhodesgrass
Chrysanthemum leucanthemum	oxeyedaisy chrysanthemum
Chrysothamnus	rabbitbrush
Chrysothamnus nauseosus	rubber rabbitbrush
Chrysothamnus viscidiflorus	Douglas rabbitbrush
Cirsium	thistle
Cirsium arvense	Canada thistle
Claydonia	lichen
Clostridium	fungus
Convolvulus arvensis	field bindweed
Coriaria	tutu
Cornus florida	flowering dogwood
Corylus cornuta	hazelnut
Cotoneaster	cotoneaster
Cowania	cliffrose
Cretraria	lichen
Cynodon	Bermudargrass
Cynodon dactylon	common Bermudagrass
Cytisus	broom
Dactylis	orchardgrass
Dactylis glomerata	orchardgrass
Danthonia californica	California oatgrass
Danthonia intermedia	timber oatgrass
Danthonia unispicata	onespike oatgrass
Delphinium	larkspur
Delphinium barbeyi	Barbey larkspur
Delphinium geyeri	plains larkspur
Deschampsia caespitosa	tufted hairgrass
Desmodium	tickclover
Digitaria	fingergrass
Diospyros texana	Texas persimmon
Discaria	
Distichlis spicata	seashore saltgrass
Distichlis stricta	inland saltgrass
Dryas	dryad
Elaeagnus	eleagnus
Elymus	wildrye
Elymus canadensis	Canada wildrye
Elymus caput-medusae	medusahead
Elymus cinereus	basin wildrye
Elymus junceus	Russian wildrye
Elymus triticoides	creeping wildrye

Scientific Name	Common Name
Elyonurus argenteus	elyonurus
Emmenanthe penduliflora	yellow whisperingbells
Epilobium angustifolium	fireweed
Eragrostis	lovegrass
Eragrostis curvula	weeping lovegrass
Eragrostis lehmanniana	Lehmann lovegrass
Eragrostis trichodes	sand lovegrass
Eremophila gilesii	false sandalwood
Erodium	filaree
Erodium botrys	broadleaf filaree
Erodium cicutarium	redstem filaree
Eucalyptus	eucalyptus
Euphorbia esula	leafy spurge
Eurotia lanata	common winterfat
Festuca	fescue
Festuca arizonica	Arizona fescue
Festuca arundinaceae	tall fescue
Festuca elatior	meadow fescue
Festuca idahoensis	Idaho fescue
Festuca octoflora	sixweeks fescue
Festuca scabrella	rough fescue
Festuca viridula	green fescue
Flourensia cernua	American tarbush
Fraxinus americana	white ash
Gale	gale
Garrya wrightii	Wright silktassel
Geum rossii	alpine avens
Grayia spinosa	spiny hopsage
Gutierrezia	snakeweed
Gutierrezia sarothrae	broom snakeweed
Halogeton	halogeton
Halogeton glomeratus	common halogeton
Haplopappus tenuisectus	burro goldenweed
Helenium hoopesii	orange sneezeweed
Helianthus annuus	sunflower
Heteropogan contortus	common tanglehead
Hilaria belangeri	curlymesquite
Hilaria jamesii	galleta
Hilaria mutica	tobosa
Hippophae	buffaloberry
Holodiscus discolor	creambush rockspirea
Hordeum brachyantherum	meadow barley
Hymenoxys odorata	bitterweed actinea
Hyparrhenia hirta	hyparrhenia
Hypericum perforatum	common St. John's wort

Scientific Name	Common Name
Ilex glabra	inkberry holly
Ilex vomitoria	yaupon holly
Iris missouriensis	rockymountain iris
Juglans	walnut
Juniperus	juniper
Juniperus osteosperma	Utah juniper
Juniperus virginiana	eastern redcedar
Juncus	rush
Koeleria cristata	prairie junegrass
Lantana camara	common lantana
Larrea	creosotebush
Larrea divaricata	common creosotebush
Larrea tridentata	common creosotebush
Lepidium densiflorum	prairie pepperweed
Lespedeza	lespedeza
Lespedeza striata	common lespedeza
Libocedrus decurrens	California incensecedar
Lolium	ryegrass
Lolium multiflorum	Italian ryegrass
Lolium perenne	perennial ryegrass
Lupinus	lupine
Lycopersicon esculentum var. *minor*	wild tomato
Madia glomerata	cluster tarweed
Medicago	medic
Medicago hispida	burclover
Medicago sativa	alfalfa
Melilotus indica	annual yellow sweetclover
Mertensia arizonica var. *leonardi*	tall bluebells
Molina caerulea	purple moorgrass
Morus	mulberry
Muhlenbergia montana	mountain muhly
Myrica	waxmyrtle
Onopordum	cottonthistle
Onopordum acanthium	Scotch cottonthistle
Opuntia	pricklypear
Opuntia arbuscula	pencil cholla
Opuntia fulgida	Sonora jumping cholla
Opuntia inermis	pricklypear
Opuntia imbricata	walkingstick cholla
Opuntia leptocaulis	tasajillo
Opuntia lindheimeri	Lindheimer pricklypear
Opuntia megacantha	mission pricklypear
Opuntia stricta	pricklypear
Oryzopsis	ricegrass

Scientific Name	Common Name
Oryzopsis hymenoides	indian ricegrass
Oryzopsis miliacea	smilo
Oxalis cernua	buttercup woodsorrel
Oxytropis	loco
Panicum	panic
Panicum antidotale	blue panic
Panicum coloratum	buffalo panic
Panicum maximum	Guineagrass
Panicum obtusum	vinemesquite
Panicum virgatum	switchgrass
Paspalum	paspalum
Paspalum dilatatum	Dallisgrass
Paspalum notatum	bahiagrass
Paspalum notatum var. *saurae*	Pensacola bahiagrass
Pennisetum	pennisetum
Pennisetum ciliare	buffelgrass
Pennisetum purpureum	elephantgrass
Petradoria pumila	rock goldenrod
Phalaris	canarygrass
Phalaris arundinacea	reed canarygrass
Phalaris tuberosa	bulb canarygrass
Phalaris tuberosa var. *hirtiglumis*	koleagrass
Phalaris tuberosa var. *stenoptera*	hardinggrass
Phaseolus	bean
Phleum	timothy
Phleum pratense	common timothy
Phragmites communis	common reed
Picea glauca	white spruce
Picea mariana	black spruce
Pinus	pine
Pinus attenuata	knobcone pine
Pinus banksiana	Jack pine
Pinus contorta	lodgepole pine
Pinus echinata	shortleaf pine
Pinus elliottii	slash pine
Pinus lambertiana	sugar pine
Pinus nigra	Austrian pine
Pinus palustris	longleaf pine
Pinus ponderosa	ponderosa pine
Pinus radiata	Monterey pine
Pinus sabiniana	digger pine
Pinus serotina	pond pine
Pinus taeda	loblolly pine
Poa	bluegrass

Scientific Name	Common Name
Poa ampla	big bluegrass
Poa arachnifera	Texas bluegrass
Poa pratensis	Kentucky bluegrass
Poa secunda	Sandberg bluegrass
Populus	poplar, aspen, cottonwood
Populus tremuloides	quaking aspen
Prosopis	mesquite
Prosopis glandulosa	honey mesquite
Prosopis juliflora	common mesquite
Prunus emarginata	bitter cherry
Pseudotsuga menzesii	Douglas fir
Psoralea tenuiflora	slimflower scurfpea
Pteridium aquilinum	western bracken fern
Purshia	bitterbrush
Prushia tridentata	antelope bitterbrush
Quercus	oak
Quercus agrifolia	California liveoak
Quecus alba	white oak
Quercus douglasii	blue oak
Quercus dumosa	California scrub oak
Quercus gambelii	Gambel oak
Quercus havardii	shin oak
Quercus marilandica	blackjack oak
Quercus stellata	post oak
Quercus turbinella	scrub liveoak
Quercus virginiana	common liveoak
Quercus wizlizenii	interior liveoak
Ramalina reticulata	lichen
Ranunculus alismaefolius	plantainleaf buttercup
Ranunculus occidentalis	western buttercup
Rhizobia	nitrifying bacteria
Rhus	sumac
Rhus glabra	smooth sumac
Rosa bracteata	Macartney rose
Rubus	blackberry
Rubus fruticosus	European blackberry
Salix	willow
Salix scouleriana	scouler willow
Salsola	Russianthistle
Salsola kali	common Russianthistle
Scarcobatus vermiculatus	black greasewood
Scirrhia acicola	pine needle blight
Scleropogon brevifolius	common burrograss
Serenoa repens	common sawpalmetto
Setaria macrostachya	plains bristlegrass

Scientific Name	Common Name
Shepherdia	buffaloberry
Sitanion hystrix	bottlebrush squirreltail
Sorghastrum nutans	yellow indiangrass
Sorghum almum	Argentine sorghum
Sorghum halepense	Johnsongrass
Sorghum intrans	sorghum
Sorghum plumosum	sorghum
Spartina	cordgrass
Spartina patens	marshhay cordgrass
Sporobolus airoides	alkali sacaton
Sporobolus curtessii	Curtis dropseed
Sterculia apetala	
Stipa	needlegrass
Stipa columbiana	subalpine needlegrass
Stipa comata	needle and thread
Stipa pulchra	purple needlegrass
Stipa thurberiana	Thurber needlegrass
Stipa viridula	green needlegrass
Stylosanthes humilis	Townsville stylo
Symphoricarpos albus	common snowberry
Taeniatherum asperum	medusahead
Tamarix	tamarisk
Taraxacum officinale	common dandelion
Tetrachne	
Themeda	kangaroograss
Themeda australis	Australian kangaroograss
Themeda triandra	Rooi kangaroograss, red oatgrass
Trifolium	clover
Trifolium hirtum	rose clover
Trifolium repens	white clover
Trifolium subterraneum	subterranean clover
Triodia	spinefex
Tristachya hispida	
Triticum aestivum	wheat
Ulex	gorse
Ulex europaeus	common gorse
Ulmus	elm
Ulmus alata	winged elm
Ulmus parvifolia	Chinese elm
Wyethia amplexicaulis	mulesear
Xanthium	cocklebur
Yucca	yucca
Zygadenus	deathcamas
Zygadenus paniculatus	foothill deathcamas

Appendix II

Common and Scientific Names of Animals

The following alphabetical list includes the common names of animals used in the text and their scientific names. The references consulted for the scientific names were as follows.

Code	Reference
B	Blair, W. F., A. P. Blair, P. Brodkorb, F. R. Cagle, and G. A. Moore. 1968. *Vertebrates of the United States.* New York: McGraw Hill.
D	Borror, D. J., and D. M. Delong. 1971. *An introduction to the study of insects.* New York: Rinehart and Winston.
P	Peterson, R. T. 1961. *A field guide to western birds.* Boston: Houghton Mifflin.
Wa	Walker, E. P., F. Warnick, K. I. Cange, H. E. Uible, S. E. Hamlet, M. A. Davis, and P. F. Wright. 1964. *Mammals of the world.* Silver Spring: Johns Hopkins Press.
W	Williams, J. G. 1967. *A field guide to the national parks of East Africa.* London: Collins.

Common Name	Scientific Name	Reference
ant	*Veromessor pergandei*	D
ant, army	*Eciton*	D
antelope, blackbuck	*Antilope cervicapra*	W
antelope, nilgai	*Boselaphus tragocamelus*	Wa

Common Name	Scientific Name	Reference
antelope, pronghorn	*Antilocapra americana*	B
antelope, roan	*Hippotragus equinus*	W
antelope, sable	*Hippotragus niger*	W
antelope, saiga	*Saiga tatarica*	Wa
aoudad	*Ammotragus lervia*	Wa
bear, black	*Ursus americanus*	B
bear, grizzly	*Ursus horribilis*	B
beaver	*Castor canadensis*	B
beaver, mountain	*Aplodontia rufa*	B
bison	*Bison bison*	B
blesbok	*Damaliscus albifrons*	Wa
boar, European wild	*Sus scrofa*	Wa
buffalo, cape	*Syncerus caffer*	W
burro	*Equus asinus*	B
bushbuck	*Tragelaphus scriptus*	W
bushpig	*Potamochoerus porcus*	W
camel	*Camelus dromedarius*	Wa
caribou	*Rangifer* spp.	B
cattle	*Bos* spp.	
cattle, Hereford	*Bos taurus*	
cattle, Indian	*Bos indicus*	
cattle, Santa Gertrudis	*Bos taurus x indicus*	
cattle, Zebu	*Bos indicus*	
cheetah	*Acinonyx jubatus*	W
chicken	*Gallus gallus*	
condor, California	*Gymnogyps californianus*	P
cottontail rabbit	*Sylvilagus* spp.	B
coyote	*Canis latrans*	B
deer, axis	*Axis axis*	Wa
deer, California black-tailed; Columbian back-tailed	*Odocoileus hemionus* ssp *columbianus*	B
deer, mule	*Odocoileus hemionus*	B
deer, red	*Cervus elaphus*	Wa
deer, white-tailed	*Odocoileus virginianus*	B
dikdik	*Rhynchotragus* spp.	W
dingo	*Canis dingo*	Wa
dog	*Canis* spp.	
dog, domestic	*Canis familiaris*	Wa
dog, hunting	*Lycaon pictus*	W
donkey	*Equus asinus*	B
duck, mallard	*Anas platyrhynchos*	P
duiker	*Cephalophus* spp.	W
eland	*Taurotragus oryx*	W

Common Name	Scientific Name	Reference
elephant, African	*Loxodonta africana*	W
elk	*Cervus canadensis*	B
elk, Roosevelt	*Cervus canadensis*	B
emu	*Dromiceius novae-hollandiae*	
fly, tsetse	*Glossina* spp.	
gazelle	*Gazella* spp.	W
gazelle, Grant's	*Gazella granti*	W
gazelle, Thomson's	*Gazella thomsonii*	W
giraffe	*Giraffa camelopardalis`*	W
goat	*Capra hircus*	
goat, Angora	*Capra hircus*	
goat, feral	*Capra hircus*	
goat, Rocky mountain	*Oreamnos americanus*	B
gopher, pocket	*Thomomys* spp.	B
grouse, ruffed	*Bonasa umbellus*	B
grouse, sage	*Centrocercus urophasianus*	B
grouse, sharptail	*Pedioecetes phasianellus*	B
hare	*Lepus capensis*	
hare, snowshoe	*Lepus americanus*	B
hartebeest	*Alcelaphus* spp.	W
hippopotamus	*Hippopotamus amphibius*	W
hog, giant forest	*Hylochoerus meinertzhageni*	W
horse	*Equus cabalus*	Wa
horse, wild	*Equus cabalus*	Wa
hunting dog	*Lycaon pictus*	W
hyena, spotted	*Crocuta crocuta*	W
hyena, striped	*Hyaena hyanea*	W
impala	*Aepyceros melampus*	W
jackal	*Canis* spp.	W
jackal, black-backed	*Canis mesomelas*	W
jackrabbit	*Lepus* spp.	B
jackrabbit, black-tailed	*Lepus californicus*	B
jackrabbit, California	*Lepus californicus*	
jay	*Garrulus glandarius*	P
kangaroo	*Macropus* spp.	Wa
kangaroo rat	*Dipodomys* spp.	
kangaroo rat, giant	*Dipodomys ingens*	B
killdeer	*Charadrius vociferus*	P
klipspringer	*Oreotragus oreotragus*	W
kob, Uganda	*Adenota kob*	W
kudu, greater	*Tragelaphus strepsiceros*	W
kudu, lesser	*Strepsiceros imberbis*	W
lemming	*Synaptomys borealis*	B

Common Name	Scientific Name	Reference
leopard	*Panthera pardus*	W
lion	*Panthera leo*	W
molerat	*Spalax ehrenbergi*	
moose	*Alces alces*	B
mouse, meadow	*Microtus* spp.	
mouse, pocket	*Perognathus* spp.	B
mouse, white-footed	*Peromyscus* spp.	B
nyala	*Tragelaphus angasi*	Wa
opossum, Australian	wide variety of genera and species	
oryx	*Oryx beisa*	W
ostrich	*Struthio camelus*	
peccary	*Tayassu tajacu*	B
Peking man	*Homo erectus*	
pheasant, ringneck	*Phasianus colchicus*	P
pig	*Sus scrofa*	B
pig, feral	*Sus scrofa*	Wa
porcupine	*Erethizon dorsatum*	B
prairie chicken	*Tymanuchos* spp.	B
prairie dog	*Cynomys ludovicianus*	B
quail, bobwhite	*Colinus virginianus*	B
quail, Gambel's	*Lophortyx gambelii*	B
quail, valley	*Lophortyx californica*	B
rat	*Rattus rattus*	
reedbuck	*Redunca* spp.	W
reindeer	*Rangifer tarandus*	Wa
rhinoceros, black	*Diceros bicornis*	W
rhinoceros, square-lipped	*Diceros simus*	W
rhinoceros, white	*Diceros simus*	W
sheep	*Ovis aries*	Wa
sheep, bighorn	*Ovis canadensis*	B
sheep, feral	*Ovis aries*	Wa
sheep, mouflon	*Ovis musimon*	Wa
sheep, Rambouillet	*Ovis aries*	
springbok	*Antidorcas marsupialis*	Wa
squirrel, ground	*Citellus* spp.	B
topi	*Damaliscus korrigum*	W
tortoise, giant Galapagos	*Geochelone elephantopus*	
tsessebe	*Damaliscus* spp.	W
turkey, wild	*Meleagris gallopavo*	B
vole	*Microtus* spp.	
walkingstick	*Diapheromera velii*	
warbler, Kirtland	*Denroica kirtlandii*	B

Common Name	Scientific Name	Reference
warthog	*Phancochoerus aethiopicus*	W
wasp, black cricket	*Chlorion laeviventris*	
waterbuck	*Kobus ellipsiprymnus*	W
wildebeest	*Connochaetes taurinus*	W
wildebeest, black	*Coanochaetes gnou*	Wa
wildebeest, blue	*Connochaetes taurinus*	W
wolf	*Canis lupus*	B
yak	*Bos grunniens*	*Wa*
zebra	*Equus burchelli*	W

Index